PROSTATE!
PROSTATE!
PROSTATE!

A Problem Of Men

PROSTATE!
PROSTATE!
PROSTATE!

A Problem Of Men

An easy to read
caring and compassionate account
for **men,** and
women who have men in their lives

Harold Usher, P. Eng., DTM
Prostate Cancer Survivor

Joseph Chin, M.D., FRCSC
Medical Editor and Co-Author of Medical Chapters

Order this book online at www.trafford.com/06-0700
or email orders@trafford.com

Most Trafford titles are also available at major online book retailers.

© Copyright 2008 Harold Usher/Dr. Joseph Chin.
All rights reserved. No part of this publication may be reproduced, stored in a retrieval system, or transmitted, in any form or by any means, electronic, mechanical, photocopying, recording, or otherwise, without the written prior permission of the author.

Literary Editor: Ellen Ashton-Haiste
Medical Editor: Joseph Chin, M.D., FRCSC
Cover Design: Rachel Dottermann
Illustrations: Sue Nham

Note for Librarians: A cataloguing record for this book is available from Library and Archives Canada at www.collectionscanada.ca/amicus/index-e.html

Printed in Victoria, BC, Canada.

ISBN: 978-1-4120-8944-9

We at Trafford believe that it is the responsibility of us all, as both individuals and corporations, to make choices that are environmentally and socially sound. You, in turn, are supporting this responsible conduct each time you purchase a Trafford book, or make use of our publishing services. To find out how you are helping, please visit www.trafford.com/responsiblepublishing.html

Our mission is to efficiently provide the world's finest, most comprehensive book publishing service, enabling every author to experience success. To find out how to publish your book, your way, and have it available worldwide, visit us online at www.trafford.com/10510

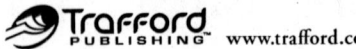 www.trafford.com

North America & international
toll-free: 1 888 232 4444 (USA & Canada)
phone: 250 383 6864 ♦ fax: 250 383 6804 ♦ email: info@trafford.com

The United Kingdom & Europe
phone: +44 (0)1865 722 113 ♦ local rate: 0845 230 9601
facsimile: +44 (0)1865 722 868 ♦ email: info.uk@trafford.com

10 9 8 7

This book is intended for inspiration, information, education and empowerment. It is not a medical manual. The information herein is intended to inspire you to take action regarding your health and your medical check-ups. It is also intended to enable and empower you to take appropriate and timely action to treat any prostate disease or condition that you might be diagnosed with, as quickly as possible. Nothing contained herein is intended as a medical directive. The ideas, thoughts and opinions are solely those of the authors, one of whom is a prostate cancer survivor, and an advocate of annual check-ups and early prostate cancer diagnosis and treatment, and the other a urologist and surgeon, who has performed many surgeries to remove the prostate. They both urge you to seek competent, qualified medical advice before undergoing any prostate treatment. They provide this account because they feel that the research and documentation that was put into gathering this information deserves to be shared with others to make a difference, not in just one life, but, rather in thousands of lives, yours included.

Some of the net proceeds from the sale of this book will be donated to prostate cancer research and education.

WHAT THEY SAY ABOUT THIS BOOK

Comments from some of those who have read the manuscript and or attended a presentation on the contents …

"This book is straightforward and simple, and will save your life."
Brenda D.
Daughter of a prostate cancer survivor

"This book is educational and informative and really helped my family."
Sarah T.
Wife of a prostate cancer patient

"Excellent! Very helpful!"
Thelma M.
Wife of a BPH patient

"Excellent! Well organized! It's invaluable, practical information for me as I move into my senior years."
Rick W.
Forty somethinger

"Good, practical information. I definitely learned some ideas I can take into consideration."
Jeorge C.
Fifty somethinger

"I feel inspired and well informed."
Duncan S., PhD (Professor of Psychology)
Experiencing prostate problems

"One of the most informative books on the subject of the prostate that I have ever read."
Dennie T.
Brother of prostate cancer survivor

"It was a great experience taking this journey. Very informative! I wish I had this before I had treatment. By far under-priced …"
George H.
Prostate cancer survivor

"Very informative material with real world experience."
Lennox P., M.D.
Performed many DREs

"Informative, inspirational, bold and very helpful! Now I think I am ready to ask questions and make my decision regarding treatment."
Danny Y.
Prostate cancer patient – until now, in denial

AUTHORS CONNECTION

"There are two ways of spreading light: to be the candle or the mirror that reflects it."

EDITH WHARTON

I first met Harold Usher professionally in 1996. He and I took a "journey," from suspicion to diagnosis of prostate cancer to decision making through surgery and finally through recovery and rehabilitation, that was NOT typical for most of my patients. I have come to know Harold as a highly intelligent man with an analytical and inquisitive mind, likely as a result of his engineering background. When Harold first approached me with the idea of a book on the prostate, after his long delay following his diagnosis of prostate cancer, which ended in surgery and recovery, my first thought was that many excellent books have already been published, both by leading urologic surgeons and by "celebrity" prostate cancer survivors, ranging from detailed surgical manuals to "moving" personal accounts. However, when I read the first draft of Harold's book, I recognized immediately that this book would make a worthwhile contribution to the area of patient information and education and I became an enthusiastic participant. I willingly accepted the role of ensuring the information was medically accurate and the scientific explanations were comprehensible for readers with various backgrounds.

The book combines personal experience from a patient's perspective with information for patients and family members who are faced with the intimidating and frightening diagnosis of prostate diseases, particularly prostate cancer, and with the daunting task of decision making regarding therapy. It is not meant as a medical manual. It does, however, provide basic background knowledge to readers to be better prepared in their consultations and discussions with their physicians and surgeons. It should facilitate, and thus help to speed-up, the all-important decision-making process.

I congratulate and applaud Harold for his initiative and his perseverance in putting this material together. His insightful book provides an invaluable service for the prostate cancer community.

Joseph Chin, M.D., FRCSC
Head of Surgical Oncology,
London Health Sciences Centre;
Associate Scientist,
Lawson Health Research Institute;
Professor of Urology and Oncology,
The University of Western Ontario;
London, Ontario, CANADA

My relationship with Dr. Joseph Chin spans over a decade, starting in 1996, when I first became his patient as a result of my physician referring me to him with a suspected prostate problem. He monitored my condition through the phases of suspicion, checking, diagnosis and finally the chosen therapy and caring for my after-effects. Throughout that period of more than three years, I came to recognize and respect him as the foremost expert that he is and a very concerned, dedicated and highly respected urologic surgeon, scientist and professor, by his colleagues, staff, residents, students, patients and me.

Along the way, I learned a lot about the subject of health, prostate and diseases of the prostate, as well as their diagnosis and possible treatments. I decided to pen that information for others' benefit and to offer men, and women in their lives, more understanding, as I needed. When I decided to publish the work, I sought Dr. Chin's concurrence that there was a place for it in the urologic world. He took some time out from his busy schedule and read the manuscript providing some constructive input to make it more complete and accurate. I was very pleased and invited him to become a co-author. Since he had made such a substantial contribution, he accepted that challenge. The result is this book – an easy to read, caring and compassionate account for men, and for women who have men in their lives.

I thank Dr. Chin for his valuable input, his partnership and for concurring that this book provides an invaluable service for the prostate cancer community.

Harold Usher, P. Eng., DTM
Prostate Cancer Survivor
City Councillor
President – "Adventures in . . ." SEMINARS & SPEECHES
London, Ontario, CANADA

DEDICATION

This book is dedicated to: all those men who experienced a prostate problem and were willing to share their stories for inclusion in this book; as well as those men who listened and acted on my persuasion to get a regular medical check-up, especially those who subsequently found that they unknowingly had prostate cancer; and also to all the women who persuaded the men in their lives to take treatment action; and finally to my wife Melba, my companion and most caring friend, who has stood by me in every endeavour that I have undertaken, supported me unceasingly during my entire challenge with my prostate, from the beginning when an abnormality was first suspected, through to the prostate cancer treatment that I opted for, and then on through rehabilitation, to the present and with whose strength and sacrifice that I went through this experience fearlessly and positively. These are the people whose inspiration showed there was a need for this book. Hopefully it will benefit thousands of others who will go through some of our experience and have this book to help them along the way.

ACKNOWLEDGMENTS

My sincere gratitude and thanks to:

My wonderful grand daughter, Sierra Nicol Usher Van Eyk, who inspires me by her own disposition to share the information in this book with others.

My enthusiastic daughter, Melanie Usher, who believes in me and unceasingly encouraged me during and after my illness to change my diet and lifestyle and later, to write this book.

The people who cared for me before, during and after my surgery and treatment, including my physician, Dr. Chawla, my urologist and surgeon, Dr. Joseph Chin, and his research associate, Nancy Pus.

All the people who tended to me in the operating, recovery and rehabilitation rooms while I was hospitalized.

All the people, especially men, who shared their experiences and knowledge, and allowed me to use their stories.

All the people from whom I have learned something for inclusion in this book, and who have encouraged me to take some positive action to share that information with others.

My many relatives, friends and acquaintances – including strangers – who wrote me words of support and encouragement throughout the time I was putting this material together,

To my friends, Emily Marcoccia and Rev. Anne Beattie-Stokes for their encouragement and many suggestions.

To my friends, Sandy Morden, Reanne Bradley, Alma Coye, Victor Sinclair, Tracey Guthrie, Dr. Kay Tillett and others for offering their invaluable critique and editorial advice in the preparation, content and format, of this book.

Acknowledgments

To my friend, Brenda Dottermann, who went above and beyond what was expected of her in encouraging me continuously and participated actively in the development of this book, took a very special interest in scoping it, and whose continuous input, contributions, friendship and support were invaluable.

To Rachel Dottermann for designing the covers and the spine.

To Shelley Markland, who made time in her busy schedule to review the book and offer significant and valuable input regarding grammar and punctuation.

To my Literary Editor, Ellen Ashton-Haiste, who painstakingly reviewed the material and contributed valuable edition.

To Jo-Ann Walsh who packaged all the final corrections and alterations.

Again, to my co-author for the medical chapters, my urologist Dr. Joseph Chin, who took time out from his busy schedule to read the manuscript and offered significant and invaluable input to validate and authenticate the material, and who ultimately prepared part of the "authors' connection."

To Sue Nham for her wonderful artistic illustrations which are incorporated in this book and Paul Van Eyk, for his original advice on illustrations.

And finally, to the many people whose material and writings were a source of information and education – I owe you a debt of gratitude and hoping that preparing this book is satisfaction for your contribution.

PREFACE

"One thing I know, that whereas once I was blind, now I can see…"

JOHN 9:25

If you are a man 40 years of age or older, you will want to read this book and always have a copy handy, because there is a 90 percent chance that you will experience a problem with your prostate sometime in your life. In fact, you have a 16 percent chance of that problem being cancer. What is even more startling is that you have the power to do something to help prevent it, and/or to treat it swiftly, so that it does not become too damaging or fatal.

The purpose of this book is to:
1) Offer sufficient information to men who have been, or may be, diagnosed with a prostate disorder, so that they can formulate appropriate questions and/or make informed decisions about their treatments.
2) Persuade men to make it a habit to get a regular medical check-up.
3) Help men dispel any fears that they may entertain regarding medical check-ups, their processes and results.
4) Inspire men who are experiencing a prostate problem to take action and have it diagnosed, and promptly treated.
5) Persuade men to care for themselves, especially their prostates, regardless of whether they have a problem.

I am a survivor of prostate cancer who opted for surgical treatment after a relatively long delay from the time I was diagnosed. My delay resulted from negligence, first because I went into denial, then I procrastinated, and then as I began to take it seriously I realized that I lacked sufficient understanding to make an intelligent decision. The latter led me into research, deliberation and experimentation with various alternative forms of treatment.

Preface

In this book I offer you the story of how I coped with my prostate cancer and what I learned in my extensive research that helped me cope. It is written for the benefit of men, and women who have men in their lives, be they a spouse, mother, sister or daughter, as well as any devoted partner or friend. I offer what I learned over the past eight years, in a logical, easy to read, format and sequence, so that you can read it quickly and easily and, I hope, avoid delay making your choice of treatment decision.

I am confident that the treatment I chose offered me the greatest potential for a long, healthy and good quality life. The treatment you opt for may be different than mine. I hope this book will help you reach an intelligent decision before the disorder spreads to other parts of your body. To that end, I am sharing with you all the things I wish I had known at the beginning, so it would not have taken me so long to reach my decision.

As you read this book, you will come to realize that it reflects your feelings and needs, and it fulfills them by being a road map to help guide you to make your own decisions or at least to ask the right questions. It was written by two people who experience prostate cancer in different ways. **Harold Usher** is a prostate cancer survivor who has already experienced it, knows how you feel, and understands your needs. **Dr. Joseph Chin** is a distinguished Urologic Surgeon who believes that it makes a worthwhile contribution to the area of patient information and education and provides an invaluable service for the prostate cancer community. Both of them understand the resulting frustration from lack of clarity, simplicity and understanding, and it is written with that in mind.

"Prostate! Prostate! Prostate! A Problem of Men" offers you some ideas of what you can expect, precautions you could take, preparations you may wish to consider, questions you may want to ask, and treatment options that are available to you. You may come to realize that having a prostate problem, and particularly prostate cancer, 'is not the end of the world.' My story may help you think past the initial shock of the diagnosis and realize that a healthy, wonderful life is still in your future.

Part I of the book (five chapters) deals with **your health** and making yourself more healthy, leading into nurturing the prostate. This addresses the use of nutritional supplementation including vitamins, minerals and trace elements.

Part II (five chapters) is about **your Prostate**, the very major role it plays in man's reproductive and urinary systems, and the different diseases that can affect the prostate and your quality of life.

Part III (10 chapters) deals with **prostate cancer diagnosis**, the process or steps you need to go through in order to confirm it is cancer, and decide on the severity of the cancer. All prostate cancers are not the same.

Part IV (seven chapters) deals with **managing the condition**, including your behaviour tendencies, breaking the news to family and friends and others, changing your lifestyle, and temptation to deny or refuse to believe, and what the woman in your life can do to help.

Part V (nine chapters) deals with the various alternative **treatment options** (several of them – ones that few people know about), and making the decision regarding treatment.

Part VI (nine chapters) deals with **the surgery experience, the** hospital admission and treatment and what to expect and post-hospital care, subsequent visits to your urologist and finally the conclusion.

Part VII includes the **glossary, resources and index**.

I hope something you read here will inspire and maybe even empower you to take better care of yourself, get a regular medical check-up, and when you have an indication that something is wrong with your prostate, take action to have it treated or corrected promptly.

Read, enjoy and act.

CONTENTS

What They Say About This Book	6
Authors Connection	7
Dedication	9
Acknowledgments	10
Preface	12
Contents	15
Introduction	17

Part I Your Health!

1. Your Health Is In Danger!	26
2. Chronic Degenerative Diseases	28
3. Causes Of Degenerative Diseases	32
4. Preventing Chronic Degenerative Diseases	45
5. Take Control Of Your Health – You Are Responsible!	59

Part II Your Prostate!

6. Understanding The Prostate Gland	64
7. Understanding "Tumour"	73
8. Prostatitis	75
9. Benign Prostatic Hyperplasia	78
10. Prostate Cancer	91

Part III Prostate Cancer Diagnosis

11. Diagnosing Prostate Cancer	98
12. The Digital Rectal Examination (DRE)	101
13. Prostate-specific Antigen (PSA)	104
14. Biopsy	111
15. When Is Biopsy Necessary?	117
16. You Have Cancer!	121
17. Grading The Cancer	126
18. Staging The Cancer	132
19. Bone Scan	137
20. Partin Probability Tables	140

Part IV Managing the Condition

    21. No Instant Decision   148
    22. Behaviour Tendencies – "DISC"   155
    23. State Of Denial   160
    24. Breaking The News   163
    25. Change Your Lifestyle   167
    26. My Search For More Understanding   172
    27. What The Woman In Your Life Can Do To Help   180

Part V Treatment Options

    28. Options For Prostate Cancer Treatment   190
    29. Watchful Waiting   198
    30. Surgery   204
    31. External Beam Radiation   226
    32. Internal Radiation Treatment   236
    33. Hormone Therapy   252
    34. Cryotherapy   260
    35. High Intensity Focused Ultrasound (HIFU)   270
    36. Chemotherapy   282

Part VI The Surgery Experience

    37. Making My Decision – Opting For Surgery   292
    38. Pre-admission Clinic   297
    39. Admission   300
    40. Surgery Made Easy   303
    41. Hospital Stay   308
    42. Post-surgery Care   321
    43. Tips For Care And Maintenance   325
    44. Post-surgery Medical Check-up   335
    45. Recurrent Prostate Cancer   342

Part VII Glossary And Resources

    Glossary Of Terms   352
    Suggested Additional Books To Read   373
    Other Resources For Prostate Conditions   375
    Index   378

INTRODUCTION

*Admitting that we don't feel well takes a great deal of courage.
We live in a society that prizes beauty, strength, and productivity, and there is
a great deal of shame and self-blame that comes with not living up to that ideal.
More often than not, when someone asks us how we are, we're likely to say 'just fine' and
change the subject. Our discomfort is compounded when our symptoms are largely invisible.*

SUSAN MILSTREY WELLS
WebMD COLUMNIST

Awareness of Prostate Cancer

Prostate cancer is a growing concern, worldwide. Next to skin cancer, it's the most common form of cancer found in men. Its incidence will continue to rise as the baby boomers age. It's, therefore, extremely important to make the public aware of its danger, its symptoms, diagnostic techniques and treatments.

We care for our eyes, teeth, nails and hair. We care for our lawns, cars, clothes, and homes. We do not seem to care as much for our heart, lungs, liver, kidney – and prostate.

Infection, enlargement, or cancer of the prostate can be painful, inconvenient, and embarrassing – even dangerous.

Prostate cancer is a very serious condition, with serious consequences, including complications, intolerable side-effects from treatment, and premature death.

Prostate cancer can happen to you. In fact, it may already be happening to you, although you may not know it, or want to admit it. One thing is certain: if you live long enough, you will have a problem with your prostate, be it prostatitis, benign prostatic hyperplasia or cancer. In fact, if you live long enough, you will likely have prostate cancer.

Currently, there are close to 90,000 Canadians and one million Americans living with prostate cancer. According to the Canadian Cancer Society and the Prostate Cancer Research Foundation of Canada, it's estimated that upward of 20,000 Canadian men are diagnosed with prostate cancer annually and about 4,200 die from it. The American Cancer Society and the National Cancer Institute estimate that some 230,000 American men are similarly diagnosed and more than 27,000 die annually from prostate cancer. These numbers are on the rise, a trend likely to continue for the foreseeable future.

Canadian cancer organizations say that 1 in 8.3 men will have prostate cancer in their lifetime and 1 in 28 (3.6 percent) will die from it. American organizations claim that 1 in 6 men will contract this cancer and 1 in 34 (3 percent) will die from it.

While numbers of diagnosed cases have risen rapidly in recent years, mortality rates have been steadily declining, probably due to both early screening and identification.

An information paper put out in 2002 by the American Red Cross, reported that 75 percent of men diagnosed with prostate cancer survive 10 years and 54 percent survive 15 years. Unfortunately, this does not indicate the characteristics of the cancer, such as grade and stage.

It's said that the risk of a man being affected with prostate cancer increases based on his family history, race, age, and lifestyle. If your father or brother had prostate cancer, your risk increases two-fold. If both your father and brother had it, your risk increases four-fold.

No two prostate cancers are the same. Each is different with its own unique set of characteristics. Therefore, the treatment you ultimately choose may be different than the one I chose. Even if it's the same, it would be for a different set of circumstances based on your cancer's characteristics. Having said that, our concerns and feelings would probably be similar.

Faith Helps

As a former member of the Jaycees, I believe their creed written by C. William Brownfield in 1946:
>   That Faith in God gives meaning and purpose to human life;
>   That the brotherhood of man transcends the sovereignty of nations;
>   That economic justice can best be won by free men through free enterprise;
>   That government is made of laws rather than of men;
>   That earth's great treasure lies in human personality;
>   And that service to humanity is the best work of life.

I believe that developing and maintaining a positive mental attitude and outlook helps awaken our personal healing potential. That's why I continuously work on nurturing my own faith and belief system and connect them with my personal mission in life, part of which is to:

"Live a life of integrity, faith and caring;
Love life and live it to its fullest, in happiness and health;
Continuously better my disposition in life, physically, socially, mentally, spiritually, and financially;
Continuously enhance, garner and harness my own wisdom, experience and knowledge, and eagerly share the resulting product with others for their individual personal development;
Inspire and empower individuals to better their personal disposition;
Honour and respect people for what and who they are, and want to become;
Enable individuals to tap their full potential;
Help individuals develop themselves into leaders for a world beyond tomorrow,

I also have a major goal to make one million friends and touch 100,000 lives before I leave this world.

It's Prudent to Learn More About Your Health

I believe one of the single most important things you can do for yourself is to learn more about your health. It's wise and prudent to live a healthy lifestyle and to be aware of any genetic risks.

I've always considered myself a fairly average person, one trying – sometimes more, sometimes less successfully – to lead a healthy lifestyle. I gave up smoking in 1979, after practicing that nasty habit for 18 years. Prior to 1998, I ate mostly home-cooked meals, and dined out only occasionally. I enjoyed chocolates and sweets. I loved hamburgers and steaks, but never overindulged with them. I kept busy with my job and volunteer work, often working long mentally taxing hours. I joined a gym, but seldom used its facilities. Being one to eat relatively few vegetables and fruits, and drink relatively little water, I supplemented my diet with vitamins and minerals supplements.

In addition to my health, being able to take care of my family was always foremost in my mind. Then in January of 1998, two things happened to change my life forever. And the result was an even stronger commitment to an even healthier lifestyle.

First, my cholesterol was misbehaving badly. It was out of control. The low-density lipoprotein (LDL), otherwise known as the bad cholesterol, was running very high, and the high-density lipoprotein (HDL), the good stuff, was too low.

In November 1997, my doctor insisted that, in order to remedy the situation, I was to start taking 400 IUs (international units) of vitamin E daily to reduce the LDL susceptibility to *oxidation* and hardening of the arteries.

I quickly examined the bottle containing my vitamins and minerals supplements and found it was providing only 30 IUs of vitamin E daily. I checked the contents of other popular supplements on the pharmacy shelves and discovered the highest concentration of vitamin E was 50 IUs.

Second, a few years earlier I was suspected of having a prostate disorder, possibly since 1995, but initial tests proved negative. However, subsequent tests and biopsies culminating in January 1998, proved positive for prostate cancer.

These two occurrences, surfacing within two months of each other, sent up a red flag in my mind and made me start thinking more about my health.

Now I wanted to learn as much as possible about nutrition and supplements. I also wanted to understand more about the prostate. I started searching for information about nurturing the body, the prostate in particular, and for any possibility of healing the cancer through the use of supplements.

As a result, I learned a whole new body of information. And it made me realize that our health – mine and yours, and that of our children and friends – is in danger.

Supplements

I learned that many of us may be nutritionally deficient, perhaps because we do not eat sufficiently balanced diets. For those of us who fall into this category – and I suspect we are in the majority – to become nutritionally sufficient, we must supplement the nutrients we get from our food with extra vitamins and minerals.

For example, in the case of vitamin E, some experts suggest that we need 400 to 1000 IUs daily, for optimal health, particularly to combat *free radicals* that bombard our *cells* with negative ions and to repair the resulting cellular damage. At the other end of the spectrum, some nutritionists and dietitians claim that if we eat very balanced meals, we do not need supplements. And there is some research to suggest too much vitamin E can be dangerous.

Many people claim that when they take supplements, they feel much more energetic and full of life. In fact many of those people feel it's not only additional vitamin E that we may need, but many other vitamins, minerals and *trace elements*.

Introduction

I learned there are many nutritional supplements on the market, but only a few that meet a standard experts consider optimal, balanced and *bioavailable*. This means the necessary active ingredients are present in specific quantities and proportions and remain available and fully effective in our systems for a requisite period of time. Most so-called optimal supplements are neither balanced nor bioavailable, mainly because they aren't manufactured to scientifically researched or pharmaceutical standards.

I embarked on a search for what I considered an appropriate selection of nutritional supplements. I knew that I wouldn't find them in regular supermarkets or pharmacies, since it appears that they carry only cheaper supplement brands containing a fraction of what I consider the optimal requirement for active ingredients. I did not find many to be balanced or bioavailable. After a long search, I found some which I considered to be relatively good supplements, in various health food stores and through individual suppliers. One of those, which particularly impressed me, I began purchasing on a regular basis.

At first, I took the supplements with skepticism. But about three weeks after I started on them, I realized that I had much more energy. Soon I felt that I was sleeping better and my appetite had improved. I introduced them to my wife, daughter and some friends. Within a year, my cholesterol was normal for the first time in many years. My wife's allergies were improved and my daughter's monthly cramps disappeared after 14 years. And a friend claimed that her frequent migraine headaches were drastically reduced. Finally, I realized that my lifelong "cold sore," that would usually attack my lips and/or my nose every three to four months, had not returned for quite a while – WOW!

Now, understand that I can only speak for myself and about my experience. I cannot say that these would necessarily work for others.

I soon realized that whenever I read about amounts of nutrients advocated for optimum health, those types and quantities were present in my supplements.

I continued to take the supplements while researching treatment options for my prostate cancer. I also began to control my diet. I altered the amount and type of food that I consumed to a controlled, balanced proportion of *carbohydrates, protein* and fat. In the process, I delayed making my decision about cancer treatment. I delayed that decision for two years.

I would not encourage you to delay treatment that long. It's one of the reasons I am writing this book – so that you will be able to make your decision sooner.

Making My Decision for Prostate Cancer Treatment

In December 1999, I finally decided on surgery as my treatment of choice. A *bilateral nerve-sparing retropubic radical prostatectomy*, was performed on March 3, 2000. Six weeks later I felt almost as good as I had prior to surgery. According to those who cared for me, I had a remarkable recovery.

I believe that two things, more than anything else, pulled me through: my positive mental attitude and my physically healthy condition.

Each of us is different. Our backgrounds, attitudes, lifestyles, diets, environments, cultures, ages and health practices make us different. Some of us are vegetarian, some do or do not consume dairy products and each of these differences may have played a part in the condition of our prostate. Cumulatively, these characteristics affect you differently than they affect me.

When it comes to making decisions regarding your prostate disorder and the treatment to pursue, there are many things to consider, including: your age, physical condition, health practices beliefs and history, test results, whether the *tumour* is cancerous, probability that it has spread (*stage* of the cancer), its aggressiveness (*grade* of the cancer), availability of medical expertise, and finally your fears and attitude, your family, and your financial situation. In addition, people you meet, books you read, risks you are willing to take, things you are prepared to give up – will all have an impact on your choice of treatment and your recovery.

My big challenge in making my choice was the fact that I didn't feel comfortable with my level of understanding about my condition. I didn't feel I had sufficient understanding to make the decision. I attributed this partly to the fact that the information that I had was limited and beyond my level of comprehension, given my state of mind, and partly to the fact that I did not ask enough questions. Unfortunately, I did not know what questions to ask; I didn't even know what I really wanted or needed to know. I couldn't see the big picture. I saw surgery as one choice, but was reluctant to succumb to it so quickly, without more understanding. I felt that I didn't know what was involved and what would be the side-effects or after-effects. I am not blaming anyone. Doctors only have so much time to spend with their patients, and patients comprehension levels vary. At the same time I felt that I had to make that decision.

I therefore embarked on my own research, mainly because I did not want to waste my doctor's time trying to educate me or make me feel comfortable. I also did not want to feel pushed into an uncomfortable decision-making situation

Let me make it clear that I'm only speaking of my feelings, but I have encountered several people who expressed the same sentiments. I have also encountered several who did not want to be bothered with the details. They just wanted to get on with the treatment recommended by their specialist. And that's alright, if you're comfortable with that.

Considering the Options

Most doctors believe that they inform their patients of the treatment options and give them enough information to make decisions. Despite that, however, many patients I have encountered with an abnormal prostate condition still feel they lack understanding. For myself, when I was diagnosed, my urologist, whom I and many others consider to be one of the best, recommended "surgery," because of my young age (59 years), and good health. He also mentioned alternatives treatment options such as "watchful waiting," "external beam radiation," and "*seeds implant.*" This information was provided after I was informed that my tumour was malignant. I left that session without realizing what I'd been told. What I did know was that I had cancer and it was being recommended that they cut me open and take it out. I also knew I was not ready to agree to that or to reject it.

Some people are comfortable in knowing the various options right away and making their decisions immediately, whereas some people want time to first digest the news and understand their options more clearly.

I Wanted More Understanding

If you are one of those who want more understanding – and there is much more to be had – you will have to take the responsibility to ask for it or research it yourself. In fact, you'd better read about it, because no one person will give you all the information you may want, or need, to have the level of understanding to make an informed decision.

This book tells you some little-known information about after-effects of treatments that no one talks about. It contains information that I wanted but did not know how to ask for.

If you think you know enough, consider this: On every subject there is information you know that you know, and there is information you know that you don't know. Then there is information you don't know that you don't know. This book may help fill some of the gaps for you.

There is a lack of consensus among medical professionals on how best to treat prostate cancer. However, in most cases the advice given is largely based on your age, general health, the characteristics of your cancer and, of course, who your specialist is. There are several different workable alternatives, and there are many competent specialists to get you through each of them. But all specialists do not have the same experience in this area.

In most cases, you will have time to research, read, ask questions, and digest information before you have to make your ultimate decision. This is not something that you are diagnosed with today and die of tomorrow. You should have a proper analysis and diagnosis by an experienced urologist. In fact, a second opinion may not hurt. It may help in making your final decision.

In the end, the decision is yours to make. I remind you not to waste valuable time waiting or doing nothing. That could lead to wasting a wonderful precious life – yours!

The best advice anyone can give you is to not focus on **treatment** initially, but rather **first** on **understanding** your condition. Then you can begin to focus on selecting the treatment and the doctor. Remember that advice as you read through this book.

Authors' Advice

As you read this book, you are encouraged to underline or write down anything that triggers a question for your urologist. In various chapters, a sample of important questions you may wish to ask are offered. Some of your questions or concerns may be answered in subsequent chapters and some may not be.

I intend to utilize every opportunity to travel anywhere in the world, and accept speaking engagements on the material in this book. I will use my knowledge, my experience and my public speaking skills to inspire you and others to take action fearlessly.

Again, I cannot emphasize enough that this is neither a medical book nor a treatment book. It's simply an information book. You must seek a qualified urologist for proper diagnostic information and appropriate treatment options for any abnormal prostate condition. But remember this: your urologist cannot instruct you as to which treatment to proceed with, he can only recommend. The final decision is yours.

Read on, and learn! And our best wishes to you.

Harold Usher
Co-Author

Part I

Your Health!

Chapter 1

YOUR HEALTH IS IN DANGER!

The health and well-being of individuals and the prosperity of the nation require a well nourished population – we all have a role to play in improving the nutritional health of Canadians.

1996 Joint Steering Committee on
Nutrition for Health: An Agenda for Action
Responsible for Development of a National
Nutrition Plan for Canada 1996

Most of us take our health for granted. We live thinking, or convincing ourselves, that we're healthy or invincible. Unfortunately, nothing is further from the truth. The fact that we feel good, look good and think we eat well is no guarantee that we're healthy. No matter how we think or feel, right now our health is in danger. You can take that to the bank.

If we are so healthy, why is it so many of us are always so tired? Why is it we are invaded again and again with vague illnesses that sap our energy? Why is it so many of us are always on some kind of medication, sometimes several at the same time? If we're as robust as we claim, why are millions of us suddenly so surprised to find we have cancer, heart disease, *diabetes*, high blood pressure, or some other terrible, or possibly terminal, disease? Why do we, in North America, spend so much more money on health care than any other nation, and still have more health problems than people of other nations? The answer is simple: most of us aren't as healthy as we like to think we are. Many experts believe it's simply that we tend to look for and treat the symptoms, but rarely do we treat the cause of the illness, or focus on prevention strategies.

In a March 2000 television report on a beauty pageant, a health reporter commented that: "the contestants all look so healthy, but they aren't as healthy as they look. Most of them are terribly malnourished." Now, understandably, beauty pageant contestants and models may look the way they do as a result of specific life choices. Sadly, that statement may also be true for many others in the western world.

We live in a world with rising levels of *toxins* in the environment, declining quality of food nutrients, and increasing amounts of hazardous substances in the products we consume and utilize. So, living in this toxin filled industrialized world, eating less than optimal quality food, breathing the polluted air, drinking the contaminated water, we may be doing more harm to ourselves than we realize. We need to eat better, but no matter how well we eat, many of us will still fall short of the recommended nutrients we need to live a really healthy and fulfilling life. So, it may be necessary to supplement our diet.

A doctor once told me that there are probably not many people alive, particularly over the age of 30, who are totally healthy. "Put them under a microscope and you'll find something unhealthy," he said. "In fact, many of them have diseases that are eating away at them right now and will kill them slowly, but they don't know it and therefore aren't doing anything about it."

Another doctor stated, "No matter how healthy we think we are or feel on any given day, the truth is that our cells are being bombarded every second by millions of free radicals that result in *oxidative stress* on those cells. These free radicals are damaging our cells right, left and centre, and it's only a matter of time before some of them and their resulting oxidative stress cause some form of irreparable damage to our cells, or cause one or more of the *chronic degenerative diseases* to invade our bodies."

Fortunately, in many instances our bodies have some built-in safeguards to fight these free radicals, although many times, they are so severe that the safeguards are insufficient.

Cancer in the *prostate gland* is one of the most common lifestyle conditions or diseases. As we saw earlier 16 percent of all North American men will discover that they have prostate cancer, and at least 16 percent of them will die from it, many because they found out and/or took action too late. In addition, studies have shown that one-third of men who died from other causes, such as accidents, military action and so on, unbeknownst to them, had cancer in their prostate. Now if that's not sobering, I don't know what is.

No doubt about it, your health is in danger, and so is mine. Our bodies are the finest engines ever created. They are potentially strong, alert, swift and flexible. The catch is that they require proper fuel to work as they were meant to.

Chapter 2

CHRONIC DEGENERATIVE DISEASES

*You gotta have guts to grow old.
To claim life, you've got to be bold.
But you've got to be smart, as well as have heart,
if you want your whole tale to be told.*

DR. WALTER BORTZ II
PAST PRESIDENT OF THE AMERICAN GERIATRICS SOCIETY
AUTHOR OF "WE LIVE TOO SHORT AND DIE TOO LONG"
"DARE TO BE 100" AND "LIVING LONGER FOR DUMMIES"

We Take Our Health for Granted – Big Mistake

The quotation above really brings home to me how so many of us take our health for granted when we're feeling good. Unfortunately, that feeling of healthiness is too often short-lived. We suffer from chronic illnesses, some of them degenerative, much too long before we die from them. But we can reverse that situation. With what we know about proper maintenance of our bodies today, we can live longer and die quicker. We can dare to live to 100. We may even be able to avoid or delay these chronic conditions. Let's admit it! And then let's do it! Let's be bold, smart and have heart and then have our whole tale told.

The leading cause of premature death in the western world has changed drastically since the early 1900s. Prior to the 1950s, people, died from *infectious diseases* such as diphtheria, polio, tuberculosis, and smallpox. Today, as a result of immunization and treatments to prevent or manage these diseases, they are seldom heard of, except in developing countries. In the Western World, more people now suffer from chronic and disabling illnesses which impose increasing burdens on hundreds of millions – physically, mentally, socially and financially.

According to the World Health Organization: "Infectious diseases will still dominate in developing countries. As the economies of these developing countries grow, non-communicable diseases will become more prevalent. This will be due largely to the adoption of our Western World's lifestyle and its accompanying risk factors, such as smoking, unhealthy diet and physical inactivity."

Chronic diseases include cardiovascular disease, cancer, diabetes, obesity, osteoporosis, arthritis and Alzheimer's disease among others.

Cardiovascular Disease: This is the number one killer in industrialized nations. In most cases you do not feel cardiovascular disease until it's too late. It accounts for 16.7 million deaths annually worldwide (29.2 percent of the total global deaths), according to the 2003 World Health Report. Of those, 7.2 million were from heart attacks, 5.5 million from stroke and 3.9 million from hypertension and other heart conditions. Another 20 million survive heart attack and stroke yearly.

Cancer: You do not feel cancer at first. It may grow for years undetected and then it explodes. Cancer is the number two killer in the world today and will remain one of the leading causes, accounting for 7.1 million deaths annually (12.5 percent of the global total), according to the 2003 World Health Report. There are more than 20 million people living with cancer worldwide and that's expected to rise to 30 million by 2020. The estimated number of new cases is expected to rise from 10 million annually in 2000 to 16 million by 2020.

Diabetes: You may start to lose feeling in your feet or recognize some deficiencies in your eyesight, then you risk losing your feet altogether. Diabetes has doubled the risk of heart attacks and strokes, and resulted in more than 20,000 amputations annually. More than 171 million people suffered from diabetes in 2000, a number expected to more than double (to 366 million) by 2030, largely because of dietary and lifestyle factors, according to the 2003 World Health Report. One of the major concerns is a growing incidence of Type 2 – often referred to as adult onset – diabetes (approximately 90 percent of all cases). About 3.2 million people die annually from this disease.

Obesity: Obesity is a new common disease of grave concern, especially in North America. It's reaching epidemic proportions with more than a billion overweight adults worldwide, at least 300 million of them obese. Obesity is undoubtedly one of the largest contributors to chronic disease and disability, particularly:

Part I   Your Health

- heart disease
- stroke
- hypertension
- arthritis (hips and knees cannot take the weight)
- type 2 diabetes

Exercise and a sensible diet, low in *saturated fat* and *trans fat*, could certainly help to reduce obesity.

There's also evidence to support the suggestion that obesity is related to prostate cancer development, perhaps due to the *hormone* status.

Osteoporosis: You don't feel osteoporosis until your first bone is broken. Then you fall, and you realize that you have very unhealthy bones. This is a disease of decreased bone mass and changes in bone structure that increase it's fragility and susceptibility to fracture – particularly of the hip, spine and wrist. This silent disease can go unnoticed for years. Many people think this is a woman's disease, but for every four women there's one man with the condition. According to Osteoporosis Canada, 1.4 million Canadians are affected. The National Osteoporosis Foundation in the U.S. reports that 10 million Americans have osteoporosis and another 34 million have low bone mass, placing them at increased risk. The International Osteoporosis Foundation estimates this disease affects more than 75 million people in Europe, the U.S. and Japan.

Arthritis: You feel arthritis. It creeps into your joints slowly until every movement becomes painful. There are several forms. The two most common are rheumatoid arthritis and osteoarthritis. The Public Health Agency of Canada reported in 1995 and again in 2000, that arthritis and rheumatism affected four million Canadians 15 years and older. That includes me and perhaps you. According to the U.S. National Institute of Health, over 40 million Americans have some form of arthritis (2.1 million with rheumatoid and 20 million with osteoarthritis).

Alzheimer Disease: This progressive degenerative disease quietly destroys vital brain cells, stealing your life little by little until you may not know your own name, or your spouse's name or a language you adopted. Your family suffers along with you. I know a man, originally from Eastern Europe, who has lived in North America for more than 50 years, and recently was stricken with this disease. During those years he learned and spoke only English. Today, he doesn't speak a word of English. He has reverted completely to his native Eastern European Language, one he had not used for more than thirty years. The Alzheimer Society of Canada reports that 290,000 Canadians, most over the age of 65, suffer from Alzheimer disease. According to the Alzheimer's Association in the U.S., 4.5 million Americans suffer from Alzheimer disease, a number that has more than doubled since 1980. It estimates that by 2025, between 11 and 16 million individuals will develop Alzheimer's.

In addition to the above chronic diseases, millions of people also suffer from other feared degenerative conditions, classified as auto-immune diseases, such as **multiple sclerosis (MS), lupus and others.**

Why are so many people suffering from these illnesses, some which weren't even on the rader until the latter half of the 20th century? For some of the answers we can no doubt look to the nutritional deficiencies, a more toxic environment, and the stream of hazardous substances we are almost forced to consume and inhale, that were discussed in the previous chapter. These are some of the same elements known to produce the free radicals that bombard our cells, resulting in oxidative stress, cellular damage and, ultimately, degenerative disease.

Chapter 3

CAUSES OF DEGENERATIVE DISEASES

One of the unfortunate consequences of poor nutrition, exposure to toxins, lack of exercise, and emotional stress is that they cause our bodies to wear out prematurely – often decades too soon.

Timothy J. Smith, M.D.
Author of "Renewal"

Our World of Food and Lifestyle

A major survey of men with diagnosed prostate cancer, conducted by a team of chemists/hygienists in Montreal and printed in the American Journal of Epidemiology a decade ago, identified 17 occupations, 11 industries, and 27 substances that showed an apparent correlation to the cancer growth. The survey resulted in an estimation that about 15 percent of the participants' cancers were related to exposure on the job.

The researchers found moderate support for risk due to occupation in electrical power, water transport, aircraft fabricators, metal product fabricators, structural metal erectors and railway transport. Topping the list of substances exhibiting moderately strong association were metallic dust, gasoline, lubricating grease, and hydrocarbon from coal.

Recognize that an association with a certain chemical does not necessarily imply that it causes prostate cancer, although it may be a contributing factor and may be considered an important public health issue.

Chapter 3 | Causes of Degenerative Diseases

It's believed by some people that many modern day chemicals burden our lives with the task of *detoxifying*, a process that uses up some of our natural stores of essential nutrients.

It's been reported in various books and articles that many foods we enjoy, such as fats (except omega fats or essential fatty acids), dairy products (including cheese and butter), meat and sugar, contribute to degenerative diseases, in particular cancers such as breast and prostate cancer. Although some may question the existence of substantial scientific proof for these assertions, there does appear to be sufficient concern to warrant caution in excessive use of such products.

We live in a world unlike that of our grandparents. Today's baby boomers, baby echoers (children of the boomers) and subsequent generation, have been exposed to a lifestyle that include ever-increasing amounts of processed, preserved and refined foods, *hydrogenated* oils, carbonated beverages and chemicals such as aspartame, exacerbated by air pollution, contaminated water and bad habits like smoking. It's feared by some that these lifestyle elements are damaging our cells and contributing to an escalation in the occurrence of cancers and other degenerative diseases.

Sugar – How Sweet It Isn't

Although I have been told many times that sugar is bad for my health, that it's toxic to my immune system, I always found that difficult to believe. But the books I've read on nutrition say the same thing: sugar is the one thing not to consume; it's a major health risk and can be called a metabolic poison.

According to Lorna Vanderhaeghe, co-author of the Canadian bestseller, The Immune System Cure, and publisher of the newsletter, Healthy Immunity:

> "**Sugar** is one food that should come with a warning label stronger than that found on a cigarette package. Sugar inactivates our *Natural Killer cells*. These Natural Killer cells are often the first cells that a *virus* or bacteria encounters, and if they are effective, the invading virus or bacteria will never be able to infect healthy cells. They are also our cancer fighting cells. As little as one teaspoon of sugar shuts off Natural Killer cells activity for up to six hours, leaving us vulnerable to the invasion and growth of cancer and infectious disease."

The sugar, sucrose, is a novelty of industrial civilization, the same as the cigarette. Some people believe that it brought cancer and cardiovascular disease to developed countries. Sucrose, when ingested, forms both glucose and fructose; this is why it's called a disaccharide.

At the turn of the 20th century, the average sugar consumption was just five pounds per person per year. Cardiovascular disease and cancer were virtually unknown then. Today we consume about 140 pounds of sugar per person per year.

Along with sugar there are cautions about white flour, white rice, processed oils, margarines and shortenings, non-dairy creamers, white flour pasta, corn starch and fried foods.

Fibre Failure

Lack of sufficient fibre is also reported to be a major cause of cardiovascular diseases and cancer.

"We do not consume sufficient fibre," says Dr. Myron Wentz, a scientist and expert in human cell research in Salt Lake City, Utah. Many other advocates agree. The National Cancer Institute maintains that the human body needs about 25 – 35 grams of fibre per day to prevent colon and rectal cancer. Most of us are lucky if we consume 15 grams a day. Of course there are those who believe fibre has no protective effect against colorectal cancer.

Refined flour, which most bread, cookies, pies and pizza crusts are made of, is our biggest culprit. It contains no fibre, because all the fibres – and with them the natural nutrients – have been intentionally removed, in order to make items cook, feel and taste better. After the fibres are removed, some artificial nutrients are added. The resulting product is called "enriched" flour. But that fibreless, enriched product plays havoc with our intestines and *colon*. In some cases, it clings to the inside walls of the intestines like putty. The molecular structure of refined or enriched flour is reported to be recognized and treated just like sugar, by the digestive system.

Many of the ailments we experience in life can be traced to an insufficiency of fibre intake. Some symptoms believed to result from this insufficiency are: constipation, acne, elevated cholesterol, headaches, hemorrhoids, chronically elevated liver enzyme system, and irritable bowel syndrome.

There are two types of fibre – water-soluble and water-insoluble.

Water-insoluble fibre is found in whole grains and vegetables. It helps to keep us regular and reduces the risk for colon problems ranging from constipation and irritable bowel syndrome to colon cancer. It's critical for the proper functioning of the colon, ensuring that undigested and indigestible food move quickly through the intestines and don't stay in one place too long, thus irritating the intestine lining. This is the type of fibre your mother used to refer to as "roughage." It also binds up bile from the liver and gall bladder which contains oil soluble wastes, such as excess hormones and pesticides residues that need to be removed quickly, through the bowels, so they aren't reabsorbed.

Water-soluble fibre is found in oat, beans and certain fruits, especially apples. It's probably what's behind the saying "an apple a day will keep the doctor away." Eating an apple a day may very well prevent you from being a patient of the cardiologist, since water-soluble fibre binds up cholesterol and removes it from the body. It helps to lower total cholesterol levels, further reducing risk for heart disease. It may also reduce the risk of gallstones.

Another type of water-soluble fibre is called "lignan," a family of phytochemicals that has antioxidant activity. This is now being studied because of its effect in lowering women's risk for breast cancer. The best food source for lignan is flax seed meal. Whereas flax seed oil contains a full range of *essential fatty acid*, which can help reduce allergy related problems and inflammations, as well as the risk for heart disease, it contains no fibre or lignan.

Caution: To prevent fibre from becoming like cement in your gut, it's advisable to drink eight glasses of water each day.

Fats in the Fire

Dr. Udo Erasmus of Vancouver, British Columbia, author of Fats that Heal – Fats that Kill, said:

> "Eight out of 10 baby boomers and baby echoers are getting too little of 23 of the 43 essential minerals, vitamins, aminos, and fatty acids that must be present in food supply for humans to sustain life. If not corrected, these deficiencies will snowball into a nationwide health crisis for the adult population."

According to Dr. Michael Colgan, internationally acclaimed research scientist in sports nutrition and on aging, and Director of the Colgan Institute of Nutritional Science in San Diego, California and Victoria, British Columbia, in his book, The New Nutrition – Medicine for the Millennium, "**fats and oils** should be no more than 20 percent by calories – 10 percent by weight – of your diet at most. And that includes what you get from high-fat meats and dairy food." It is now a common belief that diets high in fat promote obesity and increase the risk of numerous diseases, including *atherosclerosis*, *hypertension*, adult-onset diabetes and certain cancers including prostate.

Saturated fats and hydrogenated fats have been shown to increase blood cholesterol levels and cause circulation congestion problems more than unrefined vegetable oils do. Even worse for your body than saturated fats, may be the trans fat found in hydrogenated products, such as margarine and shortening.

According to studies conducted by Dr. A. Whittemore and colleagues at Stanford University School of Medicine in California, and reported in the Journal of the National Cancer Institute in 1995, prostate cancer was strongly correlated with saturated fat intake. Dr. Whittemore and his colleagues examined that association in African-Americans (highest risk ethnic group), whites-Americans (high risk), and Asian-Americans (low risk) in Los Angeles, San Francisco, Hawaii,

Vancouver and Toronto. They compared 1,600 men with prostate cancer against 1,600 men without it from 1987 to 1991. In all groups, the cancer was strongly correlated with saturated fat intake. Note: the African-American men consumed the most amount of saturated fat. The Asian-American consumed the least amount of saturated fat. Several other studies have since corroborated these findings.

One should note that there are also genetic differences amongst these groups that contribute to the differences in prostate cancer incidence.

Danger in the Dairy

In our society, we consider dairy an important component of the food groups and something that contributes significantly to bone development.

In her book, Your Life in Your Hands, author, professor and five-time breast cancer survivor, Jane Plant of the United Kingdom, advocates that eliminating dairy products completely from our diet can help avoid and even cure some cancers. She believes that giving up milk is the key to beating breast cancer. Professor Plant, a respected scientist in Britain, reported that she experienced this when she was diagnosed with recurrent breast cancer for the fifth time. She eliminated dairy products from her diet completely and, according to her, six weeks later she was cured of the cancer.

Quoted in the Daily Mail May 22, 2000, comparing the high incidence of cancer in Britain to that of China, Professor Plant observed:

> "… whatever was causing my breast cancer and the shockingly high incidence in this country (Britain) generally, it was almost certainly something to do with our better-off, middle-class, Western lifestyle."

She added that:

> "… there is an important point for men here, too. I have observed in my research that much of the data about prostate cancer lead to similar conclusions.
>
> According to figures from the World Health Organization, the number of men contracting prostate cancer in rural China is negligible, only 0.5 men in every 100,000. In England, Scotland and Wales, however, this figure is 70 times higher.
>
> Like breast cancer, it's a middle-class disease that primarily attacks the wealthier and higher socio-economic groups – those that can afford to eat rich foods."

I don't know if we would classify fast food restaurants as middle-class, rich food, but I suspect that's where many earlier African-American prostate cancer victims consumed much of their saturated and hydrogenated fats.

Here's Professor Plant's story in brief:

> "Following my insight into Chinese diet, I decided to give up all diary produce immediately. Cheese, butter, milk and yogurt and anything else that contained dairy produce. Within days the lump started to shrink. About two weeks after my second *chemotherapy* session and one week after giving up dairy produce, the lump in my neck started to itch. Then it began to soften and to reduce in size. The line on the graph, which had shown no change, was now pointing downwards as the tumour got smaller and smaller. And, very significantly, I noted that instead of declining exponentially as cancer is meant to do, the tumour's decrease in size was plotted on a straight line heading off the bottom of the graph, indicating a cure: not suppression or remission of the tumour."

Of course, this is one anecdote and we do not know what other dietary products Professor Plant was pursuing simultaneously or if this was solely responsible for her "cure." The reason for mentioning it here is to identify that dairy food, with all its important components, may have some effect on cancer, particularly of the prostate.

As noted previously, genetic and other factors also play a major role in the etiology of prostate cancer.

I clearly remember two things on this subject that my father, who was a citrus farmer in Belize, telling me when I was growing up. One was that "cow's milk is for calves, women's milk is for human babies." The other was that "the soil on which I grow my grapefruit trees is depleted of its *nutrients* and will be useless after these trees have stopped producing." Farmers in Belize did not use artificial soil nutrients or fertilizer in those days.

Salt of the Earth – Not?

According to Dr. Michael Colgan, "we are increasing our consumption of salt in our foods and decreasing our consumption of potassium, simply in order to preserve meats and dairy foods for long shelf life, and to compensate for the lack of taste in denatured, over-processed supermarket foods. We now eat 20 times the amount of salt needed for optimal health, and conversely, much less of needed potassium. The result of this is, a sodium-induced hypertension for many North Americans. This is the biggest single risk for cardiovascular disease."

Both the Canadian Heart and Stroke Foundation and the American Heart Association advocate reducing our salt intake. An article on the Heart and Stroke website states that healthy adults should not consume more than one teaspoon of salt a day. And the American Heart Association advocate that healthy adults should eat no more than 2,300 milligrams of sodium a day, which is the equivalent of about one teaspoon of salt. When you must reduce the amount of sodium (salt) you consume, be aware of both natural and added sodium content. Table salt is sodium chloride with 40 percent sodium by weight. Sodium is also included in sodium bicarbonate or baking powder, and many other products that we consume.

A Breath of Not-so-Fresh Air

Air quality has become an environmental crisis today. Never before have people been as concerned about clean air. Public health experts in Canada estimate that air pollution is responsible for 16,000 premature deaths in this country each year; at this rate, forty Canadians die from air pollution-related causes each and every day. Estimate for the U.S. is ten folds or more. Look outside. See the smog? Look at the vehicles traveling our streets or idling in our neighbours' driveways. See the carbon dioxide? Where do you think it goes? Up our nostrils! And with it comes free radicals and oxidative stress, attacking every cell in our bodies, causing degenerative diseases.

Fossil fuel emissions from automobiles, coal and diesel generating plants, are polluting our air. We try to overlook the issue, but all of us are being harmed by air pollution. Some experts attribute many preventable diseases and deaths to it. The number of infants born with respiratory sensitivities to the environment is on the rise. Asthma is rampant among our children. The health of our aging population is being seriously compromised. If you do not believe this, visit any nursing home and ask the staff about growing numbers of admission of residents with both chronic conditions and respiratory problems. There is no doubt about it, air quality contributes to several degenerative diseases, including, in some instances, cancer.

Killing the Bugs – Or Us?

People of my generation – the baby boomers – and our children are walking time bombs in terms of these diseases. We smoked – or inhaled second hand smoke – drank and grew up on saturated fat, fatty foods and dairy products. Furthermore, many of us have pesticides stored in our systems that very few of us are even aware of.

In the 1950s most of us were exposed to the dreaded pesticide DDT. It was used to control bugs and insects that caused malaria, such as mosquitoes. We inhaled DDT daily for years until it was banned. This and other pesticides penetrated our systems via our noses, mouths, ears and our very pores. I suspect many of us still have relatively high levels of this dangerous substance in our systems, only now exposing the damage it has done to our cells, surfacing as a slow killer.

Today as well, many of our fruits and vegetables look healthy and fresh because they have been sprayed with pesticides, herbicides, or insecticides to keep away bugs and blight. Do you wash away these from your vegetables and fruits before you eat them? You should do so.

In North America, we use toxic substances, and various forms of "cides," to achieve immaculate lawns, without regard for the harm they may be doing to our environment – to our children, seniors, animals, the creatures around us and to ourselves.

So, men are getting prostate and women are getting breast and ovarian cancer, and all of us are getting various cancers at an alarming rate. Could one cause be due to DDT, or other pesticides? Or could it be fat or dairy products? Perhaps it could be each or all of them. We need to intentionally cleanse ourselves of these destroyers.

Anecdotally, a friend of mine who suffered from cancer from 1997 to 2001 had extensive tests to determine the cause of her cancer and its treatment. The results showed that her body was contaminated with pesticides, which she inhaled while working on her parents' farm in the 1970s. The specialists concluded that they could clean out some of this substance, but they could not remove it all. She finally succumbed to her cancer in July 2001.

Butting Out

Let me put this mildly. I believe, as do millions that smoking is dangerous to human health. Second hand smoke, exhaled after inhaling, is even worse. It's said that when we inhale smoke from cigarette we breathe in eight dangerous toxins. When we exhale we let out six of those toxins and pass them on to others.

On one occasion, while speaking to some high school students, I suggested the danger that smoking has on optimal health. One young woman approached me afterwards and announced sarcastically:

> "Mr. Usher, despite what you say and with all due respect to you, I love to smoke, and I have no intention of giving it up!"
>
> I replied, "That's alright honey, but you don't smoke, I assure you!"
>
> She quickly responded with confidence "Oh yes! I do. I smoke a pack of cigarettes every day."
>
> I replied again, calmly, "That's great honey, but I still say that you don't smoke."
>
> I could sense she was becoming annoyed as she repeated herself.

> I once more reiterated, "That's what you think and believe, but the fact is you don't smoke."
>
> Hearing that, she pulled out a pack of cigarettes and lighter from her pocket, removed one of the cigarettes from the pack and placed it between her lips. She flicked the lighter, brought its flame up to the other end of the cigarette and sucked in to ignite it. She blew out some smoke, as she closed the lighter, with a smile on her face, as if to say she had proven her point. Quickly, she lifted the cigarette to her mouth once more and sucked in. As she did so, the burn moved up the length of the cigarette. She removed it from her mouth and blew the smoke out as she boastfully stated once again, "See, I smoke!" and as if to say, "and there is nothing you can do about it."
>
> Thereupon I smiled and responded politely, "I see indeed! You should see yourself. What I saw was the cigarette smoking and you sucking. That tells me, it's the cigarette that smokes, you are only the sucker."
>
> She quickly walked away in a huff and a puff.

The late Ann Landers reprinted the following in her April 12, 2000 column:

"According to the American Cancer Society, as soon as you snuff out that last cigarette, your body will begin a series of physiological changes, as follows:

- Within 20 minutes: your blood pressure, body temperature and pulse rate drops to normal.
- Within eight hours: your smoker's breath disappears, carbon monoxide level in your blood drops and your oxygen level rises to normal.
- Within 24 hours: your chance of heart attack decreases.
- Within 48 hours: your nerve endings start to regroup and your ability to taste and smell improves.
- Within three days: your breathing becomes easier.
- Within two to three months: your blood circulation improves, walking becomes easier, and your lung capacity increases up to 30 percent.
- Within one to nine months: your sinus congestion and shortness of breath improve; cilia that sweeps debris from your lungs grows back; and your energy increases.
- Within one year: your excess risk of coronary heart disease is half that of a person who smokes.
- Within two years: your heart attack risk drops to near normal.
- Within five years: your lung cancer death rate, as an average former pack-a-day smoker, decreases by almost half, your stroke risk is reduced , your risk of mouth, throat and esophageal cancer is half that of a smoker.

- Within ten years: your lung cancer death rate is similar to that of a person who does not smoke, and your pre-cancerous cells are replaced.
- Within 15 years: your risk of coronary heart disease is the same as a person who has never smoked."

Get Off the Couch

We have become a nation of couch potatoes. On August 31, 2000, Dr. Art Quinney, a spokesperson for The Canadian Council for Health and Active Living at Work, had this to say about the danger of lack of physical activity:

> "Canadians are fast turning into slugs as they haven't increased their physical activity in five years. In 1981, 79 percent were physically inactive to the extent that they were threatening their health. Today it's 63 percent, a statistic that hasn't changed since 1995. This is costing businesses millions of dollars in absenteeism, stress, workplace injuries and benefit claims. ... too many employees spend their days as virtual desk potatoes, sitting in front of their computer screens, on the telephones, or in meetings. We have a major health problem on our hands – some might say a major health crisis."

In fact according to data from the 2000-2001 national surveys, **more than half of Canadians are physically inactive**. Inactivity increases as people age. Women are more inactive (59 percent) than men (53 percent). And it differs from Province to Province as well as from State to State. Our congratulations to the West Coast, which has the lowest percentage of physical inactivity.

These alarming statistics can be transferred similarly to anywhere in the industrial world. Added to the above, we leave work and travel by automobile, and when we arrive home, we plop ourselves down in front of either the television or the computer screen.

It's no secret that people of all ages can improve the quality of their lives through moderate physical activity. You don't have to be training for the Boston Marathon to derive real health benefits. A regular, preferably daily, regimen of at least 30-45 minutes of brisk walking, bicycling, or even working around the house or yard will reduce your risk of developing coronary heart disease, hypertension, colon cancer, and diabetes. And, if you're already doing that, you will benefit even more by increasing the intensity or duration of the activity. You may want to consider picking up the pace.

One of the best wake-up calls to the medical community, that inactivity is a big health risk was an article published in the "Journal of the American Medical Association" in 1982, by Dr. Walter

Part I Your Health

Bortz II, from the department of medicine at California's Palo Alto Medical Clinic, an author of several books and also a past president of the American Geriatrics Society. He postulated that inactivity causes a chain reaction of cardiovascular decay. First, it reduces vital capacity. Sitting like a couch potato reduces ability to take up and use oxygen, causing vital muscles, organs, and the brain to be deprived of oxygen. Second, it reduces the ability of the heart to pump blood around the body, so that the tissues become doubly deprived of adequate oxygen and blood and thus, the essential nutrients the blood supplies.

Hundreds of subsequent studies have presented supporting evidence that Dr. Bortz was right. One of the best such studies was conducted by renowned exercise guru Dr. Kenneth Cooper, and colleagues, at his Aerobics Centre in Dallas, Texas. They followed 13,344 men and women for 15 years. Their meticulous research controlled all major interfering variables, such as age, family history, personal health history, smoking, blood pressure, cardiovascular conditions and insulin metabolism.

According to the Division of Nutrition and Physical Activity, National Centre for Chronic Disease Prevention and Health Promotions (U.S.), regular physical activity can improve health and reduce the risk of premature death in the following ways:

- Reduces the risk of developing coronary heart disease (CHD) and the risk of dying from CHD
- Reduces the risk of stroke
- Reduces the risk of having a second heart attack in people who have already had one heart attack
- Lowers both total blood cholesterol and triglycerides and increases high-density lipoproteins (HDL or the "good" cholesterol)
- Lowers the risk of developing high blood pressure
- Helps reduce blood pressure in people who already have hypertension
- Lowers the risk of developing non-insulin-dependent (type 2) diabetes mellitus
- Reduces the risk of developing colon cancer
- Helps people achieve and maintain a healthy body weight
- Reduces feelings of depression and anxiety
- Promotes psychological well-being and reduces feelings of stress
- Helps build and maintain healthy bones, muscles, and joints
- Helps older adults become stronger and better able to move about without falling or becoming excessively fatigued.

Can a lack of physical activity hurt your health? Evidence shows that those who aren't physically active are definitely not helping their health, and may likely be hurting it. The closer we look at the health risks associated with a lack of physical activity, the more convincing it's that those who aren't yet regularly physically active should become active.

If you live in Canada, you can adapt and commit to the Health Canada's "Canada's Physical Activity Guide to Healthy Active Living." If you live in the U.S. take a look at the "Surgeon General's Report on Physical Activity and Health." If you live somewhere else, follow the advice of the World Health Organization's Global Strategy on Diet, Physical Activity and Health. If you do not follow any physical activity program, you are misusing your organs and body, and "misuse is disuse." You can change that!

Don't Distress – De-Stress

Another major killer is stress. Workplace stress is the most common form, according to a Decima Research poll done for the Heart and Stroke Foundation and reported in the Globe and Mail on February 3, 2000.

Many people complain they don't have enough time for family or friends, nor for personal activities they enjoy. Often this is related to stresses at work, ranging from abuse and harassment by customers, supervisors and colleagues to physical conditions such as inadequate ventilation system, poor ergonomics and noise. Often they suffer from work overload – too many responsibilities or demands, too few breaks and too much overtime. Frequently people are afraid to complain for fear of losing their jobs.

The tragedy is that most people don't make a lifestyle change, until it's too late, after they are rushed to hospital with a heart attack, to the emergency room with palpitation, or worse, diagnosed with a serious illness.

> A woman I knew, who worked for a law firm in Manhattan, N.Y., was verbally abused by a senior officer in the firm, for what was perhaps a relatively minor incident. This woman took a lot of pride in her work, and the incident bothered her for the entire evening at home, and throughout the night. It bothered her to the extent that she hardly slept. She told her children about the incident. The following day, she decided that she would go to work early and try to rectify the situation, before the officer arrived. She left home at 6:00 a.m. to catch the early subway. While standing on the platform of the subway station, waiting for the train to arrive, she had a massive heart attack. She died right there, all alone, with no one around to help her. She left two young daughters behind. She was my sister. Stress kills! And people can heap stress upon others on the job, largely through ignorance, by harassment, intimidation, bullying and making high demands for productivity and performance.

> A friend of mine suddenly began to feel a painful pressure in his chest whenever he hurried to get to a destination. When he went for his annual check-up, he told his doctor about it. His doctor sent him to a cardiologist to have a stress test, an intense physical exercise to stress the heart and test its reactions. The results of the test indicated he had angina. The doctor told him he was lucky since more than 80 percent of angina victims discover their condition after they've had a heart attack. When known in advance, angina can be treated and a heart attack may be avoided.

It would appear that if a person has heart disease and is faced with workplace stress, that stress might place additional burden on the heart and cause it to fail sooner.
As a heart failure survivor, I believe that stress and lack of physical activity can lower the immune system and cause or worsen any of the degenerative diseases mentioned earlier.

I also believe, as someone who has experienced tremendous stress in my lifetime, that it literally poisons our bodies and makes us more vulnerable to fatigue and illnesses such as colds and flu. Some people have even experienced a raging appetite, resulting in the depositing of stress fat – the kind that accumulates around the waistline. This fat, in addition to being our main source of energy to fight or flee during stress, also increases the risk of heart disease, high blood pressure, high *cholesterol*, stroke, diabetes, and cancer.

Stress relief, avoidance and elimination are all urgent health issues, particularly in the workplace. Stress also worsens the lack of nutrition in the modern diet.

Is your job contributing to a condition of cancer, heart weakness, or other disease that could show its ugly head later on in life? No? Think again! All these conditions and factors can, and do, contribute to declining health and, ultimately, degenerative diseases.

No doubt about it, the food we eat and the lifestyle we live are killing us faster than anything else.

Chapter 4

PREVENTING CHRONIC DEGENERATIVE DISEASES

"Until quite recently, it was taught that everyone in the country gets enough vitamins through their diet, and that taking vitamin supplements just create expensive urine. I think we now have proof this is not true."

Dr. Walter Willett,
Scientist and cardiovascular expert,
Harvard University,
Newsweek, June 7, 1993

Eating for Health

Eating is one of life's greatest pleasures. It's also a necessity. As the saying goes, "We eat to live" Therefore, food should contribute to our enjoyment of life, not detract from it. A varied menu of healthy foods can enrich all stages of life. Diets containing the right balance of carbohydrates, proteins and fat can reduce risks of chronic disease and can be part of a rich, enjoyable, and energetic lifestyle.

In an article entitled "Optimal Macronutrition: Long-term Health, High Performance, and Weight Control," published in Lifelong Nutritions, Volume 1, Issue 2, March 2000, (USANA Health Sciences) Gaale Rudolph, PhD, and Tim Wood, PhD, reported:

"*Macronutrients*, carbohydrates, proteins and fat serve as the major sources of energy for the body. They also provide materials for tissue growth and repair. Optimal macronutrition requires that we consume the right amounts of carbohydrates, proteins and fat in the proper ratio. ... In simple terms, a diet, in which good carbohydrates supply 50 percent of the daily calories, high quality proteins supply 30 percent, and salutary (healthy) fats supply 20 percent, is likely to be a healthful diet."

The proportions are similar to those traditionally consumed in areas of the world where the people are known for their longevity and low incidence of chronic disease. In those areas, in particular the Mediterranean and some Asian countries including Japan and China, people generally live long and die short, without lengthy suffering. The traditional diets in those regions are relatively high in carbohydrates and fibre, and low in fats and protein. They are semi-vegetarian, low in consumption of dairy products and significantly high in certain fish, rich in essential "good" fats.

> Based on my own life experience, optimal macronutrition is a goal we should strive for. It's not something to be considered, practiced, and accomplished for just a short period of time, nor a start and stop process, but rather an important part of a healthy lifestyle.

This is achieved by supplying our bodies' natural defense systems with the nutrients needed to maintain healthy body function, from the cellular level through the entire organ and physiologic systems. The right balance of carbohydrates, proteins and fats is necessary for:

- vitality and well being,
- maintaining an even well-regulated metabolism, and
- reducing the amount of free radical activity that leads to chronic disease.

The right kinds of carbohydrates include nutrient-packed, complex carbohydrates, containing high amounts of balanced, soluble and *insoluble* fibres and starches as energy *sources*. These are best found in vegetables, whole grains and fresh fruits.

The right kinds of proteins contain essential amino acids, the body's chemical building blocks for growth and repair. They are necessary for the manufacture and repair of body tissues and organs, including skin, hair, muscles, and blood vessels. They are also essential in the formation of various hormones, enzymes and *antibodies*. Because our structural and metabolic proteins are constantly being recycled, the body needs a steady supply of new protein containing these amino acids.

Ideally, say the experts, we should get most of our protein from sources lower in fat, such as fish and plant products, which have additional benefits, such as *antioxidants, isoflavones* and *bioflavonoids*.

The right kinds of fats provide a more concentrated form of energy than carbohydrates. These include the essential fatty acids (EFAs), which are needed for growth, tissue repair and the manufacture of important chemical messengers. EFAs are major components of *cell membranes* and are especially important in neural tissue. They are precursors in the synthesis of *prostaglandins*, hormone-like compounds that play many important roles in our bodies. Among the best sources of EFAs are salmon, soybeans, flaxseed, hemp seed and walnuts.

Where have all the Nutrients Gone?

Despite our best efforts to eat foods that are healthy, much of the nutrient content in our food is lacking. Remember my earlier comments about when I was a young boy growing up on the farm in Belize in the 1950s? My father, who was a citrus fruit grower, believed that the soil on which his grapefruits grew was depleted of its nutrients. He figured that the crop at that time would be the last good crop he would get from that soil.

Also in our busy lives, it's sometimes a challenge finding the time to fit in all the necessary servings of fruit and vegetables for a balanced diet. We can boost our intake by drinking juices. However, without an appropriate amount of *micronutrients* (nutritionals), in the form of vitamins, minerals and trace elements, our immune systems will be at risk from the damaging effects of free radicals, stress and oxidation. So we may not be getting the necessary nutrition for optimal health from our food.

Thousands of reports, based on scientific research the world over, support the finding that there aren't sufficient nutrients in the food we eat to combat these harmful elements. Nutritional supplements of vitamins, minerals and trace elements can help.

Nutritional Supplements

In the 1940s, the U.S. government established recommended daily allowances (RDA) for vitamins and essential minerals to ensure people would get enough to protect them from deficiency diseases such as scurvy, pellagra and rickets. Today we have different needs for vitamins and minerals because of increasing stress, pollution and lack of nutrients in the soil.

RDA was a good start, but research and experience in the ensuing decades have shown that effective doses of vitamins and minerals are often significantly higher than the RDAs. There are thousands of studies available showing beneficial effects from higher doses of these nutrients.

It's important to understand that vitamins and minerals are not medicine or drugs. They are enhancements to diet and serve a preventive function by offering additional resistance to disease.

They provide protection against free radicals and oxidative stress, and help build the immune system.

Of course too much of a good thing can be harmful, and some doctors believe certain vitamins and minerals may, in some circumstances, be toxic. If a woman is pregnant or breast-feeding, it's recommended that she contact her health care professional before using supplements. However, specific formulations are routinely prescribed during pregnancy.

I quickly learned that my body could benefit from a balanced spectrum of vitamins, minerals and trace elements.

Vitamins

Vitamins are, as the name suggests, vital for good health. The primary source is from diet. However, due to excessive food processing, which can destroy many nutrients, plus the aforementioned problem of depleted soils, people today are often deficient in one or more vitamins.

Essential vitamins include vitamin A in the form of *beta carotene*, B complex, C, D from sunlight, and E.

The following information is based on sources, including professionals, who embrace supplementation as a vital part of an optimal nutritional program.

Vitamin A in the form of **Beta-Carotene** (converted by the body to Vitamin A as needed, preventing a toxic build-up) is very much an immune system vitamin and antioxidant. It's reported to be able to help protect us against cancer of the larynx, lungs, esophagus, gastrointestinal tract, colon, rectum, breasts, cervix, bladder, prostate and skin. Some reports even say that it can help combat hair loss. Its deficiency will make us prone to cold and flu. A good natural food source for Vitamin A would be apricots, cabbage, carrots, egg yolk, fish liver, mango, melon, spinach, squash, sweet potato, yellow bell pepper, watercress, and fish, among others. It's said that large doses of Beta Carotene will increase the body's demand for Vitamin E. A daily intake of 15,000 to 25,000 IUs or more is recommended, by professional believers in the field, for *optimum* health for an adult. Vitamin A at high intake can build up in body fats to become toxic. Large amount of Beta-Carotene shows little toxicity, but may turn your skin yellow.

The B-complex vitamins include **B1**-Thiamine, **B2**-Riboflavin, **B3**-Niacin, **B5**-Pantothenic acid, **B6**-Pyridoxine, **B12**-Cyanocobalamin and *folic acid*. These are reported to be essential, in order to maintain a strong and healthy immune system, optimal hormone levels, and proper growth and health of all of the body's *epithelial* tissues, including skin and organ linings.

Chapter 4 | Preventing Chronic Degenerative Diseases

Vitamin B1, which is water-soluble, converts carbohydrates to energy, enhances circulation and blood formation, aids digestion and has a positive effect on energy, growth, normal appetite, and learning capacity. A good natural food source for Vitamin B1 would be beans, bran, most vegetables, whole grain and yeast, among others. Considered toxic-free.

Vitamin B2, which is water-soluble, helps to release energy from macronutrients carbohydrates, protein and fat during *metabolism*. A good natural food source for Vitamin B2 would be, poultry, meat, fish, dairy food, eggs, leafy green vegetables, mushrooms, tomatoes, and wheat germ, among others. Considered toxic-free

Vitamins B3, which is water-soluble, enhances the optimal functioning of our cells, calms the nervous system, and is good for the thymus gland. A good natural food source for Vitamin B3 would be cabbage, cauliflower, mushrooms, and tomatoes, among others. Low toxicity.

Vitamins B5, which is water-soluble, also enhances the optimal functioning of our cells, calm the nervous system, and is good for the thymus gland. A good natural food source for Vitamin B5 would be alfalfa sprouts, avocado, broccoli, cabbage, celery, eggs, lentils, mushrooms, squash, and tomatoes, among others. Considered toxic-free.

Vitamin B6, which is water-soluble, helps reduce homocystine levels, inhibits platelet aggregation and blood clotting, helps build body tissue and aids in metabolism of protein. A good natural food source for Vitamin B6 would be banana, broccoli, brussels sprout, cabbage, cauliflower, lentils, nut, onion, squash, among others. Large amounts for months may cause reversible nerve damage in some sensitive people.

Vitamin B12 has been known to strengthen the immune system, prevents nerve damage, helps in the functioning of the nervous system and metabolism of protein and fat, as well as aids in cell formation, development and longevity. A good natural food source for Vitamin B12 would be eggs and meat, among others. Considered non-toxic.

A daily intake of 10 to 50 mg of B6 taken together with 5 to 8 mcg of B12, around 25 to 200 mg of each of B1 and B2, 30 to 100 mcg of B3, 20 to 500 mcg of B5, and 800 to 3400 mcg of folic acid, is recommended by professional believers in the field, for optimum health for an adult. Taken with food is preferred. Note that if the B-complex vitamins are being absorbed, your urine will be bright yellow with a probable pungent smell as a result of the riboflavonoids presence.

Folic Acid (Folate), another B-Vitamin, controls amino acid metabolism in the body. Its deficiency inhibits cell growth. The best sources of folate are fresh dark-green leafy vegetables, beans and egg yolk. Food-processing destroys lots of the folate.

Results of a study reported to the American College of Cardiology's 52nd Annual Scientific Session on March 30, 2003 suggest that a super combination of folate (folic acid) plus vitamins B1 and B6 were likely to cause *stent* failure or new narrowing in the stented arteries. It should be noted that, the fact that these people would have stents, like me, would be because we already have coronary artery disease – narrowing of the lumen for blood flow due to deposits of cholesterol and other materials. The stents, in my case – 4, have been inserted to keep the narrowed parts of the arteries open.

Vitamin C (absorbic acid), which is water-soluble, is reported to have antiviral, antibacterial, anticancer and anti-aging properties. It was studied extensively by the late double Nobel Laureate, Dr. Linus Pauling, who strongly advocated it as a fighter of the common cold and more serious diseases such as cancer. According to Dr. Pauling, the vitamin's versatility in illness prevention arises from its role in the manufacture of collagen, the protein that gives shape to connective tissues and strength to skin and blood vessels. Dr. Pauling also noted Vitamin C's connection with lipoprotein-a, a substance whose levels in the blood have been linked to cardiovascular disease. Lipoprotein-a is also a major component of the plaques found in the blood vessels of *arteriosclerosis* patients.

Vitamin C is an anti-oxidant that's reported to increase the level of "immunoglobin," which helps to stop invaders from entering our digestive tract, and helps to boast the immune system in general. Vitamin C also protects us against the damaging effects of stress and oxidation. It maintains connective tissue, boosts wound healing and resists scar formation. It also protects against infections of various sorts, and helps to lower cholesterol. It's essential for the structure of bones, cartilage, muscle and blood vessels. A good natural food source for Vitamin C would be citrus fruits, broccoli, cabbage, cauliflower, kiwi fruit, melon, papaya, peas, pepper, sprouted seeds, strawberries, and tomato. It may be a problem in patients with a tendency to kidney stone formation. A daily intake of 1,000 mg (one gram) or more is recommended, by professional believers, for optimum immune health for an adult. It also needs to be taken over a long period of time.

Vitamin D, which is fat-soluble, is found in food and is also manufactured in the body after exposure to ultraviolet (UV) rays from the sun. Vitamin D exists in several forms, each with a different activity. Calciferol, is the most active form. Other forms are relatively inactive in the body. Once it is produced in the skin or consumed in food, a chemical conversion occurs in the liver and kidney to form 1,25-dihydroxyvitamin D, the physiologically active form of vitamin D. The liver and kidney help convert it to its active hormone form. Active vitamin D functions as a hormone because it sends a message to the intestines to increase the absorption of calcium and phosphorus. By promoting calcium absorption, vitamin D helps to form and maintain strong bones. The major biologic function of vitamin D is to maintain normal blood levels of calcium and phosphorus. Vitamin D also works in concert with a number of other vitamins, minerals, and hormones to promote bone mineralization. Without vitamin D, bones can become thin, brittle, or misshapen. Vitamin D sufficiency prevents rickets in children and osteomalacia (softening of the bones) in adults. Research also suggests that vitamin D may help maintain a healthy immune system and help regulate cell growth and differentiation, the process that determines what a cell is to become.

Several researches regarding vitamin D's benefits have been undertaken. In June 2007, the Canadian Cancer Society suggested that, based on research, adults should consider increasing their daily dosage of vitamin D during the fall and winter months to 1,000 IUs, in consultation with a health-care provider. In September 2007, the result of a study, published in the Archives of Internal Medicine, which reviewed research analysis of 18 randomized controlled trials involving 57,311 people over the age of 50, reported that people who took at least 500 IUs of vitamin D daily, had a seven per cent lower risk of death, compared to those given a placebo. Lead researcher Dr. Philippe Autier said it was not clear how the supplements lowered risks of mortality, but he suggested that Vitamin D may block cancer cell proliferation or improve blood vessel and immune system functions.

Other researchers have studied how the sunshine vitamin affects other forms of cancer. Researchers at the University of California, San Diego, suggested in the March 2007 issue of the American Journal of Preventive Medicine that a daily dose of 2,000 IUs of vitamin D along with 10 to 15 minutes in the sun and a healthy diet, could reduce the incidence of colorectal cancer by two-thirds. The same authors found that breast cancer rates were 50 per cent lower in people with high levels of vitamin D in their blood, and suggested that the average person could maintain those levels also with a daily dose 2,000 IUs of vitamin D and spending 10 to 15 minutes in the sun.

Several research suggest vitamin D may help prevent prostate, breast and especially colon cancer. Some report vitamin D stifles abnormal cell growth, curbs formation of blood vessels that feed tumours and has many other anti-cancer effects.

A study, led by Dr. Pamela Goodwin of Mount Sinai Hospital in Toronto, involving taking blood from 512 woman at three different hospitals in Toronto when the women were first diagnosed with early-stage breast cancer, released in May 2008 by the American Society of Clinical Oncologist, reported that "Breast cancer patients with low levels of vitamin D were much more likely to die of the disease or have it spread, than patients who get enough of the nutrients." The researchers wanted to see whether it made a difference in survival. A decade after the blood were taken, 83 percent of the women who had adequate vitamin D, blood levels were alive and without extensive spread of their cancer, versus 79 percent of those whose vitamin D were considered insufficient and 69 percent of those who were deficient. It should be noted that the few women with very high levels of vitamin D seemed to have worse survival.

Vitamin D is found in salmon and other oily fish and certain foods, such as cow's milk and margarine, are fortified with it. Cod liver oil is an excellent dietary source.

Part I   Your Health

Vitamin E, especially when combined with Vitamin C and selenium, is a key player in providing optimal health. It acts as a *free-radical scavenger*. It's reported to increase our resistance to infection and to protect us against the damaging effects of stress and oxidation, including *cancer, cardiovascular* disease, such as hardening of the arteries, *angina*, heart attack, and stroke, and inhibits the formation of cataract. It enhances the release of some immune factors, and improves antibody production. It protects blood cells, body tissue and essential fatty acids from harmful destruction. A good natural food source for Vitamin E would be beans, broccoli, raw leafy vegetables, peas, pine nuts, sunflower and sesame seeds, unrefined corn oil, wheat germ, whole-grain cereals, among others. A daily intake of 400 IUs is recommended by professional believers for optimum health for an adult. Vitamin E is reported to be more effective when taken before a meal. Recent reports of deleterious effects on the heart, pertaining to excessive intake of Vitamin E (800 IUs or higher per day), are yet to be confirmed. Consult your physician before taking high doses of Vitamin E on a regular basis, especially if you have a history of high blood pressure.

A multi-centre coordinated study on the combined effect of vitamin E and selenium, on men who have never had prostate cancer, is underway across North America. Its purpose is to understand how a combined daily dose of 400 IUs of vitamin E and selenium, or either compound alone, can resist or prevent prostate cancer.

The body also needs other nutrients such as coenzyme Q10 (CQ10), essential fatty acids and essential amino acids.

Coenzyme Q10 (CQ10) is vital for energy. This vitamin-like antioxidant destroys free radicals and boosts the immune system. Our bodies manufacture CQ10 up to age 30, beyond which the production declines markedly. CQ10 has been reported to halt tumours and improve heart function. It's said to produce energy in the cell, prevent oxidation of LDL (bad) cholesterol, help lower blood pressure, strengthen heart function, improve blood flow, and reduce the risk of heart failure, angina and cardiomyopathy. It has antibacterial and antiviral properties. Its deficiency opens the door to chronic oxidative stress leading to degenerative disease. High dosage has also been reportedly used to treat breast cancer with very good tumour inhibiting action. A daily intake of 30 to 60 mg/day is recommended. No *toxicity* is found at this level. Consult a physician prior to use, if you're taking blood thinning medication or if on *radiation therapy*.

The essential fatty acid omega-3 (alpha-linolenic acid) is sometimes called uncommon essential fat – "uncommon" because it and omega 6 (linoleic acid) are the only fats that the body cannot manufacture, and "essential" because the body needs them to function at its best.

This is the fat that helps, among other things, to build superior cell membrane structure in the prostate, brain and other organs. It's reported to support the synthesis of hormone-like chemical messengers called prostaglandins, which influence the activity of the immune, nervous, circulatory endocrine (hormone), excretory and *reproductive systems*. More than 80 percent of our diet is deficient in omega-3 fat. Certain fish, including tuna and salmon, are rich in it. A daily intake of one to two tablespoons of omega-3 is recommended.

Amino acids, the end products of protein digestion and the building blocks of all protein, are contained in various organs and glands in differing proportions. Although not totally understood, they are believed to provide certain curative functions. Three of these amino acids – glycine, alanine and glutamic acid – have been found to help with relief of urinary symptoms due to an enlarged prostate. Since amino acids are a byproduct of protein, one must be cautious not to embark on a very low protein diet.

Those Precious Minerals

Minerals are the keys to the vitamin engine. No vitamin can be absorbed or carry out its intended function without the presence of specific minerals in very particular amounts.

In an article, "The Importance of Minerals in Your Overall Health," published in the Physicians Choice E-newsletter, Issue 33, September 2, 2000, Michael Tiplisky MD, wrote:

> "Minerals are often overlooked because most people, including medical doctors, do not commonly recognize their significance. But minerals function as important co-factors, which activate and regulate various enzymes that are responsible for all the functions of the body cells, tissues, and organs. While all the minerals are necessary for good health, calcium and magnesium are by far the most important. Unfortunately, these are the minerals in which most people are deficient."

Fundamentally metals, they are separated into major minerals, required in amounts greater than 100 mg per day, and trace elements, required in much smaller daily quantities. Major minerals include: calcium, magnesium, phosphorus, potassium and sodium. Trace elements include: boron, chromium, cobalt, copper, florine, germanium, iodine, manganese, selenium, silicon, vanadium and zinc.

It's well known that adequate **calcium** will prevent, and maybe even reverse, osteoporosis and the risk of dangerous fractures. It's also essential for normal hormonal balance. A study of 500 women, performed at Columbia University and published in 1998 in the American Journal of Obstetrics and Gynecology, showed that calcium is effective against a wide variety of premenstrual syndrome (PMS) symptoms. A daily calcium supplement has been shown to reduce the occurrence of mood swings, headache, food cravings, and bloating by as much as 50 per cent. Other benefits include: stronger bones and teeth, healthy gums and normal blood clotting, heart function, blood pressure, muscle contraction, sleep pattern and function of the nervous system and nerve impulses. Studies have shown that deficiency of calcium can lead to heart rhythm irregularities, insomnia, high blood pressure, cramps, growing pains in teenagers, brittle nails and joint pain. Calcium is better absorbed in the presence of vitamins C and D. Food sources include almonds, brewer's yeast, cabbage, dried beans, green vegetables, nuts, sunflower seeds. A daily intake of 800 to 1000 mg is recommended, particularly to support bone health in seniors.

Magnesium is one of the most important minerals in the body, necessary for normal functioning of more than 300 different *enzymes* with a broad range of activities. Because of this, a deficiency can lead to a wide range of symptoms, such as irritability, fatigue, insomnia, poor digestion, palpitation, cardiovascular problems, high blood pressure, pain, depression, asthma, PMS, muscle weakness and cramps. Studies show that magnesium is necessary for energy; nerve impulse transmission; pH balance; maintenance of blood pressure; normal heart function and rhythm; relaxation of the arteries and muscles; carbohydrate metabolism; balance of minerals in the body; protection against kidney stones (together with vitamin B6); prevention of osteoporosis and PMS symptoms; improved mental function and cellular activity; and amelioration of chronic fatigue syndrome. The best source of magnesium is green leafy vegetables, but since most of us do not eat the recommended amount of fruit and vegetables, magnesium deficiency is probably more common than we realize. A daily intake of 280 to 300 mg is recommended.

The combination of calcium and magnesium improves the quality of sleep, thereby enhancing the body's natural rejuvenation process, thus they are best taken at bedtime.

Selenium is an essential trace mineral believed to play an invaluable role in the prevention of cancer, heart attack, and stroke caused by hardening and clogging of the arteries. Food sources are Brazil nuts, broccoli, cabbage, lentils, mushrooms, wheat germ, and zucchini. Selenium may synergize the effects of Vitamin E. Because of our increased need for selenium, and its growing deficiency in our produce, a daily intake of 100 to 200 mcg/day is recommended.

Zinc is an important mineral that boosts the immune system at the cellular level and fights infection. It's essential for cell growth and accelerates the healing of wounds. It's reported to play a significant role in the development and function of the male reproductive system, particularly sexual organs and the prostate. In fact, it's been reported that the normal prostate gland contains about 10 times more zinc than any other gland in the body, but a diseased prostate is quite deficient in this mineral. It may help prevent cancer, particularly of the prostate; however, it's also reported to help speed up the growth and multiplication of cancer cells. So it may be good for some conditions and bad for others. Food sources include almonds, Brazil nuts, brewer's yeast, egg yolks, oats, oysters, pumpkin seeds, rye, whole wheat. A daily intake of 50-100 mg/day is recommended.

Nutritional Supplementation – No Diet Should be Without Them

In a survey of 21,500 people conducted by the United States Department of Agriculture (USDA), none of the participants were found to be consuming 100 percent of the minimum recommended dietary allowance of 10 essential nutrients.

One family practitioner from Rapid City, South Dakota, said in a lecture at a USANA Health Sciences convention: "It's simply amazing to me to see the benefit that my patients have received by taking good quality supplements. No diet should be without them."

Just as women need certain nutrients to protect themselves from osteoporosis and breast cancer, men need certain nutrients to protect themselves against prostate cancer.

Studies from the National Cancer Institutes, Harvard Medical School, U.S. Department of Health and Johns Hopkins University, concluded that nutritional supplementation produces positive changes in a person's health throughout their entire body.

Changes due to supplementation		
Category	**Change**	**Percent**
Overall death rates	down	33 percent
Heart Attacks	down	50 percent
Cancer deaths	down	50 percent
Infections	down	70 percent
Cataracts	down	80 percent
Bone fractures	down	30 – 40 percent
Bone loss	down	30 – 40 percent

Although general, the above data signifies that there are benefits to be achieved by using vitamin and mineral supplements. It's time to take a proactive approach to our health, and judiciously supplement the food we eat with the proper vitamins and minerals.

Extra! Extra! Read all About It!

An apple a day may do more than keep the doctor away. It might also keep death at bay. A recent Swedish study found that middle-aged and elderly men who ate the most **fruits** tended to live longer than those who ate fewer fruits. This suggested that high fruit intake is associated with reduced risk of death among men.

While increasing intake of fruits is essential to good health, a **grapefruit** a day may not, in fact, keep the doctor away, especially when combined with certain medications. Several substances in grapefruit or its juice can interfere with the way our bodies handle certain drugs – increasing or less commonly decreasing their effects – including some used in the treatment of cardiovascular disease. Consult your physician when prescribed any drugs and report to him any adverse reaction or interaction with grapefruit.

Lycopene is the substance that gives colour to fruits such as tomatoes, guavas, watermelon and pink grapefruit. It's a class of plant antioxidant from the bioflavonoid family. Bioflovonoids are largely responsible for the colours of many fruits and flowers, as well as their medicinal properties/actions.

In 1995, Harvard Medical School released a report about the effect of tomatoes on cancer. It followed the eating habits of 47,000 men for six years. According to the report, these men, who had at least 10 weekly servings of tomato-based foods, were up to 45 percent less likely to develop prostate cancer.

In an analysis published in February 2000, Dr. Edward Giovannucci of Harvard Medical School reviewed 72 studies that looked for a link between cancer risk and tomatoes. He found that 57 of the studies linked tomato intake with a reduced cancer risk. In 35 of these, the association was strong enough for them to be considered statistically meaningful. The data were most compelling for cancers of the prostate, lung, and stomach.

Reports are becoming more and more compelling that the nutrient responsible for this is lycopene. However, one should realize that associations suggested by epidemiologic studies do not necessarily establish a causal relationship – although they offer food for thought.

There is a secret ingredient missing from your diet: **SOY**. For meat eaters, I admit it might seem inconceivable but this bland, humble bean and its processed incarnations have super powers that may be able to help prevent two deadly diseases – heart disease and prostate cancer.

Soy is a product that's has become popular as a functional food with significant nutritional benefits. Used as a main source of protein in Asian countries for hundreds of years, it's now being recognized in the Western world. Soy is considered to be a great source of protein and a supplier of essential amino acids. It has a high content of *phytonutrients*, as well as being high in fibre (76 per cent), which is essential to help reduce cholesterol and decrease risk of diabetes, colon cancer, heart disease and *gastrointestinal* problems. Soy is cholesterol-free and low in saturated fat.

Research has shown that eating about 47 grams of soy protein a day can reduce "bad" LDL cholesterol levels by 13 percent and triglycerides by 10 percent. Some studies suggest it can inhibit the growth of prostate cancer cells. Now that's a health food! Here's the kicker: You can reap all those benefits without ever having to taste the stuff. You do not even have to know the soy is there. It will be whatever you tell it to be. Put it in chili and it turns hot and spicy. Put it in spaghetti and it speaks Italian. Soy has the ability to disappear into the flavour of any other food.

I would not do this chapter justice if I did not include something about what some researchers consider to be the most potent antioxidant – **proanthocyanadin**, sometimes referred to as oligomeric proanthocyanadins (OPCs).

OPCs are also a class of plant antioxidant from the bioflavonoid family. Some research suggests they may be useful in the treatment and prevention of certain health conditions and may act as anti-inflammatory, anti-allergy, antiviral and anticancer agents. The most common suggestion is that OPCs can act as powerful antioxidants and provide remarkable protection against free radicals.

Grape seed, as well as white pine bark, are excellent sources of proanthocyanadin. An extract of good grape seed is said to contain 95 percent proanthocyanadin.

According to a report, entitled "Free Radicals and Grape Seed Proanthocyanadin Extract: Importance in Human Health and Disease Prevention," by D. Bagchi, M. Bagchi, S.J. Stohs, D.K. Das, C.A. Kuszynski, S.S. Joshi and H.G. Pruess, of the Department of Pharmaceutical and Administrative Sciences, Creighton University School of Pharmacy and Allied Health Professions, in Omaha, Nebraska:

"Oligomeric proanthocyanadins, naturally occurring antioxidant widely available in fruits, vegetables, nuts, seeds, flowers and barks, have been reported to possess a broad spectrum of biological, pharmacological and therapeutic activities against free radicals and oxidative stress."

Results of clinical research studies have shown that OPCs may be effective in treating varicose veins, *capillary fragility* (easy bruising and rupture of small blood vessels), and disorders of the *retina*, including *diabetic retinopathy* and *macular degeneration*.

As antioxidants, OPCs are said to be roughly 50 to 200 times more powerful than the antioxidant vitamins C and E.

Generally, as a preventative measure and antioxidant support, a daily dose of 50 mg of proanthocyanadin is considered satisfactory. If used for therapeutic purposes, a daily dosage of 150 mg to 300 mg is suggested as more effective. I take a daily dose of 180 mg of grape seed extract, containing 95 percent proanthocyanadin.

No significant side effects or adverse drug interactions have been observed as a result of taking OPC. However, some people, taking large amounts of grape seed extract daily have initially experienced diarrhea for a short period of time.

Summary

In summary, food alone is not enough. Today's choices have short-comings, which can be overcome by a supplementation of micronutrients consisting of vitamins, minerals and trace elements; activities, consisting of various exercises; and avoidance of toxins, stress, and the likes. I suspect that if we were to eat only fruits and vegetables, we would probably get all the nutrients that we need, but we would have to eat a substantial amount, more than our stomachs can accommodate. A minimum of 6 to 9 servings of fruits and vegetables daily is generally recommended for optimal health.

Chapter 5

TAKE CONTROL OF YOUR HEALTH – YOU ARE RESPONSIBLE!

It's the action, not the fruit of the action, that's important.
You have to do the right thing…
You may never know what results from your action
but if you do nothing, there will be no results.

MAHATMA GANDHI

Life is a Gift

It's no secret that good health is a requirement for a long and happy life. Life is a gift, and we ought to make the most of it. My life's mission borrows a line from Dr. Myron Wentz: "Love life and live it to its fullest, in happiness and health." One of the ways I fulfill this is to get a regular medical check-up.

If you are a male, 50 years or older, and aren't getting a yearly check-up, then you're doing yourself – as well as your loved ones – a disservice and an injustice. I urge you to start getting checked annually. Pick up that telephone, right now, call your doctor, and make an appointment.

I have spoken to men throughout Canada, the United States, Central America and the Caribbean, individually and in groups, on this subject. Many of these conversations were conducted in the presence of wives and loved ones. I soon realized there are a large number of men who do not avail themselves of regular check-ups. Even some male doctors are known to neglect this critical requirement. In some cases, I get nods from the spouses, as I impress upon the men to go.

Part I   Your Health

For years, from 1998 to 2008, I conducted an informal survey among the men I encountered. What I learned led me to realize there are a number of reasons why many men put off regular check-ups. Predominant among these is male ego. Although this borders on stupidity, they do not want the doctor performing a *digital rectal examination (DRE)* on them. Some, like my relative Joe, say they don't want anyone putting a finger through their anus and up their rectum, which is a necessary, albeit an uncomfortable part of the medical check-up for men. Joe, by the way, suffered from urinary problems, and refused to return to the doctor for a long time. He later had to be operated on – TURP. There are other reasons. Many men fear not only the procedure itself but also the resulting diagnosis, possibly of prostate cancer. They don't want to learn of any ill-health condition, thinking that such knowledge, and condition, will make them feel or appear helpless, powerless or less manly. That was the case with Tom, who wanted to die rather than be diagnosed. He suffered for a long time until his pain became unbearable. His doctor found his problem to be an enlarged prostate and treated it. That was in 1996. He has been happy, pain-free, and active ever since. He's now over 80.

Thus men have differing reasons for avoiding the regular check-ups. Some, like Joe, would rather die than succumb to a DRE. He calls it pride. I call it ego. Tom would rather have died, but succumbed because of excruciating pain. He calls his "fear of the unknown."

For your own peace of mind, quality health and longevity, it's better to put pride, ego and fear aside and put up with the discomfort to know your overall health condition, particularly that of your prostate. If you don't have that check-up done regularly, one day your prostate will begin to enlarge, and will continue to do so until it becomes uncomfortable, painful and embarrassing – or even fatal. By getting a regular medical check-up, you will know when this change begins to take place, find out the condition, and start treatment early and appropriately. It may not necessarily be of cancer. In fact, almost every other man will experience a prostate problem before they turn 60; and nine out of every 10 will experience a prostate problem by the time they reach 80. About 15 percent of those nine will be diagnosed with prostate cancer. More than likely, you will be one of the nine. Will you be one of the 15 percent?

Of those who will be diagnosed with prostate cancer, about one-fifth will die from it. Early diagnosis can enable you to determine the steps to treatment and healing, and perhaps avoid death.

A digital rectal examination (DRE) is essential to determine the health of the prostate. If your doctor doesn't perform one during the check-up, then ask him to do so.

He will insert a single gloved-covered index finger through your anus and into your rectum, and press it against the wall of the rectum, adjacent to the prostate, for about five to 15 seconds. By doing so, he can feel the gland and make some quick assessments about it, whether it's larger than it should be or if it has a lump.

A medical check-up may include other tests including urine, blood and stool. The blood sample can be tested for the amount of *antigen* released from the prostate into the blood, a relatively good indicator of prostate health.

After the check-up, your doctor may be quite satisfied. Or he might be suspicious as a result of something he felt or observed, or heard you say. If there is concern, he will order additional tests, or refer you to a specialist. On one occasion, my doctor recommended I get a *bone scan,* to determine any cancer *hot spots* or other degenerative bone disease. On another occasion, as a result of a complaint that I relayed to him about pain in my chest, he sent me for a stress test, which resulted with my being diagnosed with angina.

After one of my annual medical check-ups, which included a blood test, my doctor referred me to a urologist, for further specialized diagnosis of my prostate condition. He did so because during the DRE, he felt a lump or hardness on my prostate, and from subsequent blood tests he observed that there might be some abnormal condition. But note, he did not come to any conclusion – just a suspicion.

Your doctor may also make some recommendations, perhaps regarding exercise, weight control, nutritional supplementation, or diet. On one occasion, when my cholesterol was getting too high, my doctor recommended that I start taking 400 IUs of vitamin E daily.

It was soon after the cholesterol discovery, that I re-evaluated my lifestyle, including my diet and activity level. I concluded that I needed to make some drastic changes.

There are many advantages to a medical check-up. You may walk away with a clean bill of health. But you can't be sure of that without being checked. Even then there is no guarantee that there may not be some undiscovered health issues.

The message bears repeating. Everyone would be wise to have a medical check-up, performed by a reputable physician, on a regular basis. That's every two years before age 40, and yearly thereafter. I discovered that, unlike women, few men do this.

I started going for a regular check-up at the age of 33. At 40, I started going yearly. As a result of those visits, my prostate problem was discovered early, allowing me time to seek the right information and take treatment action accordingly.

If you do not have access to a family physician, go to a neighbourhood clinic and ask for a medical check-up. However, understand that doctors are busy and set aside specific times when they do complete physicals. So be prepared to make an appointment up to six months in advance. If you cannot find a doctor to do this, ask a friend or a neighbour. Somewhere there is someone who can help you. Once you do this, you will never regret it.

> Let me close this chapter by telling you a true story about my childhood friend, Melvin. In early August 2000, Melvin and his wife Geraldine, along with my wife's cousin Diane and her friend Eugene visited us in London, en route from Chicago to Toronto for the annual Caribbean carnival, Caribana. They spent a half a day at my home. Eugene had undergone a radical prostatectomy a few years earlier, and I was anxious to chat with him. During the visit, Melvin and I discussed health and prostate cancer and getting regular *check-ups*. He assured me that he got an annual check-up. You can imagine how shocked I was when, in November of that same year, Diane called me to tell me that Melvin had died that morning, from pancreatic cancer that had spread to his liver. This cancer was discovered in September of that year, less than two months after we chatted in my home.

We cannot leave anything to chance. We must take control of our own health.

Part II

Your Prostate!

Chapter 6

UNDERSTANDING THE PROSTATE GLAND

There is no room or reason for ignorance or lack of patient's knowledge and information regarding what is involved or what we are dealing with when it comes to disease of the prostate.

HAROLD USHER,
... IN CONVERSATION WITH
PROSTATE CANCER PATIENTS.

What is the Prostate?

The prostate is one of a man's most prized possessions, although too few realize it. In fact, it is sometimes called the "second heart of man."

The prostate is not essential to sustain life, but it does play a major role in a man's reproductive capability and can significantly affect his urinary function. Therefore, it's no surprise that every man should want to nurture and protect his prostate from harm.

Unfortunately, most of us never think about our prostate until something goes wrong with it, or it begins to cause inconvenience. However, if you have a prostate problem, you should know as much as possible about its structure and function, as well as its contribution to quality of life, so that you can make informed treatment decisions.

The prostate gland is situated directly below and adjacent to the bladder, surrounding the upper part of the urethra, and sandwiched between the *pubic bone* and rectum. It consists of many elements, including various types of tissues and thousands of tiny, fluid-producing glands that drain into ejaculatory ducts, which in turn drain into the *urethra*.

Normally, the prostate is about the size of a chestnut and shaped like an apple. The top is referred to as the base and the bottom is called the apex. It's encased in a fibrous cover or sheath, referred to as the capsule. In its normal shape and size, it's about two centimetres or 3/4 of an inch thick, three centimetres or 1 1/4 inches long, and almost four centimetres or 1 1/2 inches wide.

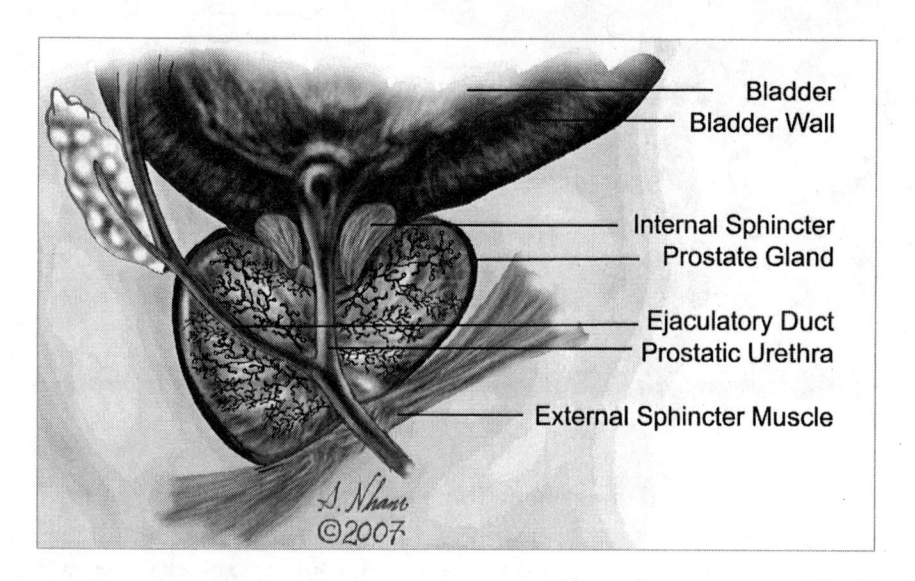

The entire gland usually weighs in at about 3/4 of an ounce or 20 grams. However, it can sometimes grow to the size of an apple, weighing as much as 2 ounces (50 grams), or more.

Losing or damaging the prostate, may cause any or all of the following: sterility; erectile dysfunction (*impotence*); loss of sexual desire; shrunken penile tissue; inability to ejaculate during orgasm; inability to achieve orgasm; pain; incontinence; bladder problems; weak or slow stream when urinating; and a myriad of other inconveniences that interfere with or reduce the quality of life. As a result self-confidence may be negatively affected.

Structure and Zones

The prostate gland is divided into four zones, in spherical layers, one within the other like layers of an onion. Each has a different glandular fluid production pattern and drainage system. They are:

- The **peripheral** zone, which occupies about 70 percent of the total volume of the prostate, is directly adjacent to the encasement capsule, and surrounds the entire periphery of the other zones. It consists of loose tissues, thousands of tiny glands which secrete prostatic fluid, and excretory ducts which drain this fluid through to the central zone and into the urethra at ejaculation. This is the predominant zone for prostate cancer development – 70 percent of cancers develop in this zone.

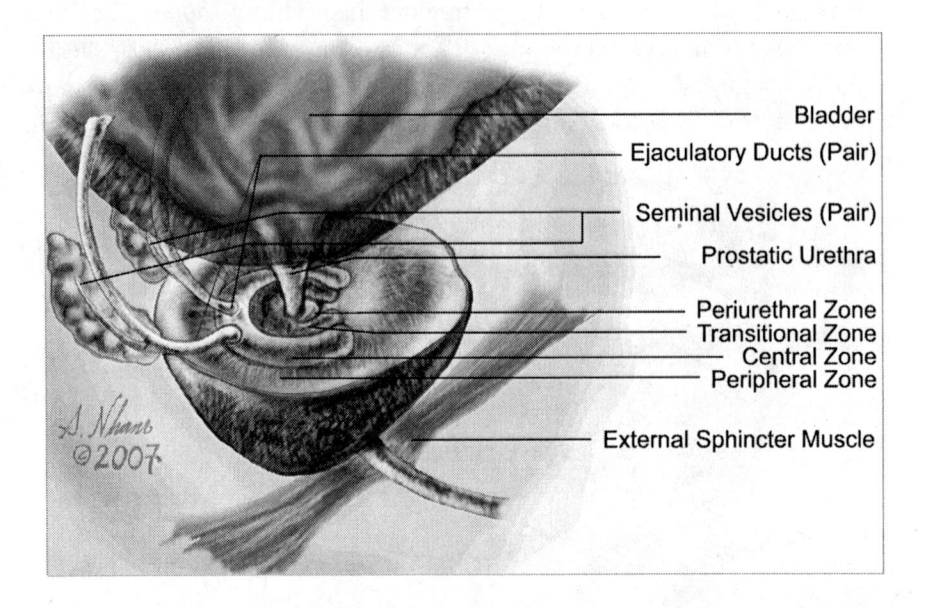

Diagram labels: Bladder; Ejaculatory Ducts (Pair); Seminal Vesicles (Pair); Prostatic Urethra; Periurethral Zone; Transitional Zone; Central Zone; Peripheral Zone; External Sphincter Muscle

- The **central** zone, which occupies about 20 percent of the total volume of the prostate, is situated within, and adjacent to, the peripheral zone, in an almost spherical, cup-like shape. It surrounds the two inner zones at the back, the sides, and toward the front without closing the cup. It consists of dense tissues and drainage ducts. It's through this zone that the *ejaculatory ducts* enter the prostate gland and exit at the urethra. Some eight to 10 percent of cancers develop in this zone.

- The **transitional** zone, which occupies about seven percent of the total volume of the prostate, is within, and adjacent to, the central zone, also in a spherical cup-like shape. It surrounds a narrow strip of tissue that's fixed to the prostatic urethra at the back, the sides and toward the front, without closing the cup. About 20 percent of cancers develop in this zone, but more significant is the fact that this is the predominant area for *benign prastatic hyperplasia* (BPH), or prostate enlargement.

- The **periurethral** zone, which occupies about one percent of the total volume of the prostate, hugs the front half of the narrow strip of tissue that surrounds the other half of the prostatic urethra. Prostate cancer generally does not develop in this zone; however, it's a dominant zone for BPH.

The whole prostate is encapsulated in a relatively strong, tough skin called, the capsule. Spreading out on two sides of the external surface of the capsule are neurovascular nerves. They look like fine red fibres, are cobweb-thin, and are referred to as neurovascular *nerve bundles,* or *nerve bundles.* These nerve bundles originate from the brain, traverse down along the spinal cord to, around and alongside the prostate (two sides), to the apex (lower end) of the prostate, to the urethra, and terminate in the shaft of the penis. Included among those nerve bundles are *cavernous nerves,* which are the specific nerves responsible for the erection and enter the penis accordingly – during the erection process, they cause the penis to become engorged with blood, enlarged and elongated. As the nerve bundles traverse across the prostate, they splay out and wrap themselves around the surfaces of two sides of the capsule, like fingers cupping a baby's face.

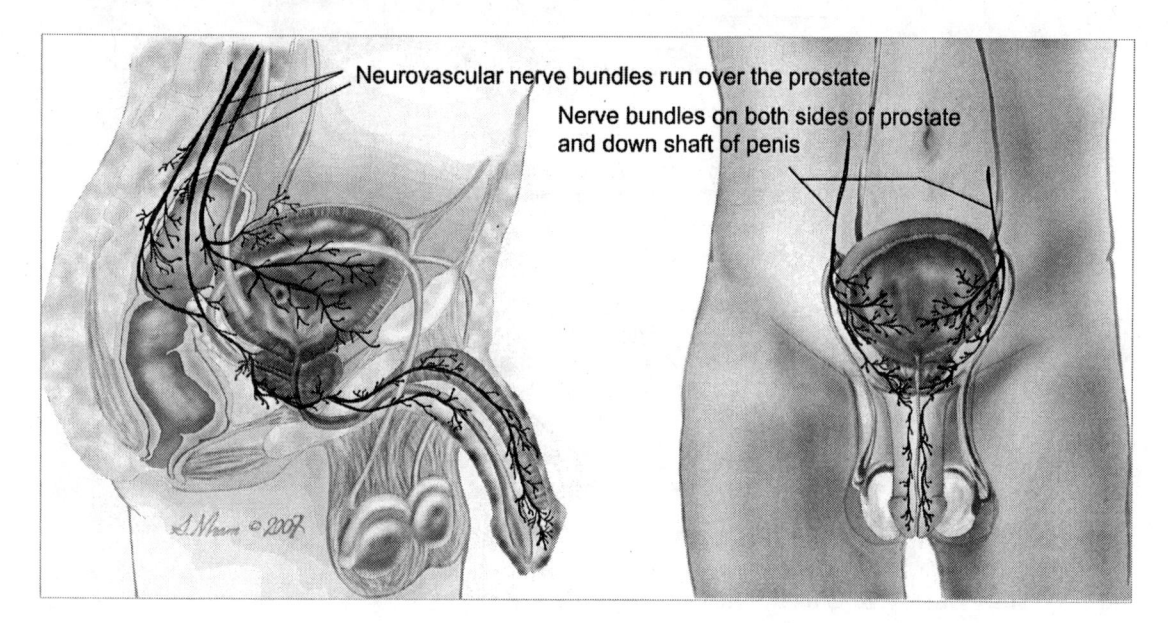

Neurovascular nerve bundles run over the prostate

Nerve bundles on both sides of prostate and down shaft of penis

The Reproductive System

As part of the reproductive system, the prostate gland forms a partnership with the testicles, the *epididymis,* the *vas deferens,* and the *seminal vesicles.* Together, these glands, tubes and pouches are marvels of baby production.

The testicles manufacture millions of *sperm,* about 50,000 per minute and in excess of 70 million per day, which are deposited in the epididymis. The epididymis is a very long tube, wound tightly in thousands of hair-pin turns and shaped together like an arch over one side of the testicle, which if stretched out would span several metres. In this tube the sperm collect and mature for up to two weeks.

The epididymis sends the sperms to the vas deferens, a pair of sperm transportation tubes, one from each testicle. They connect from the epididymis, up, over, and around the bladder, and

Part II   Your Prostate!

down to the ejaculatory ducts that are located inside the prostate gland. The vas deferens are each about two feet long. These are the tubes that are cut, and tied or knotted, to accomplish sterilization in a vasectomy. Sperm can remain in the testes and epididymis for up to a month. If they aren't released through ejaculation, they are absorbed by the body.

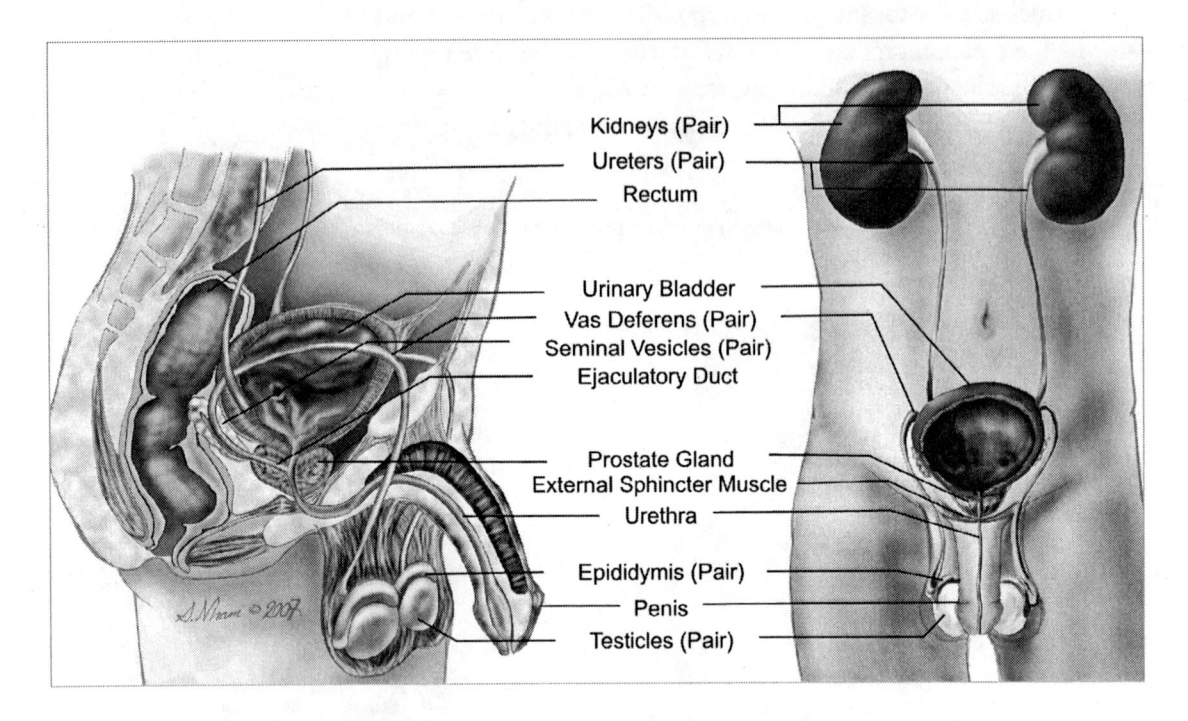

The ejaculatory ducts lead directly into the prostatic urethra.

The seminal vesicles are a pair of glands, resembling small bags or pouches, situated above and behind the prostate gland, at the base of the bladder. They manufacture and secrete a thick liquid called *seminal fluid* that contains fructose and other nutrients, which discharges upon ejaculation, into the ejaculatory ducts.

The prostate gland also contains thousands of tiny, fluid producing glands which produce and secrete a thin alkaline liquid, called *prostatic fluid*. This is drained through *excretory ducts* within the prostate and, upon ejaculation, shoots into the prostatic urethra.

Other glands that play a role in the development of *semen* and its ejaculation are the prostatic utricle, and the *bulbourethral or Cowper's glands*. The latter are located below the prostate within the *urogenital diaphragm*, a sheet of muscle lining the floor of the pelvis, which secretes a fluid that forms part of the semen.

Upon ejaculation, the bladder is shut off by the contraction of the *internal sphincter muscles* at the neck of the bladder. The prostate gland and muscle grow tense and squeeze the ducts, and the sperm are squirted into the ejaculatory duct simultaneously with the thick liquid from the seminal vesicles and the prostatic fluid from the excretory ducts. The resulting semen shoots in *spasm* and travels with tremendous force to the prostatic urethra, through the membranous urethra, picking up secreted fluid from the bulbourethral glands, and through the length of the penile urethra along the erect elongated penis to the outside.

So, without the neurovascular nerve bundles, more specifically the cavernous nerves, the penis would not be able to experience an erection. Without the testicles, no sperm could be manufactured. Without the seminal vesicles, there would be no thick liquid nutrients to move the sperm onward after they are deposited from the epididymis and vas deferens to the ejaculatory duct. Without the prostate, there would be no prostatic fluid for the sperm to swim in, during ejaculation. Without the internal sphincter muscles at the neck of the bladder, which blocks the semen from entering the bladder and directs it instead in the other direction, it would be impossible to prevent *retrograde ejaculation*. When the prostate is removed, as a cancer treatment, the seminal vesicles and ejaculatory ducts are removed along with it.

It should be noted that semen and sperm are not the same thing. Sperm are the seeds that impregnate. Semen is a combination of the various fluids and the sperm, which facilitates easy transportation of the sperm through the ejaculatory ducts and then into the urethra, a sort of launching pad to shoot the semen out of the body. Each ejaculation releases about 200 million sperm.

The Urinary System

As part of the urinary system, the prostate gland forms a partnership with the urinary bladder, it's muscles, the internal sphincter muscles, the urethra, and the *external sphincter muscle*.

The "urinary bladder" is a reservoir that collects, holds and supports urine until you are ready to discharge it through the urethra and penis. It's positioned directly above the prostate gland and shares a common juncture with the mouth (or tail end) of the urethra and the prostate.

The internal walls of the bladder are lined with "muscle fibres" that terminate at the juncture of the bladder, the prostate and the urethra. These muscle fibres are called 'bladder detrusor muscles' and blend in with the internal sphincter muscles at the junction of the bladder, the prostate and the urethra. When difficulty arises as a result of pressure against the urethra due to BPH, or blockage in the urethra due to obstructions, a man might apply pressure to the bladder to force the urine out. This type of constant pressure to the bladder tends to build up the bladder detrusor muscles, making them thicker, thus reducing the size (volume) of the reservoir of the bladder. This causes the bladder to fill-up quicker and more frequently and thus require emptying more frequently as well.

Part II   Your Prostate!

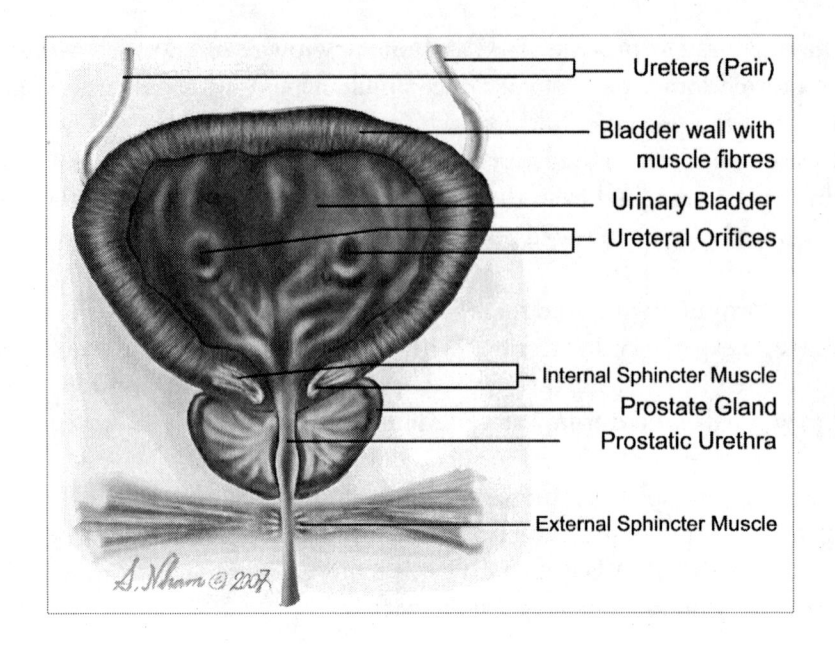

The "internal sphincter muscles," sometimes called "preprostatic sphincters" or "muscular sphincters," are tissues that surround the urethra at the juncture of the prostate gland and the neck of the bladder. They form one with the bladder and the prostate. They squeeze tight to help control the escape of urine from the bladder, as well as to prevent semen from entering the bladder during ejaculation (retrograde ejaculation). When viewed in cross-section, the internal sphincters appear as a tightly contracted set of muscles in a circular formation, similar to those at the anus. These muscles are smooth and require no effort to contract. They constantly maintain tightness until they are relaxed by nerve impulses and are critical mechanisms in urinary control.

When the prostate is removed by surgery, this sphincter is also removed and the control of urine movement is transferred to a different, rarely used, muscle called the external sphincter. This is one of the causes of incontinence, after surgery.

The urethra is the tube that leads directly from the bladder down through the prostate membrane and the penis, to the outside.

So the length of the urethra is made up of three segments, namely:
- Prostatic urethra, that part surrounded by the prostate gland;
- Membranous urethra, that part that adjoins the prostatic urethra and extends through the membrane to the base of the penis;
- Penile urethra, which extends through the length of the penis from its base to the tip of the head.

Actually, it's all one urethra. It's just that different segments are sometimes referred to with a different name for specific purposes.

The urethra is long and flexible enough that the penis can stretch during erection. Together the urethra is used as a conduit for the transport of urine and discharge of semen. When the prostate is removed as a result of surgery, the prostatic urethra is removed along with it, leaving behind the membranous and penile urethra.

The "external sphincter muscle" is situated just below the prostate around the membranous urethra. It's generally not put to much use unless the internal sphincter muscle malfunction or are removed. This is a relatively small muscle that has to be exercised regularly in order to be in continuous control. They contract upon voluntary impulse and generally can only retain that contraction for about 25 seconds. Regular *Kegel exercises* can help to strengthen and lengthen the contraction.

So, in removing or destroying the prostate, there is a strong possibility that the internal sphincter muscles could be removed or damaged, transferring control of urine flow to the little used external sphincter, thus probably causing incontinence for a period of time. Likewise, when experiencing conditions such as BPH, the urethra could malfunction, severely limiting the passage of urine and causing some damage to the bladder and the urethra and thus the urinary system.

Development of the Prostate

The prostate gland is affected by male sex hormones. All the cells in the four zones are dependent upon *androgens*, for normal growth and development, or more specifically the male hormone known as *testosterone*, which is manufactured almost entirely (90 percent) by the testicles or by cells in the *testes*, called Leydig cells.

Testosterone maintains and stimulates growth and development.

After puberty (11 to 14 years of age), a man's prostate gland grows gradually in size and volume until about age 30. At that time, its size is what is considered normal. However, it starts growing again when the man is about 45. That's a natural process. It undergoes this process of enlargement because of hormonal changes and some nutritional deficiencies. At some time in a man's life, this enlargement can, and more than likely will, become troublesome, because it begins to infringe on other organs. It may also become infected, or degraded, with a malignant tumour. There are some symptoms in most cases, but some may be so subtle that they aren't readily detected.

There are three possible conditions associated with the prostate that necessitate treatment: *pros-*

tatitis, benign prastatic hyperplasia (BPH), and *malignancy* (cancer). These are explained in the remaining chapters of this section.

Chapter 7

UNDERSTANDING "TUMOUR"

Man is so made that whenever anything fires his soul, impossibilities vanish.

Jean de la Fontaine

Cell to Tumour

Tumour generally means swelling; however, when it's used in the context of cancer, it means a growth of abnormal cells or abnormal growth of tissue.

The human body is made up of trillions of cells. Cells function for a while, replace themselves, then they die. In fact, cells grow and divide to produce more cells and keep the body healthy. Each cell performs specific functions individually and/or in groups. Good health is dependent on the effective performance of well-organized cells carrying out their specific functions.

Frequently, cells are replaced in ways that lack organized structure and normal functioning. Like tiny computers in our bodies, they can go faulty, produce out of control and lose their normal functioning capabilities. They may be damaged by bombardment from by "free radicals," for example, causing oxidative stress.

Sometimes, when new cells are formed, the body does not get rid of the old ones, or some old cells do not die when they should. When this happens, the cells which continuously survive may exceed the capacity of the tissue, causing a growth or abnormal lumps to be formed. Some of these lumps may grow larger and grow their own vessels to keep themselves supplied with blood. We call this type of growth "tumour," because when they multiply and grow into clusters, they form a tumour.

Part II   Your Prostate!

There are two types of tumour, namely, *benign* and *malignant*.

Benign tumours are non-cancerous, as in "benign prostatic hyperplasia" (BPH) or enlargement of the prostate. These tumours aren't life threatening and can be treated successfully.

Malignant tumours are cancerous and usually fast growing since cancer cells reproduce at a much higher rate than non-cancerous ones.

Tumours grow in size and volume, squeezing against nearby tissues or organs, causing periodic pain and interfering with the body's normal functioning. In the case of prostate, the tumour squeezes the urethra, and sometimes bulges into the bladder and rectum, causing *urinary problems*. However, BPH would result in this condition only at an advanced stage or if neglected. Cancers are usually found much earlier.

The Prostate – A Place Where Tumour Forms and Grows

When doctors speak of prostate cancer, they typically speak of "prostatic *adenocarcinoma*," which means cancer of the glands in the prostate, which secrete prostatic fluid. Occasionally, the cancer may be a different type, and may have spread to other areas of the body. These may be more difficult to detect and/or treat.

Most men will have a prostate problem if they live long enough.

As many as 50 percent of men, by the time they reach age 50, will experience some form of a prostate problem, including unpleasant or unwanted growth in their prostate glands. More than 90 percent of men, 80 years and older, will experience some form of enlargement of their prostate. One of every six to seven men will experience prostate cancer in their lifetime and nine out of 10 will have a problem related to enlargement.

Remember what was said in Chapter One, that studies have shown one third of men who die from other causes such as accidents or military action, were found to have undetected cancer in their prostate. Many more had a benign enlargement.

Chapter 8

PROSTATITIS

Fear defeats more people than any other one thing in the world.

RALPH WALDO EMERSON (1803-1882)
PHILOSOPHER, POET, ESSAYIST

What Is Prostatitis?

Prostatitis is an inflammation of the prostate gland and may result from bacterial infection, although evidence of infection is not always found. It can be short or long term. Although it's not easy to diagnose, prostatitis must be identified and treated. It's not cancer, nor does it cause cancer; however, you will know something is wrong because of the symptoms.

Prostatitis can affect men of any age and it's estimated that by the time they are 80 years of age, 50 percent of men will have experienced the disorder. It rarely occurs before puberty and is the most common urological disorder in men over the age of 50 and the third most common disorder in men younger than 50. Five to eight percent of men are thought to have prostatitis at any given time. According to the National Institutes of Health, prostatitis accounts for 25 percent of all office visits involving the *genitourinary system* by young and middle-aged men.

Renown Canadian prostatitis expert, Dr. J. Curtis Nickel of Queen's University, Kingston, Ontario, and W. Weidner, reported in an article entitled "Chronic Prostatitis: Current Concepts and Antimicrobial Therapy" published in Infect In Urology 13:S22-S29, 2000, "In the early 1990s, there were as many office visits for prostatitis as there were benign prostatic hyperplasia (BPH) or prostate cancer – more than two millions annually." These accounted for one percent of all visits to family physicians and eight percent of visits to urologists, and the number continue to rise. Overall, the prevalence of prostatitis is between five and nine percent of the male population aged 18 years and older. In Canada, the average urologist sees close to 300 patients annually for prostatitis of which close to 40 percent have newly diagnosed disease.

According to data collected by urologist Harold Wheeler, MD of Durango, Colorado, U.S.A., prostatitis is on the rise in the U.S. I suspect that it's the same for the entire Western world.

An infected or inflamed prostate can result in painful urination and ejaculation and serious complication.

There are four types of prostatitis:

- *Acute Bacterial Prostatitis* (ABP) – intense, but time limited.
- *Chronic Bacterial Prostatitis* (CBP) – indefinite duration and characterized by repeated urinary tract infection.
- Non-bacterial Prostatitis – indefinite duration with no evidence of bacteria in urine nor urinary tract infection.
- Prostatodynia – painful prostate.

Acute Bacterial Prostatitis (ABP) presents as an acute urinary tract infection, believed to be caused by bacteria. It's easy to identify because of its uniform presentation. Often related to enlarged prostate or obstruction, it occurs in both sexually active young men and older men with enlarged prostates. Acute bacterial prostatitis comes on suddenly, and may include chills and fever, painful bloody urination, burning, urgency or difficulty urinating, and extreme pain in the lower back and lower abdomen, groin and testicles. It will clear up with appropriate short-term (14 days minimum) antibiotic therapy.

> An acquaintance, one day suddenly experienced chills and fever. His symptoms were accompanied by painful, bloody urination. The passing of blood was a one-time occurrence, while the fever lasted for two days. The man immediately contacted his family physician who diagnosed the condition as (Acute Bacterial) prostatitis and prescribed antibiotic treatment. The man followed the fully prescribed course of the antibiotics. His prostatitis disappeared for good.

Chronic Bacterial Prostatitis is caused by infection in the form of a bacteria-filled abscess. Symptoms may include deep pelvis pain, or difficult, painful or frequent urination. These may occur singly or in combination and are usually progressive, leading to eventual urinary obstruction, erectile dysfunction and/or incontinence. The condition requires long-term antibiotic therapy, lasting four to 12 weeks, and sometimes longer. Repeated urinary tract infections often occur, if antibiotics aren't taken for the whole prescribed period.

According to Dr. Daniel Shoskes, Associate Professor of Urology at the University of California, Los Angeles School of Medicine, "Chronic Prostatitis is an enormous problem in our country and around the world. It's one of the most common reasons why men visit urologists, and it's one of the most discouraging conditions doctors face, because oftentimes there is very little we can do to alleviate the pain."

There are doctors in other parts of the world, however, who use a technique called "*prostatic massage*" to drain the prostate. Dr. Antonio Novak Feliciano of the Philippines reports that he utilizes this treatment for Chronic Bacterial Prostatitis. He inserts an index finger gently into the anus until it reaches the prostate gland, then pushes against it with increasing pressure toward the midline on both sides. The procedure is done several times, as many as the patient can tolerate. The prostate will yield a few drops of the prostatic fluid each time. According to Dr. Feliciano, the procedure results in instant relief of back pain and restoration of erection capability. I have found no evidence that this has ever been duplicated by other physicians treating this frustrating condition.

The cause of **Non-bacterial Prostatitis** is not known, but it's an inflamed prostate without bacterial infection. It may be due to other organisms, such as mycoplasma. Symptoms include pelvis and lower back pain, painful erection and pain after ejaculation. Antibiotics may be used but they do not always help.

Prostatodynia means painful prostate. Its symptoms are pain in the *perineum* (the area between the scrotum and the anus), prostate and penis. Antibiotics have no effect on it. However alpha-blockers, muscle relaxants, and anti-inflammatory agents have had varying degrees of success. Dietary and lifestyle modifications such as cessation of smoking, avoidance of caffeine, alcohol, and spicy foods and minimizing stress, may also help.

Seek the Advice of a Doctor

According to a Gabe Merkin, M.D., author of "The Merkin Report for Healthier Living," and also a popular radio talk show host on medical activities who keeps current on medical research, "Prostatitis can very easily be detected by massaging the prostate and extracting some of the white blood cells that's secreted from it and testing these cells under a microscope." Conversation with several doctors indicates that this may not be as easy a procedure as is implied. All of the doctors were knowledgeable about this procedure, but reported that it's not routinely done and may not be at all helpful.

If you begin to experience any of the symptoms mentioned above, you are advised to seek the advice of your doctor and follow his directives.

Chapter 9

BENIGN PROSTATIC HYPERPLASIA

*You aren't here merely to make a living.
You are here in order to enable the world to live more amply,
with greater vision, with a finer spirit of hope and achievement.
You are here to enrich the world,
and you impoverish yourself if you forget the errand.*

THOMAS WOODROW WILSON (1856-1924)
28TH PRESIDENT (D) OF THE UNITED STATES

What is Benign Prostatic Hyperplasia?

Benign prostatic hyperplasia (BPH) is enlargement of the prostate gland, one of those inevitable consequences of aging. It can be considered as the manifestation of *climacteric* changes in men. It's inconvenient and, occasionally presents a major health threat.

BPH is not cancer, nor does it cause cancer, although the two can occur simultaneously. Neither does BPH treatment prevent cancer. In fact, as mentioned in Chapter 6, BPH occurs mostly in the transition and periurethral zones of the prostate, where only 20 percent of cancers develop.

Although it's not cancer, BPH is a wake-up call. It's problematic, and can and should be quickly treated. Left untreated, it can lead to more serious problems.

Who is Susceptible?

Every male over 40, with normal male hormones, is susceptible to BPH.

Most men will experience prostate enlargement at some time during their lives. Half of those over 50 already suffer from BPH, even if they experience no symptoms. And the number increases with age. Almost every man, by the time he reaches 80, will have some level of BPH, whether he is symptomatic or not.

To put this into perspective, randomly select 100 men, all of whom are 50 years of age, 25 of them will have an enlarged prostate to some degree. Bring them all together again 10 years later and 50 of them will have experienced some degree of enlarged prostate. Ten years later at age 70, as many as 75 of them will have experienced this condition. In another 10 years, most, if not all of these 80 year-olds will have had an enlarged prostate to some degree. Shocking? Yes, but true!

To compound this even further, many men who have BPH will not experience any symptoms. They will get along quite well since it may not cause any harmful side effects. On the other hand, many men who do not have enlargement may experience symptoms and require treatment.

Symptoms

As the prostate grows, it presses against the urethra, like a clamp on a garden hose. It also pushes up into the bladder, affecting the *urethral sphincter muscle*. As a result, urination becomes more difficult and the bladder stops emptying completely.

The most common recognizable symptoms of BPH are:

- *Urinary frequency* – need to urinate often during the day, at least every two to three hours. This is generally one of the earliest symptoms, caused by the bladder not being completely emptied, each time. Since there is so much fluid remaining in the bladder, it fills up more quickly.
- *Nocturia* – getting up frequently at nights to urinate. This is easily recognized, but most men are afraid to admit it and do nothing about it.
- *Urgency* – an intense urge to urinate, accompanied by the inability to "hold it in."
- **Incomplete emptying of the bladder** – you feel you aren't finished, but the flow has stopped, so you tend to squeeze your bladder, and squeeze and squeeze. This can damage the bladder's muscle and does nothing good for the prostate. See a doctor immediately.
- *Hesitancy* – delay of several seconds before the flow of urine begins. This is definitely cause to see a urologist. Checking it here could prevent serious treatment later, including surgery.
- *Incontinence* – loss of urinary control.
- *Decreased urinary stream (or flow strength)* – you experience a decrease in the force and magnitude of the flow of your urine. Most men consider this to be a sign of 'old age.' It's not. It can be treated.

- **Erectile dysfunction** – The inability to achieve and maintain an erection sufficient for vaginal penetration or satisfactory sexual performance – sometimes referred to as impotence.
- **Pain during ejaculation.**
- **Infection in the urinary tract** – this can damage the kidney and lead to kidney failure.
- *Hematospemia* – blood in the ejaculation fluid or semen.
- *Hematuria* – The passing of abnormal quantity of blood in the urine.

Any of these symptoms is cause to visit your doctor.

The main symptoms of BPH can be broken down into two categories: irritative, such as *lower urinary track symptoms* (LUTS), and obstructive, such as *bladder outlet obstructions* (BOO). Distinguishing between LUTS and BOO allows the urologist to treat the patient more effectively. However, many men who have some degree of BPH aren't even aware of it and therefore aren't seen by a physician.

Why Worry About BPH?

When the prostate gland is enlarged by BPH, it's not a proportional enlargement. As we already have learned BPH is largely confined in the transition zone (seven percent of the volume of the entire gland), and the periurethral zone (one percent of the volume of the entire prostate gland). Between these two small zones, BPH enlargement squeezes the prostatic urethra inward and pushes the central zone and the peripheral zone upward into the bladder and backward toward the rectum. This may cause a bulge, and a valley inside the bladder, a small bulge out into the rectum, and reduced passage inside the prostatic urethra. The extent of the resulting inconvenience will depend on the size of the enlargements.

Causes

No one understands fully what controls or triggers BPH. However, it's known that it results from certain activities of an enzyme called *5-Alpha Reductase* which converts testosterone into the active compound, *dihydrotestosterone* (DHT). It's DHT that causes the prostate to become enlarged. Unfortunately, it's still not clear why some men have more problems with an enlarged prostate than others.

Diagnosis

By performing a Digital Rectal Examination (DRE) (See Chapter 12), your doctor will determine if you have some indication of BPH. Prostate cancer may present with some of the same indications, but with some slight differences and only at a later stage. During the DRE, your doctor can detect simple soft enlargement (sign of BPH), or lumps (possible sign of cancer), or firm areas (possible sign of cancer). It should be noted that a lump or firmness does not necessarily indicate cancer, but it could be. Regardless of the indications, a blood test would follow to determine the level of *Prostate Specific Antigen* (PSA) and to help diagnose the condition. Depending on that determination, ultimately a biopsy could be required.

Your doctor may also put you through a simple two-minute test utilizing a series of multiple-choice questions to identify your American Urological Association (AUA) symptom index.

When symptoms of BPH exist, your doctor or urologist will recommend blood tests to check kidney function, and a urine specimen to detect infection or presence of blood. Other tests may also be required, such as:

- **Intravenous Urography** – an *X-ray*, following an injection into the blood stream, to allow visualization of the kidneys and bladder.
- **Abdominal** *Ultrasound* – a simple test by which a probe is placed on the abdomen, to visualize the kidneys and bladder, as well as the aorta, liver, spleen and other abdominal organs.
- *Cystoscopy* – a small telescope is passed through the urethra via the penis into the bladder, permitting examination of the bladder and prostate.
- **Urine Flow Study** – measurement of the strength of the urine flow, to determine the severity of the blockage.

Assessing Prostate Symptoms

An easy way to evaluate the severity of your BPH and whether you need treatment for it is to answer the International Prostate Symptom Score (IPSS) questionnaire developed by the American Urological Association. This self-administered IPSS test is based on your urinary symptoms and can help you and and your doctor determine which type of prostate treatment is needed, if any.

Using this key to answer each question:

- Not at all = 0,
- Less than 1 time in 5 = 1,
- Less than half the time = 2,
- About half the time = 3,
- More than half the time = 4,
- Almost always = 5.

you may respond to the following questions and score them accordingly to assess your BPH severity.

Over the past month:

- how often have you had the sensation of not emptying your bladder completely after you finished urinating?
- how often have you had to urinate again less than two hours after you finished urinating?
- how often have you found you stopped and started again several times when you urinated?
- how often have you found it difficult to postpone urination?
- how often have you had a weak urinary stream?
- how often have you had to push or strain to begin urination?
- how many times did you most typically get up to urinate from the time you went to bed at night until the time you got up in the morning?

Your total score offers an assessment of your BPH severity and recommended treatment, as follows:

- 1 to 7 - Mild BPH, no treatment is needed;
- 8 to 19 - Moderate BPH, some form of treatment may be needed; and
- 20 to 35 - Severe BPH, surgery would most likely be effective

Treatment

Once it's determined that you need treatment, a plan will be recommended by your urologist.

Currently, a variety of treatment choices are available, dependent on the severity of the condition.

If the BPH is severe, treatment might be beneficial, otherwise it may be deferred in favour of *watchful waiting*.

Watchful Waiting

Practicing watchful waiting means no active treatment is performed. The practice comes from the experience that more than a third of the BPH cases are mild enough that the symptoms improve without treatment.

Generally less than 50 percent of men with BPH require immediate treatment for their symptoms. The others opt for watchful waiting and are advised to:

- Limit fluid intake before bedtime.
- Limit beverages containing caffeine and alcohol.
- Empty the bladder as completely as possible when urinating.
- Urinate as soon as the urge is felt.

- Reduce, and if possible avoid, intake of caffeine-containing beverages (coffee, tea, cola and other soft drinks)

Watchful waiting requires frequent check-ups. If symptoms begin to worsen, treatment is recommended. Its advantage is that you do not experience side effects. The disadvantage is there may be no symptom relief.

If it's decided that active treatment is necessary, there are several options available, including:

- Medication (or Drug) Therapy
- Transurethral Resection of the Prostate (TURP)
- Transurethral Needle Ablation (TUNA)
- Transurethral Microwave Thermotheraphy (TUMT)
- Transurethral Incision of the Prostate (TUIP)
- Open Prostatectomy
- *Laser* Prostatectomy

It's highly recommended that you quickly proceed to choose a treatment option with the help of your urologist

Medication

This is appropriate for mild to moderate cases of BPH and is usually the option of choice. But it must be realized that most medications can only treat, not cure, the condition.

Some medications are based primarily on *alpha blockers*, such as **terazosin** (commonly known as Hytrin), **doxazosin** (Cardura), **tamsulosin** (Flomax) and **alfuzocin** (Xatral). These alpha blockers achieve success by relaxing the muscle fibres of the prostate and bladder neck (internal sphincter muscle), thereby allowing easier urine flow.

Some common side-effects of the alpha-blockers include: dizziness, fatigue, headaches, and occasionally ejaculation difficulties.

Other medications include **finasteride** (Proscar) and **dutasteride** (Avodart). These are 5-alpha reductase inhibitors, which work by inhibiting production of the hormone DHT, derived from testosterone. By doing so, these drugs have been shown to reduce the size of the prostate.

Drug therapy requires a lifelong commitment to taking daily medication.

Its advantages lie in the fact that it's non-*invasive* and does not require hospitalization.

Its disadvantages include:

- Lifelong use of the medication.
- Waning effectiveness, eventually necessitating other interventions.
- Some erectile dysfunction (8.1 percent incidence) and problems with ejaculation (3.7 percent incidence) resulting from the use of Proscar.
- Side effects such as dizziness (9.1 percent to 17.1 percent), and low blood pressure (1.7 percent to 19 percent) from the use of Hytrin, Cardura, and Flomax.

TURP (TransUrethral Resection of the Prostate)

Next to medication the most common treatment option for BPH is TURP, utilized by 90 percent of patients who do not, or cannot, use drug therapy.

TURP is usually recommended for men who did not achieve much relief by medication. Many men who have had very painful BPH achieved satisfactory relief through TURP.

The procedure which takes about 30 to 60 minutes to perform, involves removing parts of the tumour or tissue from around the urethra within the prostate gland. The outer tissue and capsule are left intact.

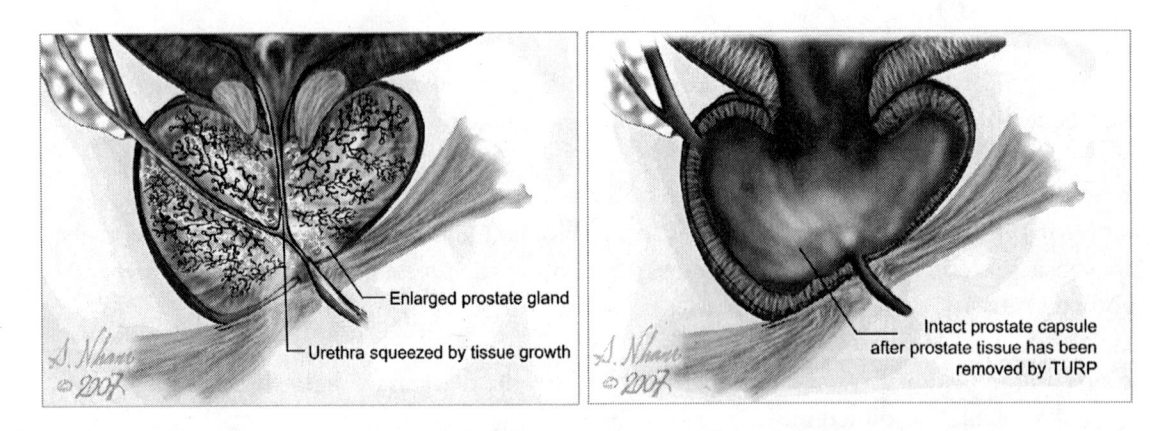

Enlarged prostate gland
Urethra squeezed by tissue growth

Intact prostate capsule after prostate tissue has been removed by TURP

The surgeon uses an instrument called a *resectoscope* (a special kind of *cystoscope*), about 12 inches long and fitted with special lens, a light, a wire loop for cutting tissues and sealing blood vessels, and a valve for controlling irrigating fluid. The patient is placed under *general* or *spinal (epidural) anaesthesia*, and the resectoscope is inserted through the head of the penis and up the urethra, to the location where the prostate presses on the prostatic urethra passage. This is the section where the prostate is blocking urine flow. The surgeon then scrapes away the blocking tissues bit by bit, using the wire loop, irrigating the area as he works. This results in a hollowing out of the passageway, widening it to allow more room for urine to flow more freely through the larger caliber passage. Thus the symptoms of BPH are alleviated; however, if the symptoms were mainly irritative LUTS, they may persist.

TURP may also be accomplished using the "High Intensity Focused Ultrasound" (HIFU) procedure as described in Chapter 35.

At the end of surgery, a catheter is inserted through the urethra into the bladder to drain urine. It's left in place for a few days, to allow the urethra time to heal.

Advantages and Disadvantages of TURP Treatment

The major **advantage** of the TURP is that most patients experience relief almost immediately.

One **disadvantage** is that unavoidable damage is done to the internal sphincter muscle and the prostatic urethra, which can result in incontinence (about one percent of the time), or sterility (68 percent).

Sterility is more likely due to retrograde ejaculation, or semen backing up into the bladder. In additional, the contribution of the semen content by the prostate is significantly compromised following the TURP procedure. Erectile dysfunction is experienced much less (15 percent).

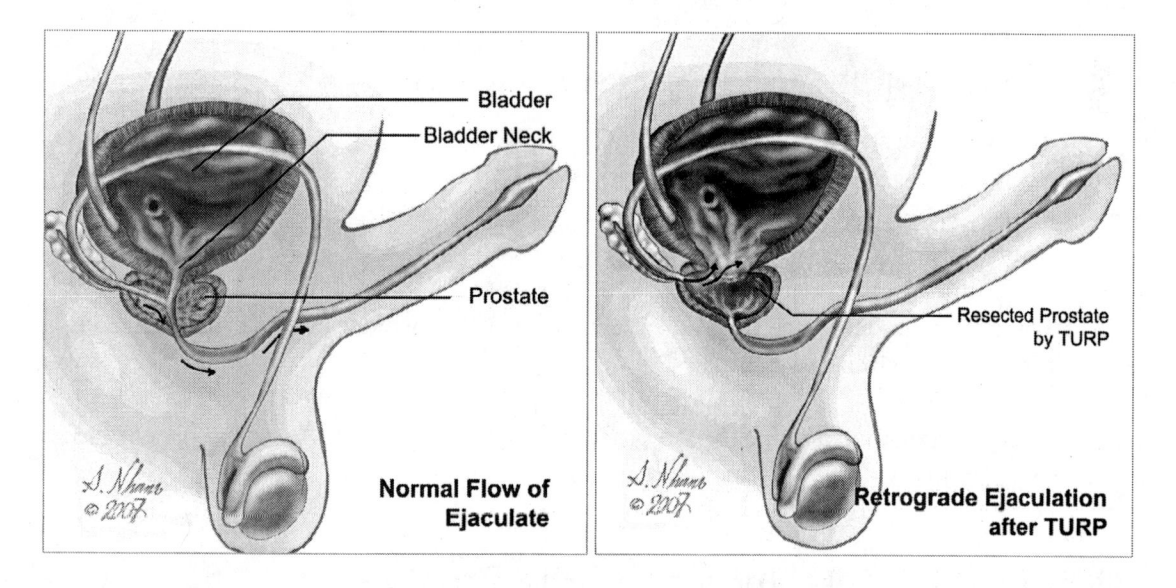

Normal Flow of Ejaculate

Retrograde Ejaculation after TURP

Libido is not affected by retrograde ejaculation, and orgasms and erections are still possible (85 – 90 percent), although the man is incapable of siring children.

Part II   Your Prostate!

TUNA (Transurethral Needle Ablation)

TUNA is a minimally-invasive treatment in use for approximately 20 years, although it has never really caught on very well. It's performed in an out-patient setting or doctor's office. Under local anaesthesia, a catheter is inserted into the urethra. The catheter contains needles that transmit radio frequency (radio waves) energy to the prostate, simultaneously heating and destroying excess cells. Another catheter may be inserted and remain in place for a period of time after the procedure to help with urine discharge.

TUNA is appropriate if

- The prostate is not too large,
- The man does not want to take medication forever,
- Medication becomes ineffective.

TUNA results in relatively few side-effects; however, it's not recommended for men whose bladders are malfunctioning.

TUMT (TransUrethral Microwave Thermotherapy)

TUMT works much like TUNA, except that it uses microwave energy to heat and destroy the excess tissue.

TUMT does not cure BPH; however, it may reduce the symptoms of:

- *Frequency*
- Urgency
- Straining
- Interrupted flow

TUMT corrects the condition of incomplete emptying of the bladder in some men, but long-term results aren't very impressive, so far.

Studies are continuing to determine the long-term effect of TUMT, and who might benefit most from this treatment.

TUIP (TransUrethral Incision of the Prostate)

TUIP, done under general or spinal anaesthesia, works by widening the urethra. A couple of small *incisions* are made in the neck of the bladder and in the prostate tissue. These reduce the pressure on the urethra and help to increase urine flow.

TUIP results in few risks and side effects, although its advantages and long-term side effects aren't fully known. Many of the risks are related to infection and bleeding, albeit uncommon, as with all surgical procedures.

Open Prostatectomy

Open prostatectomy surgery, performed under general or spinal anaesthesia, may be utilized when the transurethral procedures cannot be used. It's an open surgery that requires an incision on the outside and is utilized when complicated factors exist, such as stones in the bladder that need to be removed, or when the prostate is overly large.

In open prostatectomy surgery, the incision is made through the stomach below the navel, and the enlarged tissue is scooped out from inside the prostate gland. In dealing with very large prostates – 100 or 200 grams – there often is more bleeding and the procedure may be challenging.

It requires two or three days stay in the hospital.

The advantage of open prostatectomy surgery is that it usually provides long-term relief.

The disadvantage is that its after effects include incontinence, erectile dysfunction, and retrograde ejaculation. Occasionally a blood transfusion may be needed.

Laser Prostatectomy

Laser is an acronym for "light amplification by stimulated emission radiation." As a treatment for BPH, it's basically the same procedure as TURP, but using a different instrument.

Recent advances in the use of laser technology for tissue *ablation* (destruction) and relief from urinary obstructions are providing benefits for BPH patients. The vast majority of laser applications are for those with significant bladder outlet obstructions (BOO).

Laser technology is based on the application of a blast of high energy through optical fibre. The blast destroys or ablates the oversized prostate tissue.

Newer Holmium and Green Light lasers offer more advanced techniques although they require special training.

Not all men are candidates for this technique. Qualification depends on the condition of the prostate and severity of the condition.

In treating a large prostate, the procedure may be prolonged since some lasers only nibble a little piece at a time. Other laser techniques, which include "enucleanation" of the large adenomas, do require more advanced skills and the procedure may be prolonged.

Advantages of laser treatment are that it:

- Is less invasive,
- Is usually associated with minimal damage to surrounding tissues, and
- Results in very little bleeding.

Disadvantages may include prolonged post-operative irritative symptoms.

It should be noted that laser equipment is still very expensive, with many costly prohibitive disposable parts such as the fibres and thus, may be unaffordable for some treatment centres.

Factors Involved in Treatment Decisions

Deciding which treatment to utilize will depend on several factors: the severity of the symptoms, age, general health condition, prostate size, and the availability of the treatment.

Some people will go to any lengths to avoid surgery, especially simply for BPH. Many have used other treatment methods, with what appears to be some degree of success. However, as was said before, BPH often does not need any type of treatment.

My experience is that the amount of information covered here is what most people feel is appropriate for their needs or understanding.

However, if you need to know more about this subject than what is covered in this book, you are advised to do more in-depth research. A good place to start is a reputable site on the Internet. A list may be found in the resources at the end of this book.

Alternate Treatments

There are also some alternate ways of treating BPH, such as herbs, vitamins and minerals and oral medication, that are finding considerable favour with patients and some doctors. Some of these include:

- Saw palmetto extract;
- Pygeum Africanum;
- Lycopene (from tomato);

- Zinc (from pumpkin seed);
- Selenium (from a credible nutritional supplement supplier);
- Omega 3 (from cold water fish or flax seed);
- Soy products;
- Vitamins;
- Garlic;
- Green tea extract;
- Grape seed extract (with proanthocyanadin);
- Beta carotene;
- Others, all of which are believed to help keep the prostate healthy.

It should be noted that, currently, most Western doctors are reluctant to recommend or encourage the use of these products, in particular saw palmetto, for prostate cancer. Their rationale is that there are ingredients in saw palmetto that may alter the prostate's physiology, and give a false PSA reading. So your PSA might appear to be lowering, but your cancer might be worsening. That was the situation in my case, as well as others.

Saw Palmetto Extract comes from the berries of the saw palmetto palm trees, found along the South Atlantic coastline of North America and the Caribbean. Amongst other less understood actions, the extract reduces the activities of the 5-Alpha Reductase, that converts testosterone into dihydrotestosterone (DHT).

Several studies have found saw palmetto extract to be effective in reducing symptoms as noted above. This reduction in activity supposedly stops the growth of the enlarged prostate, and even shrinks the prostate to its natural size. When I took saw palmetto extract, it appeared to have relieved my urinary symptoms within three months.

Pygeum Africanum is Europe's most popular prescription to fight BPH. Derived from an African evergreen tree, it acts synergistically with saw palmetto extract to reduce the size of the enlarged prostate and resultant symptoms.

All the products mentioned above are marketed for their apparent treatment advantages, although those have never been proved conclusively by Western medical experts. In fact, some studies have concluded that they work as well as a placebo or sugar pills. The saying "let the buyer beware!" applies with purchase of such supplements, as there is little or no regulation on the quality or quantity of the "active ingredients" in the multitude of preparations, brands and labels being sold at pharmacies, "health products" outlets and independent distributors. Consulting your physician is advised.

Another commonly reported important nutrient for the prostate is lycopene. This antioxidant found in naturally reddish fruits, such as tomatoes, guavas, watermelon and pink grapefruits,

Part II   Your Prostate!

is believed to protect the prostate from developing cancer. It's reported that lycopene is most effective when mixed or cooked with warm or hot oil and that it can reduce the risk of cancer. Perhaps that's why some men who consume high quantities of tomato sauce have lower incidence of prostate cancer.

Currently there is an extensive North American study being conducted on the effect of Vitamin E and selenium on men, to detect if either substance alone, or working together, may have any positive effect on the prostate, including prevention of cancer.

Chapter 10

PROSTATE CANCER

*If you have prostate cancer, you are going to need some answers.
More importantly, you are going to need some questions.*

HAROLD USHER
ADAPTED FROM MERCEDES BENZ COMMERCIAL

Prostate cancer is the existence of a tumour in the prostate that's malignant. Diagnosis brings with it myriad of fears, concerns, questions and decisions. Dispelling those fears and concerns, formulating the appropriate questions and finding the proper information for making decisions can be challenging. When you are diagnosed with this condition, it's suggested that you deal with it as quickly as possible. We'll address this in greater detail later.

As stated in the introduction in this book, based on reports from the Canadian Cancer Society for statistics of several previous years, more than 20,000 men in Canada will be diagnosed with prostate cancer yearly, and more than 4,200 of them will die from it each year. These numbers have been relatively steady on an annual basis for a number of years. Similarly, based on reports from the American Cancer Society for statistics of previous years, more than 230,000 men in the United States will be diagnosed with prostate yearly, and more than 27,000 will die from it each year. These numbers have also been relatively steady on an annual basis for a number of years.

Although it appears the incidence and death rates for prostate cancer have been declining since 1994, the growing demographic of baby boomers hitting mid-life and beyond has caused the incidence to continue to rise. Some say this results from the advent of the rapid increase in use of early detection techniques, such as measurement of the Prostate Specific Antigen levels. As such it's predicted to stabilize with time, although the trend can be expected to continue as the boomers – born between 1946 and 1964 – grow into old age. Baby boomers currently represent a large percentage of the population of Canada and the United States.

Lifetime probability of developing prostate cancer is 12 percent chance or one in 8.3 among Canadian men and of dying from it – over a lifetime – their risk is 3.6 percent, or one in 28. In the United States the probability of developing it is a little more than 16 percent or one in six, and of dying from it is three percent or one in 34.

Health Canada's projections for prostate cancer in Canada, are as follows:

Year	Annual new cases	Annual Death
2010	26,900	6,300
2016	35,200	7,800

One can deduce that a good projection for the U.S. would be at least ten-fold.

Death rate reached a peak in the early 1990's and has been declining since. Incidence rates also reach a peak in the early 1990's and started to decline, but is now showing signs of stabilizing.

Just because you have prostate cancer is no cause to give up on life. First, get more information. After all, we may all have cancer cells in our bodies but fewer people are actually dying from it than ever before. Second, decide on a treatment as quickly as possible. Third, have it treated. You need to treat it to prevent local problems and subsequent spread of the cancer and to survive.

How does Prostate Cancer Spread?

Cancer spreads when individual cancer cells escape from the confines of the prostate gland and travel to other parts of the body. Sometimes, they lodge themselves on the bones of the spine or the pelvis, and surrounding *lymph* glands. That spread is referred to as *metastasizing*, and can occur via the blood stream or the *lymphatic system*.

The Need to Understand Information

The information you require can be broken down into three, equally important categories:
1) Information that you know you already know;
2) Information that you know you don't know;
3) Information that you don't know you don't know.

Chapter 10 | Prostate Cancer

Prostate cancers come in different stages and grades and these must be determined as quickly as possible. This determination will be made by your urologist, based his observation and/or on information from a *pathologist* who analyzes your *biopsy* samples. Some urologists do their own analysis of the biopsy samples.

Understand what the stage and grade of your cancer mean, in order to make the best treatment decision.

My suggestion is that you do not make any decision about treatment until:

- You fully understand the information given to you.
- You get answers to your questions – to your satisfaction.
- You know what treatment options are available.
- You are aware of the after-effects of the various available treatments.

Your age, overall health condition, the value that you and your significant other place on your virility, how you can cope with incontinence, erectile dysfunction, a reduction in penis size, your financial disposition and your state of mind, will all have a bearing on your decision. Until you are armed with the appropriate information, you will not be able to intelligently and confidently decide on a course of treatment.

The Right Questions to Ask

In analyzing the options, it's worthwhile to find out exactly how the various treatments are carried out and their consequences. You will have to ask a lot of questions, because all the information that you want may not necessarily be provided by your doctor. Or if it is, you may not catch it, or comprehend it, the first time around.

Here is a list of questions you may wish to consider asking. Get a book and write down everything. Understand that some of these questions may not be relevant and there may not be specific answers.

1. What did your doctor feel during the DRE? A lump, hardness, or mushiness?
2. What is the significance of what was felt during the DRE?
3. Did your doctor send you for blood test(s) to check your PSA level(s)?
4. What are the levels from each of your *PSA tests*? Ask each time and record them each time!
5. Will you need a f-PSA test? If yes, then, what is its reading? This is a procedures which might be able to tell, with some degree of certainty, that you do not have cancer. Understand what this is telling you. (See Chapter 15 for full explanation of f-PSA)
6. How many biopsy samples were taken during each visit, and how many were found to be positive and/or negative?

7. What size is your cancer? Is it the size of a pin head, a nail head, a sugar cube, or larger?
8. What is the grade or Gleason score (a tool used to grade the aggressiveness of the cancer) of your cancer?
9. What is the stage of your cancer?
10. Is the cancer contained within the prostate gland or has it penetrated the walls of the gland?
11. Has the cancer spread (*metastasized*) to other parts of the body?
12. How does your age and health condition factor into the equation for treatment choice?
13. What are the traditional treatment options available?
    (In depth information on individual treatments is provided in Part V of this book.)
14. Which treatment option does your *urologist* or *oncologist* recommend?
15. Exactly how is the recommended treatment performed?
16. What are the after-effects of the recommended treatment, including chance of recurrence, incontinence, and erectile dysfunction?
17. What is the experience level of the urologist or oncologist who is diagnosing you?
18. What is the experience level of the urologist or oncologist who will treat you?
19. Should you get a second opinion?
20. Will it be necessary to remove your *lymph nodes*?
21. Should you begin to follow a special diet?

I cannot promise that you will get answers to all these questions, but you should ask some of them anyway. The more you know, the better position you and your family will be in to make a decision.

Now you are probably saying, "I do not even understand these questions." That's precisely why they are presented here for you. Like most men, I would have liked to have had answers to these questions much earlier. By the time you finish reading this book, you will understand why you may want to ask these questions.

You may feel, as I did and many others have, that you respect your urologist or oncologist so much that you do not want to question them. Well, let me put you at ease – you aren't questioning them, you are merely asking them questions in order to try to understand your condition. This is an important distinction. I discovered that any concerned and reputable professional, including me, will be happy to respond to any question that concerns the patient or client.

I reviewed these questions with over a dozen men and each reported that they wished they had asked some of them before making their decision. Some even reluctantly admitted that they might have chosen a different treatment if they had answers to these questions.

If you do not know the answers to these questions, you will be allowing someone else to make decisions for you. Those decisions may or may not be the ones you would have made had you the necessary information.

Keep a Level Head and Work as a Team

Stay alert and be rational. There aren't only questions to be asked, but also decisions to be made and actions to be taken. You also have to decide whether you are going to do these on your own, or if you will make it a team effort, thus involving your spouse, urologist, and anyone else you may wish to include, such as your family physician and other family members. If at anytime you need to remind yourself of what you need to know, refer back to this chapter and review the questions.

In order to appreciate and understand the questions, you may have to read this book completely. It will not give you personal answers, but it will help you understand what the questions mean and why you need to ask them. It will definitely help other members of your family understand what you are going through.

My experience has taught me that people with an optimistic outlook survive better. Optimism works! A positive mental attitude works! You have been through challenges before and survived them. You will get through this one.

Your Responsibility

It's your responsibility to seek more information so that you can make informed decisions. Here you have been given the basics. It's what I needed. If you need more, refer to the reference material at the end of the book, or go to the Internet.

The Rest of This Book

The rest of this book will focus specifically on the diagnosis and treatment options of prostate cancer, based on this survivor's experience and knowledge and expertise from his urologist.

The goal is to help reduce the anger, fear and pain you may experience and to help you to take control and think clearly. Many men who have gone through the diagnosis and treatment process, believe that the after-effects are important considerations in deciding upon and accepting treatment.

Part III

Prostate Cancer Diagnosis

Chapter 11

DIAGNOSING PROSTATE CANCER

Our lives are molded by the daily flow of our energy, not by luck, fate, circumstance, or even a rich uncle. Whatever is in our lives at this minute… is simply the result of how we've flowed our energies in days gone by.

LYNN GRABHORN
FROM "EXCUSE ME, YOUR LIFE IS WAITING"

The Process of Diagnosis

Diagnosing prostate cancer is currently a three-step process:

1. The Digital Rectal Examination (DRE). Many family physicians mistakenly skip this step.
2. The blood test to identify the level of what is known as the Prostate-Specific Antigen (PSA).
3. The biopsy.

This process is neither simple nor swift. However, sometimes it's completed in short order and action taken quickly, particularly if evidence is so alarming as to dictate it. At times, individual steps may be inconclusive and may have to be repeated or complemented by other tests.

> In my case, which was not typical, I had several DREs, several PSA blood tests, a bone scan, a six-sample biopsy that were all negative, a cystoscopy (done by my urologist in his office), and finally a seven-sample biopsy in which five were negative, one was positive and the seventh borderline. These were done over a three-year period. Only then was there a conclusive diagnosis of prostate cancer.

Chapter 11 | Diagnosing Prostate Cancer

The Need to Understand More

In order for me to understand and appreciate my situation, I felt that I had to understand a little more of my specific condition and what prostate cancer really meant to my life. I also wanted to know what treatment options were available, and how the selected treatment would affect my life.

Unfortunately, nobody could afford the time needed to provide all that information for me to understand. Even worse, I did not know what questions to ask in order for me to get there. In fact, I did not even know what else I wanted to know. I just knew that I was not comfortable with the level of information I had. I definitely did not feel that I knew enough to say 'yea' or 'nay' to any form of treatment.

I have since spoken to many people in a similar situation, who invariably expressed similar sentiments. Many were not aware of what they went through, or why they opted or received their particular treatment. In fact, some of them did not even know where the prostate was located or its function.

In my case, it seemed that each time I visited my doctor, I became tongue-tied and left feeling that I lacked information to make a treatment decision. I could not put my finger on what was missing, but I did feel that I did not yet sufficiently understand. So I decided to learn more about the condition, its implications, and what I could do about it.

A Case in Point

In April, 2000, Rudy Guiliani, then mayor of New York City, stated publicly that he had just been diagnosed with prostate cancer. Two weeks later he held a noon-hour news conference, to further announce that he had spent 2 1/2 hours with one doctor that morning and that he would be spending an hour with another doctor that afternoon.

Most of us would rarely be fortunate enough to have any doctor spend that many hours or minutes with us to explain what we have, how it would affect us, its impact on quality of life, and available treatments alternatives. What we really need is for the information to be presented to us in a timely fashion and with empathy. In fact, based on observations and discussions with several men, it seems that we need to be informed in detail, and more than once. Our doctors really do not have that kind of time. So it's up to us, the patients, to seek out more information.

What I Did to Learn More

To learn more, I attended seminars, read numerous books, listened to many people and viewed documentaries. Each time I learned more. In some cases, I also learned more about alternative treatment options. I even learned that some of the traditional medical experts have limited knowledge about alternative treatments. It's as though some experts, do not have the time to learn about these, or perhaps just do not want to talk about them.

Do not Underestimate Self-Knowledge

There is much more than meet the eyes in understanding the prostate and prostate cancer. There are many good resources, groups and places to turn to for help and guidance as you begin to learn more about the diagnosis and its impact. And without a doubt, it will have an impact – on you and on your family.

If I learned anything from this experience, it's that having prostate cancer was not the worst thing that can happen. It was not the bottom of the pit for me. I did not have to die from it; and I was not going to let that happen. I also learned that the after-effects could be devastatingly stressful, something I think is very much under-appreciated and misunderstood. But I was certainly not going to sit back and start feeling sorry for myself.

Chapter 12

THE DIGITAL RECTAL EXAMINATION (DRE)

*If you put a small value on yourself,
be assured that the world will not raise the price.*

Anonymous

In a Digital Rectal Examination (DRE) the doctor inserts a glove covered finger up your rectum and presses it against the wall of the rectum, adjacent to the prostate gland. It's usually performed as part of a medical check-up, and takes approximately 10 seconds.

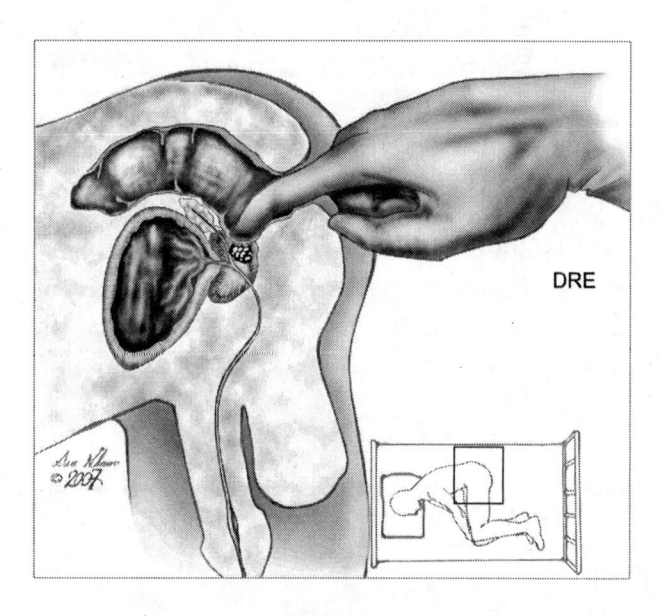

Part III Prostate Cancer Diagnosis

In performing the DRE, your physician asks you to slip off, or lower, your trousers and lay on your side, with your buttocks toward him and your knees bent upward toward your chest – some physicians prefer to have you stand and lean over the examination table. Simultaneously, he puts on a thin, non-latex, rubber glove and lubricates the index finger. He then inserts the index finger through your anus and up your rectum and presses it against the wall of the rectum adjacent to the prostate gland, applying pressure against the prostate a few times to feel for anything suspicious, such as roughness/smoothness, hardness/lumpiness (induration), discrete nodules, areas of irregularity, or asymmetry of the gland. When finished, he pulls out the finger, wipes your buttock, removes the glove, dumps it into the garbage and it's done – quicker than it took you to read this paragraph.

Often your physician will not discover anything abnormal during the DRE, or he may feel something that he considers a cause for concern, as mine did. It might just be an infection, a stone, or a scar tissue, or it might be BPH or prostate cancer. At this stage, your physician would not know for certain if there is cause for alarm. But he would know if further investigation and analysis is needed.

Feeling of an enlargement or mushiness is rarely an indication of prostate cancer, but may very well be an indication of BPH; the feel of a hardness or lump is more likely an indication of prostate cancer rather than BPH, although it could also be a stone or scar tissue.

When cancer develops in the peripheral zone (70 percent), it's usually easier to feel its induration, or hardening, from inside the rectum. However, it may not be as easy for those cancers formed in the central (10 percent) and transitional (20 percent) zones.

It's also possible you may have a cancer so small that no hardness or lump can be felt; therefore, it may not be detected by the DRE. In such cases, a blood test, taken for a different purpose, may show a high PSA reading even though there's no indication of cancer from the DRE.

Utilizing the DRE to screen for prostate cancer is really only worthwhile if radical therapy is contemplated following a positive result. That means that your doctor would probably only perform it if you have at least 10 years of remaining life expectancy. If you are well over the age of 70 and have other severe health problems your physician may choose not to do this test or for that matter any screening for cancer. That premise led one prominent urologist to remark that he "would not examine anyone over 80 years of age for prostate condition, unless he comes in with his parents."

Questions

As noted in Chapter 10, ask your doctor:

- What did he feel during the DRE, a lump, hardness, mushiness, or anything suspicious?
- Will he recommend a blood test to identify your PSA level?
- How does your age and health condition factor into the equation?
- Should you begin to follow a special diet?

Warning

If you are over 40 years of age and aren't getting a yearly medical check-up, get one now. I said this to a man I met in October 2000. He was 62 years old. He quickly got a check-up, including a DRE. The results raised some concerns for his doctor. He was therefore sent for a blood test to identify his PSA level. That identified a high PSA level of 18 ng/ml. He was then sent for a biopsy, which indicated an aggressive cancer.

If you are under 70 and your medical check-up does not include a DRE, demand one. It's harmless and could make a difference. If you are in your mid 70s to late 80s, perhaps you do not even want to know. You will probably pass away as a result of something else, unless you have a very aggressive cancer.

Chapter 13

PROSTATE-SPECIFIC ANTIGEN (PSA)

*If future generations are to remember us with gratitude rather than contempt,
we must leave them more than the miracles of technology.
We must leave them a glimpse of the world as it was in the beginning,
not just after we got through with it.*

Lyndon B. Johnson, 1908 – 1973
36th President of the United States
(Upon signing The Wilderness Act, 1964)

Antigen

Following the DRE, if your doctor feels there is cause for further examination, he will send you for a blood test to determine the level of the prostate-specific antigen (PSA) in your blood.

Antigens are proteins produced by cells. They are *biological markers* like finger-prints that are unique and specific to their gland. They can be used to distinguish gland cells from which they originate, which makes it possible to track an antigen to its gland of origin, in this case the prostate gland. Unfortunately, they aren't condition or disease specific, and therefore cannot identify a condition or disease the prostate is experiencing, such as prostatitis, BPH or cancer.

An antigen that's prostate-specific is a protein (or enzyme) produced by the prostate gland cells.

Both cancerous and non-cancerous cells produce this antigen, which leaks into the blood stream via the small blood vessels, or capillaries. However, cancerous cells are more porous and allow larger quantities to leak into the blood stream than non-cancerous cells do. Thus, the proportionate amount of PSA in the blood increases with the amount of cancer in the prostate – the more cancerous the prostate, the more leaking from the cells, and the higher is the PSA level. Having said that, it's also recognized that some prostate cancers, usually the more aggressive types, may not produce as much PSA as might be expected.

PSA is measured in nanograms (ng) per millilitre (ml) of blood mixture, (ng/ml), or in microgram (UG) per litre (l), (UG/l).

The blood sample taken for the PSA analysis is taken from the arm. Your doctor may extract the blood sample himself and send it to a laboratory, or he might send you to the laboratory to have it extracted there. In either case, the report on the PSA level will be revealed to your doctor.

Interpretations of PSA Levels

The PSA level becomes higher when cancer is present, because:

1) Cancerous prostate cells are more leaky than normal ones.
2) Cancerous cells may produce a more elevated level of PSA than non-cancerous cells.
3) A large prostate simply produces more PSA.

When cancer is present and growing, the amount of leaked antigen increases proportionately with the growth of the tumour. Thus, the amount of PSA in the blood increases also. Likewise, when prostatitis exists, the gland becomes inflamed and the blood vessels leak even more, but only temporarily. This causes the PSA to elevate to a high level fairly quickly and come down quickly as the infection is treated. In the case of BPH, the PSA level rises proportionately with the increased size of the prostate.

The PSA level resulting from BPH rarely goes beyond 15 or 20 ng/ml, unless the prostate becomes extremely large. An infection resulting in prostatitis would go beyond 10 ng/ml, but it would be temporary. PSA level as a result of cancer may start as low as 2.0 ng/ml and continue to rise, usually faster than it would rise in the case of BPH. From there, it generally does not decrease, until it's properly treated.

History of the Use of PSA

Determination of PSA level in the blood was initiated in the late 1970's. In 1986, a commercial blood test was approved as a tool for monitoring the status of already-diagnosed prostate cancer. However, the medical community also recognized its potential value for early detection of cancer, and began to use it for that purpose. In 1994, PSA was approved for prostate cancer **detection**, but not **screening** (See section on "Differing Opinions," later in this chapter).

Part III   Prostate Cancer Diagnosis

"The number of patients diagnosed with prostate cancer has increased as a result of PSA screening," says Jonathan Epstein, Professor of *Pathology*, Urology and Oncology at Johns Hopkins Hospital in Baltimore, Maryland. Until 1989, 60 to 70 percent of all prostate cancers had already metastasized, or spread, beyond the gland, by the time they were diagnosed. Today, by measuring PSA levels, more than 75 percent of all prostate cancers are diagnosed while still localized within the gland.

On the down side, however, an analysis at a prominent U.S. hospital, of 300 patients who had early cancer diagnosis and their prostate removed, found that 25 to 33 percent of those patients had such small tumours that they were insignificant and would probably never have caused a problem if they were not removed. It's reported that four to five percent of these tumours were too small to be found in pathology.

There is an ongoing *clinical trial*, which began in 1993, of 75,000 men in the United States, to see if PSA screening prolongs life. Half of the men are being screened and the other half aren't. Results are still years away.

Relationship Between Age and PSA

At about age 45, when the second phase of the enlargement of a man's prostate begins, a relationship between the age and the level of PSA circulating in the blood becomes a factor.

The generally accepted normal range for PSA in the *serum* or *plasma* of the blood is 0-4 ng/ml. However, because PSA is *synthesized* in the *epithelial cells*, which increase as the volume of the prostate increases, and simultaneously with age, PSA levels also increase. As a result, many practitioners now use age-specific PSA normal reference ranges as a guide. Levels above these ranges are cause for concern and further tests. The age-specific normal ranges are:

Age	Age-specific normal PSA Reference Ranges ng/ml or UG/l
up to 49	0 – 2.5
50 to 59	2.5 to 3.5
60 to 69	3.5 to 4.5
70 +	4.5 to 6.5

Theory of Probability of Containment Based on Lower PSA

Urologists generally agree that the more cancer a man has in his prostate, the higher will be his PSA level. They also generally agree that the higher the PSA level, the greater the chance that cancer has started to spread. One can broadly classify PSA levels into four groups to provide a probability that the cancer is fully contained within the capsule, as follows:

PSA	Probability that the Cancer Is Contained Within the Prostate Capsule
0.0 to 4.0 ng/ml	75 percent chance
4.1 to 10.0 ng/ml	50 percent chance
10.1 to 20.0 ng/ml	25 percent chance
> 20.0 ng/ml	Almost all of these men have cancer cells spreading outside the prostate

Some studies have concluded that the higher the PSA level, the more cancer a man is found to have. However, there are exceptions to these findings, as you will see below.

Differing Opinions

There are some differences of opinion regarding the use and interpretation of PSA levels for prostate cancer screening.

Urologists, in general, favour PSA testing, although it's recognized that it sometimes gives a false impression.

Some physicians misinterpret PSA levels, believing that when they are high, cancer is definitely present. The key is that PSA levels should not be interpreted in isolation. Many other factors must be taken into consideration.

There have been reports of men with low PSA levels who were thought not to have cancer, only to find out later that cancer was present. Conversely, there have been reports of men with high levels who were assumed to have cancer, only to discover later, none was present.

It's generally accepted that a patient with a PSA level greater than 10 ng/ml has a higher likelihood of cancer. Remember, however, that prostatitis can cause the PSA level to go above 10 ng/ml or even 100 ng/ml temporarily, and BPH in large prostates can cause elevations of near 20 ng/ml.

> Bob, aged 57, had a PSA reading of 32 ng/ml for a few days during one period of his life. He did not have cancer. He was correctly diagnosed and treated with antibiotics for prostatitis. His PSA level is now down to 2.1ng/ml.

Many specialists feel that a single PSA reading should not be the basis for a biopsy. Also, not all regulatory bodies endorse the use of the test. Some remain silent about its use. One thing that's certain, however, is that PSA in its present format cannot distinguish between prostatitis, BPH and cancer.

In general, PSA tests do help to monitor the prostate condition and can precipitate timely biopsy.

PSA is not perfect by any stretch of the imagination. In fact, in about 20 percent of the time, or more, it may be wrongly interpreted and lead to an inaccurate conclusion. Nevertheless, it appears to be a good tool that's currently available for early detection of prostate cancer.

PSA is Only One Step in the Process of Diagnosis

Given the foregoing information, it's clear that PSA is only one step in the diagnostic process. It's estimated that the combination of a suspicious DRE together with an elevated PSA, is predictive of cancer in 40 to 70 percent of cases; however, until a biopsy is performed, there is no conclusive evidence of the presence of cancer. No credible urologist would assume there is cancer unless the results of a biopsy confirm it.

PSA and Early Detection

As a result of PSA facilitating the early detection of the prostate cancer, the average age of men being diagnosed with prostate cancer had dropped from 72 to 69 years of age by 1994. It's expected, when more current data is analyzed in the future, it may show a further drop.

Some data suggest, not without controversy, that the number of men dying from prostate cancer has been dropping by approximately 2.5 percent per year since 1992 and further, that the number of those whose cancer has metastasized before it's diagnosed, has dropped to half of what it was in the 1980s.

The jury is still out as to whether these improvements are due to earlier detection as a result of PSA screening. Nevertheless, if you have prostate cancer, your chances are good of having it detected and treated much earlier than during pre-PSA days.

As we approach the time when more and more baby boomers will be reaching the age of 55 to 65, you can expect to see a corresponding increase in the number of men being diagnosed with prostate diseases.

There are also activities that can elevate the PSA level. These include: having sex in the previous 24 hours; riding a bicycle, motorcycle, or horse, prior to having the blood test; as well as recent tests, such as ultrasound or biopsy. It's advisable to avoid any of these activities for a day or two prior to having your blood taken for PSA purposes.

Taking Action

If your blood test came back with a PSA reading that's cause for concern, depending on the reading, it may need to be monitored, or it may require other tests or treatment. Your physician and urologist will decide on the next appropriate step.

My Story

> "My first encountered with PSA level was as a result of a bizarre series of incidents one week-end in July 1995. I was 56 years old. I had gone for a visit one Friday afternoon to my family doctor at which time he did a routine check of my prostate via a DRE. I developed a fever that evening, and later that night I passed a clot of blood in my urine. That was the first time that I had ever passed blood in my urine, and I was concerned. I called my doctor at his home and he prescribed an antibiotic. On the Monday I visited him at his office and was immediately sent for a blood test to check my PSA level. It turned out to be a high 21 ng/ml. Wow! I was then sent for a bone scan and later referred to a urologist. By the time I had my appointment with the urologist, my PSA level had fallen as dramatically as it had risen, to below 10 ng/ml. Within two months, it fell to just over 7 ng/ml. Over the subsequent year, it hovered around the 7 ng/ml. In fact, on one occasion it even went down to 2.9 ng/ml. To this day, no one can explain that drastic temporary drop.
>
> My earlier level of 21 ng/ml was obviously a one-time infection. The question is, what caused it to surge that high? Was it an irritation from the DRE? Probably. Or maybe it was acute bacterial prostatitis. By the way, there are people with PSA levels as high as 1000 ng/ml or more. I've even heard of cases over 5000 ng/ml. More than likely those are reflective of advanced cancer.

> My urologist monitored me every six months for a year and simultaneously observed my PSA. In October 1996, when my PSA level was 7 ng/ml, he sent me for a biopsy. Did I really need the biopsy? The signs – firmness on the prostate as indicated by the DRE and a PSA of 7 ng/ml – suggested that I did."

Having said all of the above, one must be reminded of two things:

1. The PSA is a *tumour marker*, not a tumour specific identifier. That means that it can tell you that something is wrong in the prostate, but it cannot tell you what is wrong.
2. We must treat the condition, not the PSA levels. So beware of treatments, such as saw palmetto that, according to some doctors/urologists, might mask the PSA, particularly if you are dealing with cancer.

Some remedies that work well for BPH may not necessarily work well for cancer. Zinc, for example, is very good for a healthy prostate and even for BPH; however, prostate cancer thrives on zinc. Always check with your physician, when you are considering the use of various non-conventional remedies.

Chapter 14

BIOPSY

Let others lead small lives, but not you.
Let others argue over small things, but not you.
Let others cry over small hurts, but not you.
Let others leave their future in someone else's hands, but not you.

JIM ROHN

What is Biopsy?

A biopsy is a procedure that involves obtaining a tissue specimen for microscopic analysis to establish a diagnosis. In the case of a prostate biopsy, a small sliver of tissue is removed from the prostate gland and examined for the presence of cancer cells. If cancer cells are found, the sample is further analyzed to determine the grade of the cancer.

A prostate biopsy is commonly preceded by a *transrectal ultrasound (TRUS)* examination, a procedure used to project a visual image of the gland on a monitor. The ultrasound is conducted and then, guided by the ultrasound picture, tissue samples are taken. The samples are sent to a pathologist for examination and analysis. This procedure may be conducted by a urologist or a *radiologist*.

The TRUS requires a clean rectum. So you will need to have an enema prior to the procedure. You will also need to take antibiotics to protect you against infection, for a few days before and after the procedure. As well, you will be given instructions about medications to take and avoid.

Part III Prostate Cancer Diagnosis

In performing the TRUS, the urologist or radiologist uses an instrument called an ultrasound probe. This is essentially a thin, lighted tube which houses a transducer that sends out sonar signals to a computer terminal and monitor.

The urologist or radiologist will lubricate the probe and have you lie on your side, knees curled up or flexed to your chest in a fetal position. He will insert the probe through your anus and up into your rectum. Initially, it may feel uncomfortable or even painful. However, once the probe is in place, you have more than likely experienced the worst of the discomfort.

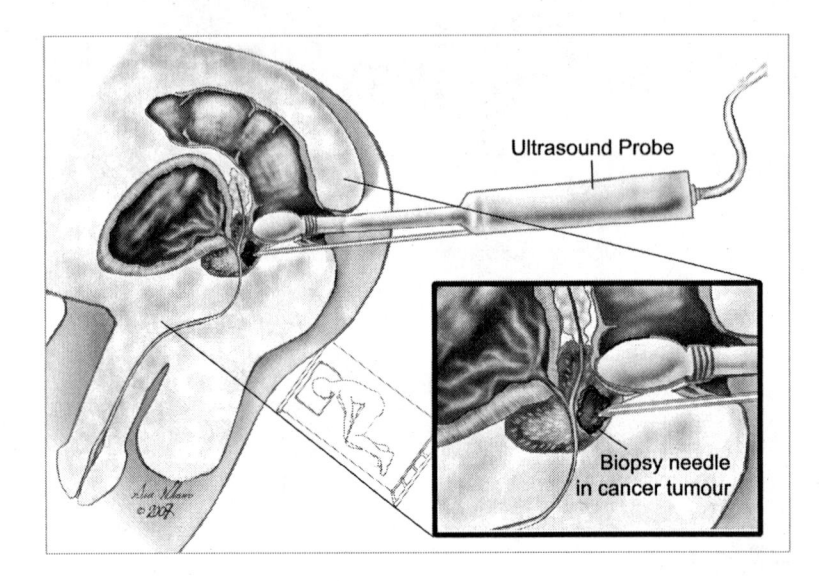

The probe will then be activated, sending out high-frequency sound waves. These are either absorbed or reflected, depending on the nature of the tissue. The ultrasound signals from prostate tissue are different from surrounding fat tissue, blood and the *bladder*. The reflected sound waves are converted into visual images that can be seen on the monitor. The urologist or radiologist can see where the prostate is located and may even identify some abnormal growth, based on the difference in the texture and the consistency of the tissue. This image is used to decide the exact location that the tissue samples will be taken from.

The Biopsy Procedure

The biopsy needle is a hollow, cylindrical needle attached to a spring-loaded gun. It's inserted alongside the probe into the rectum and manually guided toward the adjacent prostate gland. Once in place, the gun shoots the needle into the prostate at a tremendous speed and for a specific distance to a pre-planned location. You will feel a quick jab, and hear a pop as the needle passes through the wall of the rectum and into the prostate, where it grabs the small sliver of tissue and retreats almost instantly. The pain is sharp and fleeting.

In most instances, eight samples are taken, four from each side of the prostate at various strategic locations. There might be more, particularly from the central and the anterior areas. However, care is taken to avoid passing the needle through the urethra, as such an action would cause bleeding, which would be seen in the urine.

After each sample is taken, a new needle is inserted for the next one. Each sample is about the size of a half-inch of thread.

My Experience

At the request of my urologist, my radiologist, who was very experienced, performed my biopsies. My radiologist fully understood and empathized with his patients, and so understood my fears. He performed the procedure with compassion, empathy and expediency, explaining each step as he was performing them, which made me feel comfortable also.

> In November, 1996 six tissue samples were taken from my prostate gland. In those days, six samples was the norm; today it's eight, and could be as many as 12. On my follow-up visit to my urologist, he informed me that all six samples were negative. That meant that there was no evidence of cancer. I was instantly relieved. I thought: "Thank God, no cancer. So we are dealing with something else more curable and less terminal." But, did that mean that there was no malignancy in the entire gland? Absolutely not! It only meant that there was no malignancy found at the locations where the samples were taken. They could have unknowingly missed a small malignant growth, particularly if it was small enough, like say the size of a pin head.
>
> Studies have shown that biopsies miss the cancer about 30 percent of the time, even when there's known cancer in the gland. I have spoken to many men whose first, and sometimes even their second, set of biopsy samples were all negative, only to find a positive sample the next time around.
>
> I should add that I had no problems, nor adverse reactions, resulting from these biopsies. I had no bleeding, either in my urine or semen. And after the very brutal invasion of my rectum, I was certain that I would not even be able to walk and would be sore for a long time. None of these things happened. I walked away feeling very comfortable.
>
> My urologist continued to monitor my condition every six months. After the first six, he performed a cystoscopy to examine the condition of my bladder, urethra, prostate and urine flow.

Part III Prostate Cancer Diagnosis

Performing Cystoscopy

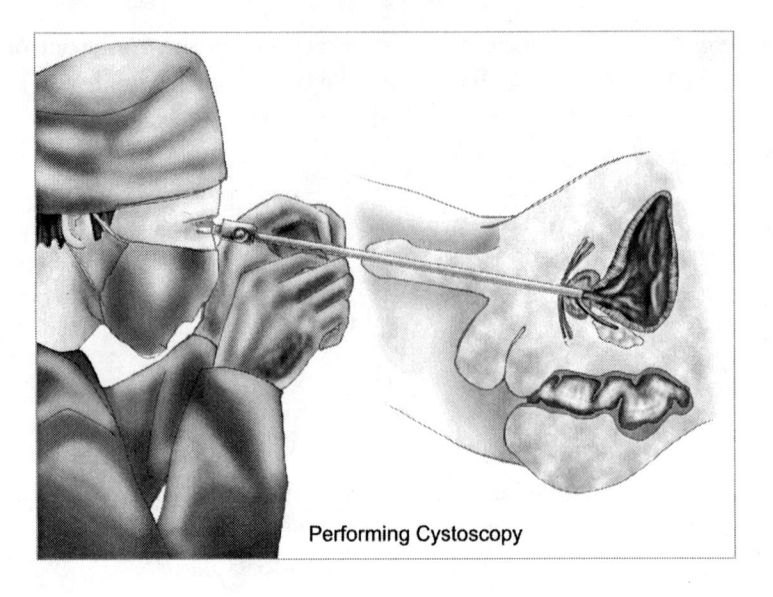

> By the end of the second six-month period, in January 1998, my PSA had risen to 11.5 ng/ml. As a result of that, my urologist sent me for another biopsy.
>
> The second time around, they took seven tissue specimens. I was not so lucky that time. Up to the sixth specimen, everything seemed to feel just like the previous occasion. But the seventh jab was excruciatingly painful. I felt as if I had just been injected with a needle from the prostate up through the length of my penis. I felt a pain from my *scrotum* straight up through my penis to its head. I was sure, for a moment, that my penis was damaged forever. That pain took more than a day to subside. That night, I had a frightening experience when I passed blood, or so it seemed, through my penis. It took about three days for it to completely clear. Hindsight tells me that my radiologist may have jabbed the needle through a blood vessel, or perhaps through the urethra.
>
> Three weeks later, I visited my urologist to receive the biopsy results. He added to that painful and bloody experience by casually informing me that one of the samples showed positive signs of malignancy and another was borderline positive. The other five samples were negative. This was stunning information as I had expected that if I had cancer, all the specimens would be positive. Then I realized that's the reason they take more than one sample. If out of 100 samples only one proves positive, that's the basis on which a cancer diagnosis would be made.

Cancer Cells and Oxygen – A Myth?

It's believed that cancer cells thrive on oxygen for survival and growth. Unfortunately, they have access to oxygen through the bloodstream. But if exposed to another source, or supply, they might grow faster. When cancer cells are deprived of oxygen, they do not grow so quickly. In the case of prostate cancer, as long as the cells are confined within the gland, they are far removed from oxygen other than from the blood stream.

However, if a pipeline was created, from outside the prostate, chances are it might act as a tunnel for additional oxygen, which would help the cancer cells to grow, and possibly even spread along the pipeline to the rectum.

There's a school of thought that believes every jab of the biopsy needle creates such a pipeline. According to internationally acclaimed research scientist, Dr. Michael Colgan, ". . . to those cancer cells, those pipelines or tunnels that happen to terminate on a cancerous tumour are like six lane highways for the supply of oxygen."

Most urologists believe this is a myth, pointing out that, of the millions of biopsies that have been conducted over the years, there has never been a documented case of such resulting spread or growth.

Some years ago, November 1999, I attended an educational seminar on prostate cancer in London, Ontario, presented by a prominent urologist, professor, and author, from Vancouver. During the question and answer period, I asked him: "There is an unproven concern that since oxygen helps the cancer cells to grow more rapidly, a biopsy needle may leave behind a potential oxygen pipeline, from outside the capsule to the cancer cells. Is this a concern when calling for biopsy samples?" He replied: "That's a very good question. We do not have any proof that this tunnel concept is so, but it's something we are studying."

Urologists are very conscientious when making decisions and recommendations regarding biopsies. They know the potential complications and that cancer cells thrive on oxygen. They see the only source of oxygen to the cancer as through the bloodstream. In fact urologists generally will use *repeat-PSA* and other tests to cut down on the number of biopsies. Some may even use *free-PSA* (referred to as f-PSA), urine tests, and other tests, as they become more acceptable. These will be discussed in the next chapter.

Final Word

Currently, without the positive result of a biopsy, a condition cannot be decisively diagnosed as cancer. Unquestionably, it's a necessity. There are three reasons why other tests, such as repeat-PSA, f-PSA or urine tests, are reasonable before finally considering biopsy:

1. Biopsies are expensive
2. Biopsies are painful and uncomfortable

Part III   Prostate Cancer Diagnosis

3. Biopsies penetrate the rectal wall and sometimes puncture a blood vessel within the prostate gland, thus opening up opportunities for bleeding, scar tissues, and/or infection.

The bottom line is that your urologist will ensure that there are good reasons for the biopsies, such as a lump or hardness or induration felt during the DRE; repeat-PSAs being above normal; a more rapid rise than expected in PSA level; or an f-PSA or urine-test which indicate a probability of cancer.

Ask your urologist and do not be reluctant to debate, demand, or express your concerns.

Chapter 15

WHEN IS BIOPSY NECESSARY?

We need time to dream, time to remember, and time to reach the infinite. Time to be.

GLADYS TABER (1899-1980)

The f-PSA

Toward the end of chapter 13, I posed the question "Did I really need the biopsy?" I posed that question because there are a couple of potential intermediate procedures that could discriminate between BPH and cancer at an early stage in the diagnostic process. Utilizing these would reduce the number of biopsies, since it would be possible to determine earlier if a condition is cancerous.

One of these procedures is called "f-PSA," and the other is a "urine-based test." Either might be able to tell, with some degree of certainty, that you do not have cancer.

If you can tell with relative certainty that you have cancer, through a relatively safe, painless test, why not go through that test before you embark on a biopsy that may prove negative?

PSA exists in the blood in three forms:

1. PSA-ACT, attached to a protein called alpha1-antichymotrypsin.

2. PSA-AMG, attached to a protein called alpha2-macroglobulin.

3. f-PSA, not attached to any protein, thus referred to as free-PSA.

Part III   Prostate Cancer Diagnosis

The attachment of PSA to the alpha 2-macroglobulin (AMG) results in a portion of the PSA being undetectable by any current methods. That fraction of the PSA, therefore, is a complete loss in the calculation of the total detectable PSA (t-PSA).

In cancerous prostate cells most, if not all, of the PSA is attached to the protein molecules. So there is less f-PSA detected in a cancerous prostate.

Current methods of distinguishing between BPH and prostate cancer use ratios of PSA-ACT to t-PSA or f-PSA to t-PSA.

If the value for f-PSA is very low in comparison to the t-PSA, it's a good indication that cancer is present. If the value is relatively high in comparison to the t-PSA, it's an indication that cancer is likely not present and a biopsy less likely to be needed.

If the ratio of f-PSA to t-PSA is equal to or less than 0.15, or one to seven, there is considered to be a high probability that cancer is present. The next step is biopsy for confirmation.

If the ratio of f-PSA to t-PSA is between 0.15 and 0.25, or between one to seven and one to four, it can be read as "*equivocal*" and it can't be used to strongly predict the presence or absence of cancer. The urologist may decide on proceeding with biopsy or continue with observation, using other factors to help him make the decision. Many cancers actually have this ratio range.

If the ratio of f-PSA to t-PSA is equal to or greater than 0.25, or one to four, there is considered to be a low probability that cancer is present. It's probably safe to take no action, just observe it (watch and wait), unless other clinical factors raise the level of suspicion for cancer.

To sum up, it has been observed that many cancers actually have a ratio between 0.15 and 0.25. That would be in the equivocal or borderline range. Few cancers have greater than 0.31. In practice, most specialists take free versus total at 0.15 and 0.16 as the cut-off ratio for high probability and low probability.

If the presence of cancer is still suspected, a biopsy would still be necessary to conclusively confirm it.

Chapter 15 | When is Biopsy Necessary?

My Case

> On one occasion, 21 months after I was diagnosed with prostate cancer, I requested a f-PSA calculation of my blood sample. My t-PSA was 6.79 and my f-PSA was 1.14, and my f-PSA to t-PSA ratio was 0.17. According to my family physician, that ratio implied that there was a good probability that cancer was present in my prostate. Actually, in my opinion and according to the ratios above, it was equivocal, meaning we could read it either way and we had to depend on other factors – not very convincing from my perspective. However, the range was between 0.10 and 0.25 and that along with my above normal PSA reading was an assurance that I was likely dealing with cancer and I had to do something about it. I already had the conclusive biopsy, but was still, to some extent, in denial. My f-PSA result prompted me to quickly seek the necessary treatment.

Continued Investigation

There is ongoing investigation and research in this area, which may ultimately help avoid the need for biopsies.

A f-PSA test uses the same blood sample as the t-PSA test.

If cancer is present, it's not going to go away if you don't have it treated. In fact, chances are it will get worse. The last thing you want is for one or more of those cancer cells to escape from your prostate through the blood stream and get latched on to your lymph nodes, pelvis, spinal column, or some other part of your anatomy. In many cases, that's how "*recurrence*" occurs. You will read more about that in the last chapter.

The Urine-Based Test

Another test on the horizon for prostate cancer that has potential is a urine-based test. Although still not widely used at the moment, one of these – the uPM3™ test – was introduced by Bostwick Laboratories of Richmond, Virginia, in September 2003.

The uPM3™ test is considered the first urine-based *genetic* test for prostate cancer. It has been reported in one study to predict cancer in the prostate with 81 percent accuracy, compared to 47 percent for PSA.

Part III Prostate Cancer Diagnosis

The uPM3™ test is based on PCA3, a specific gene found in the prostate tissue, which is thought to be 34 times greater in cancerous than non-cancerous tissue. The gene is added to urine to determine its proportionate amount.

The procedure to acquire urine for the test involves massaging the prostate – a similar routine as with the digital rectal examination (DRE). In this case the doctor massages the prostate to make it secrete the PCA3 genes into the urethra, where it mixes with the urine. A sample containing secretions is tested for proportion of the PCA3 genes in it. If the sample is positive for large proportion of the genes, then there is a very high likelihood of prostate cancer. Again a biopsy would then be required to conclusively confirm it.

Although Bostwick Laboratories introduced uPM3™ test, it's licensed from DiagnoCure Incorporated of Quebec, which holds the worldwide patent for diagnostic and therapeutic applications of PCA3 genes. The test was developed by Dr. Yves Fradet, a world-renowned urologist at Laval University in Quebec City. However, currently, the uPM3™ test is available only in the United States exclusively through Bostwick Laboratories.

We are almost certain to hear more about this in the future. Perhaps as f-PSA, urine or others tests, become more available, there might be less needs for biopsies.

Chapter 16

YOU HAVE CANCER!

"We all have cancer in our bodies; it's just that our immune system is keeping it in check… It's the breakdown of our immune system that allows cancer to grow … if you maintain a strong and healthy immune system, your chances of ever getting cancer are virtually nil."

Dr. Virginia Livingston-Wheeler
The Conquest of Cancer, pp 101-2

Cancer – Not Death

We have been conditioned to think that cancer means the end of life. I was determined to think otherwise. I was determined to think that there is life after prostate cancer. I was definitely not ready to give up, or even slow down. And I certainly did not expect to die. I just have too many things to accomplish in life. My intention is to inspire you to think the same way.

The word "cancer" is frightening. We hear it all the time, but when it's to do with us, or someone close to us, it becomes petrifying. For some of us it means "the end;"' for some, it means "fight;" for others, like me, it means "there is life after cancer."

A smaller percentage of men are dying from prostate cancer today than ever before, and the options for treatment are increasing and improving. Unfortunately, most treatment options still carry a significant risk of incomplete cure, erectile dysfunction and incontinence, among other less debilitating after-effects.

As it Affected Me

> The result of my last biopsy test was not what I wanted to hear. I was not angry, but I was disappointed. I had enough time to prepare myself for whatever the results would be. Once you go for the biopsy, brace yourself, because the result could be positive or negative.
>
> What surprised me was that I felt and looked healthy. I was not in any pain, I did not have any symptoms or discomfort, and I did not feel that I was in a terminal condition. In fact, most of the time, I really did not even consider that I had cancer or was in need of tests. Unfortunately, my slowly rising PSA was telling the tales.
>
> I was determined to remain calm and think straight in order to absorb what my urologist was telling me. But at that point, everything seemed to be happening so fast. I felt that I needed education on all the things I was hearing: words such as, malignant tumour, *metastasis*, grade, stage, options, and many others, all coming at me at once.
>
> I had a malignant tumour in my prostate, meaning I had prostate cancer. Now I had to deal with it and, frankly, I did not want to do that. I was not ready to jump to any hasty decisions, either. I had never known anyone who had to deal with such a condition. Cancer? Yes! Prostate cancer? No! My mother died of cancer, so did one of my sisters, and several of my wife's relatives. It seems that everyone I know who has died, did so as a result of cancer, diabetes, or heart failure.

Making a Decision

Depending on the characteristics of the cancer, doctors will probably advise you to decide on the method of treatment quickly, although that does not mean a rush to decision. "Quickly" does not mean tomorrow, or next week – it does not even necessarily mean next month. How quick is "quickly" depends on the characteristics of the cancer – the aggressiveness or grade, the stage, size of the tumour, PSA level, age, health condition, values regarding quality of life and family.

But remember that for most treatments, there is a long waiting list, upward to three months, at least in Canada. Therefore, you do not want to leave this decision for too long, considering that you may have to add those months to the time frame.

Chapter 16 | You Have Cancer!

Listen and Understand

Having discovered that there is cancer, your urologist will obtain information regarding its grade. He will also decide on the stage, based on results of the bone scan, *CT scan*, PSA level, and other tests. He will explain these to you but if he does not, then ask him. You must understand what these mean. The next two chapters will help to explain them.

Grade, stage, and PSA level are critical pieces of information to plan appropriate treatment options for prostate cancer. But more is needed. Refer back to the list of questions in Chapter 10, and ask them until you get answers you can clearly understand. Your urologist may not volunteer this information. Understand that it's not because he is trying to hide anything from you but, rather, because he does not want to confuse or bombard you with a lot of information all at once.

What you have to do at this moment is to make a concerted effort to listen and make notes. Write down what you hear. You will want to know, remember and understand:

- What is the size of the tumour? – Is it the size of a pinhead, a pea, a sugar cube, or a finger tip?
- What is the grade or aggressiveness?
- What stage is the cancer? Or, how far has it progressed? Has it metastasized?
- What treatment options are being recommended? Why?
- What are the after-effects of each option?
- How much time do you have, before you have to make your decision?

You may not think that you want or need this information right now, but later on you will. Your decision-making will be dependent on your grasp of the situation, and it's up to you to get a firm grip on that.

It's the responsibility of every prostate cancer patient to become an active partner in the decision-making process to select a treatment option. Some urologists or *radiation oncologists* will tell you this; some will not. Mine told me. There is absolutely no way that you can be a partner in decision-making if you do not have an understanding of your condition. Every man's condition is different. You need to have some information about your condition.

> When I was diagnosed, one of my major challenges was my difficulty in believing that I had cancer. Then I had difficulty understanding my condition. This was because I was not experiencing any symptoms related to the prostate or urethra. So I really felt that I was not well-informed. I needed somebody to sit down with me and slowly, clearly and empathically explain everything I am explaining here.

> I also felt that I wanted a second opinion, someone else to analyze my situation, in particular my biopsy test, and give me his opinion, or to confirm what my urologist had told me. Do not misunderstand: I trusted my urologist, but I have always felt that a second opinion is important.

Look at it this way. If you were planning to renovate your bathroom, would you not shop around for ideas, materials and quotations? Would you not be interested in what others know or how they feel? Would you not be interested in obtaining references? Why should we not shop around for the best treatment for our prostate cancer, and for the best therapist?

I have talked to several men who went through this process of diagnosis and treatment. Nearly all were unaware of how much information was available. Some expressed disappointment that they did not have the information in making their decision. Several were not even aware what was done to them in their surgery or *radiation* treatment. A few told me that if they had access to more information, they probably would have opted for another form of treatment, or would be more confident of the treatment that they selected.

In all fairness to the physicians, there are some men who do not want to be bothered with details, nor do they want to prolong the waiting period. They just want to get it over with. They do not want to think about it. Many of these men take the word of the urologist or radiation oncologist at face value and say "just get it done." Many of these men are happy with their decision. Some are not.

Some of those who aren't happy appear to be those who have had their treatment from free enterprise health care system, where they jockey for business with hard-edged marketing. These are mostly outside of Canada.

When all is said and done, some men still wonder if they opted for the best or most appropriate option, and some are still bitter with the results of their chosen treatment, mainly as a result of after-effects. So, it's wise to become a partner in the treatment decision from the outset, no matter how much this may feel like an extra load, or an intrusion on your doctor's domain..

Cases in Point

My friend, Romeo, discovered he had prostate cancer in 2001 and, at the time, all he wanted was to get rid of it. He had some other personal problems nagging at him and this was an extra load he didn't want to carry. He put his faith in his urologist, had a bilateral nerve-sparing radical prostatectomy. Then he could not have an erection for three years. Of course, Romeo was not a young man and had personal problems, which could have been contributing factors.

He tried various drugs, to no avail. Then he tried injections, which he found to be a nuisance. Later, he tried a suction pump, which he hated. Finally, he settled for a penile erectile implant. That's the implantation of a gadget in his scrotum and penis. It offers an instant erection just by the squeeze of a little bulb, anytime, anywhere. His continence is 98 percent and his PSA level is steady at less than 0.002 ng/ml.

Romeo does not understand everything that happened, nor does he care. However, he did buy and read a book that offered some information on prostate cancer and surgery. He was lucky. His major concern was living without being able to enjoy sexual intercourse. Some men would have said, "To heck with sexual intercourse, I am healthy otherwise." Others would say "If I cannot have sexual intercourse, I might as well die. The last time I saw Romeo, in December of 2007, he was smiling from ear to ear, as he boasted about his satisfied sex life, and the quality of the rest of his life. He even looked 10 years younger.

Some men tend to put a lot more value on the quality of their sex life than on their actual life. One man of 62, who decided to not accept any of the traditional Western methods of treatment expressed it this way: "I prefer to continue having quality sex and die prematurely. My life itself does not really matter, because I have a relatively substantial fortune, and my wife and grown children will be well taken care of for the rest of their lives." There is a man who lived only to provide for his family! He has resorted to alternative treatment consisting of herbs, vitamins and exercise. His wife is a 52 year old beauty who will most likely attract another husband after he passes away. His three children are 25, 27, and 29 years of age. You figure it out. He could probably extend his life another 10 to 20 years by having traditional treatment, such as surgery or radiation. But he will not go for those treatments, simply because he is not prepared to give up the quality of sex he currently enjoys. The quality of sex that he is referring to is to have a strong elongated erection, coupled with ejaculation, during orgasm. Before you jump to conclusions or decide to be critical of him, you are advised to read up on the after-effects of the various treatments.

When my urologist, based on all the necessary tests, concluded that I had prostate cancer, he gave me his analysis and suggested treatment option. He also sent me for a second bone scan. I will deal with that in a later chapter. I hesitated to act on his suggestion for "fairly prompt" treatment, mostly because I did not understand what I was dealing with. I needed more time to think and to learn. But I will repeat, my cancer was relatively slow growing. Yours may not be so slow growing. So do not delay your decision for too long.

Chapter 17

GRADING THE CANCER

A determined soul will do more with a rusty monkey wrench than a loafer will accomplish with all the tools in a machine shop.

Robert Hughes (1938 –)
Australian Art Critic,
Writer and Documentary Broadcaster

Grade – Aggressiveness

Grading the cancer is determining its aggressiveness or speed of growth. Some cancers grow or spread faster than others.

The grade of the cancer is important because, it correlates with the stage and the PSA reading to determine the overall *prognosis*.

When we talk about "grade" we refer to the difference in the formation or architectural arrangements of clusters of cells within the tissue, *gland* or tumour, and not the individual cells.

Some tissue cells are well formed and arranged, whereas others are less so. The organization and arrangement, based on the shape, size and arrangements, is referred to as *differentiation*. Description of these differentiations ranges from "normal" for the well-formed and non-cancerous cell arrangements, to "abnormal," which denotes cancerous cells. Thus, normal cells differ from abnormal cells by their shape, size and arrangement.

Normal cells are well-formed in tiny tubular shapes, in an orderly structure, and arranged close together.

Abnormal or cancerous cells look irregularly-shaped, distorted, undisciplined, haphazardly arranged and separated away from each other. The more aggressive the cancer, the more irregularly-shaped, distorted, undisciplined, and haphazardly arranged the tissue cells are.

The abnormal or cancerous cells are scored based on the degree of their differentiation or abnormality. The pathologist studies tissue slivers taken in the biopsy and recognizes and grades them, from 1 to 5, according to their degree of abnormality or level of differentiation. Normal, healthy portions are graded "1," while at the other end of the spectrum, very distorted-looking aggressive portions are Graded "5."

The Gleason Grading System

Pathologists have developed various systems for identifying the grades. The most commonly used is the "*Gleason grading system*," named after pathologist, Dr. Donald F. Gleason, who was the first to describe it.

The *"Gleason score"* is the term or unit used to express the aggressiveness of your cancer and has been shown to be one of the most important factors considered in the prognosis prostate cancer. An accurate Gleason score can help to determine the best treatment and even how quickly it's necessary to take action.

When you have cancer, everyone who knows anything about the subject wants to know your Gleason score. Most of those with whom I spoke about my condition, invariably asked me, "What is your Gleason score?" It's not, "What is your grade?" but always "What is your Gleason score?" At first I could not respond! I had no idea what they were talking about. In fact, I have met people who had the surgery and still did not know what their Gleason score was, or even what it meant.

You should know your Gleason score and understand what it means, if for no other reason than the fact that it's an expression of the aggressiveness of your cancer. You may wish, after reading this chapter, to ask your urologist what your Gleason score is. He will tell you. In fact, he may already have told you, but it may not have register in your brain.

The diagrams on the next page are an adaptation of Dr. Gleason's original diagram depicting the five grades.

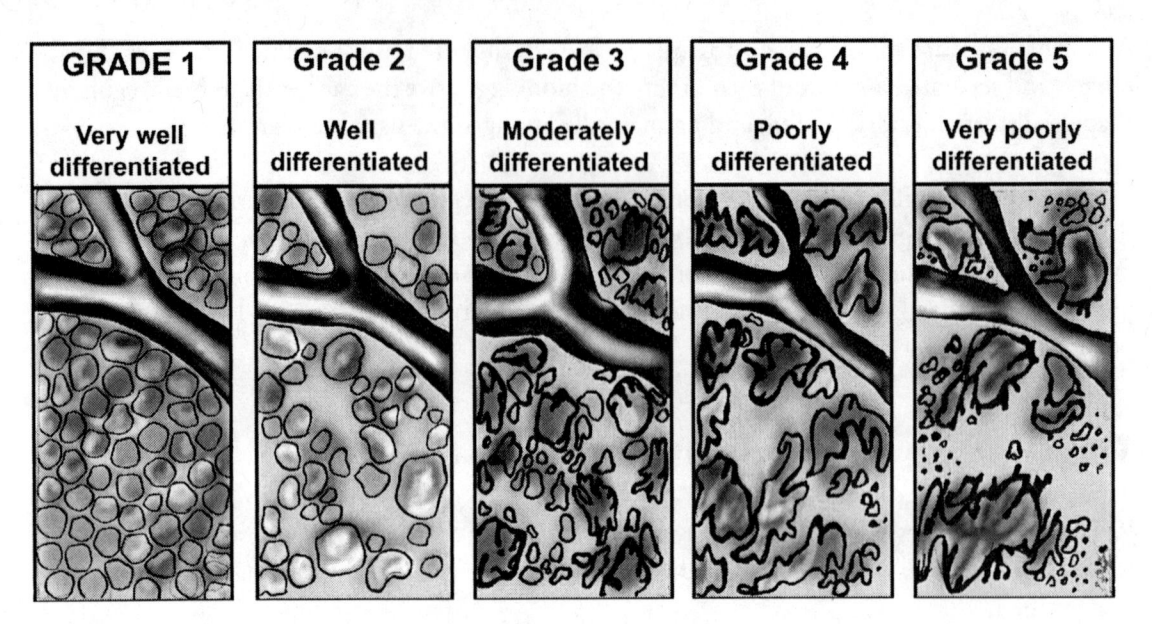

Part III Prostate Cancer Diagnosis

GRADE 1	Grade 2	Grade 3	Grade 4	Grade 5
Very well differentiated	Well differentiated	Moderately differentiated	Poorly differentiated	Very poorly differentiated

Grade 1 is considered very well-differentiated. These cells are small, fairly uniformly shaped, and tightly packed.

Grade 2 is also well-differentiated, but the cells display a more varied and irregular shape that are loosely packed. There may be some cancer cells interspaced between many normal cells.

Grade 3 is moderately-differentiated. These cells are even more irregular in size and shape and more dispersed. Some are fused so that their boundaries are less distinct.

Grade 4 is poorly-differentiated. Many of these cells are fused into irregular masses. Some blend into surrounding connective tissues.

Grade 5 is very poorly-differentiated. Most of these cells consist of irregular masses with no recognizable cellular arrangement.

The Gleason Score

After the pathologist has evaluated the sample, distinguishing the various cell formations, and graded them accordingly, he looks to see which grade is most prevalent. The most prevalent, or dominant, is called the "primary" grade. Then he looks for the second most prevalent grade and assigns it "secondary" status. He then adds the number of the primary grade to the number of the secondary grade to come up with a Gleason score. For example, if the pathologist finds many grade 3s and many 4s, he adds those two most prevalent grades (3 + 4) to get a Gleason score of 7.

If most of the specimen or tissue is composed of only one arrangement, the corresponding grade is considered twice and added as 3 +3 = Gleason score of 6, or 4 + 4 = 8.

The best Gleason score is 2, meaning the cancer is very well-differentiated and the glands normal-looking, that's Grade 1, (1 + 1 = Gleason score of 2). However, we rarely see this. The worst score is 10, indicating an overwhelming number of abnormal or very poorly-differentiated cell structures or Grade 5, (5 + 5 = Gleason score of 10).

As a rule of thumb, a Gleason score between 2 and 4 (low grade), means that your cancer is considered well-differentiated; a score of 5 and 6 (medium grade) means that your cancer is moderately-differentiated; a score of 7 is considered intermediate; and a score of 8 or higher implies that your cancer is poorly-differentiated and that you have a very aggressive cancer.

One should not jump for joy or be too careless in, or hesitant about, making a decision or taking action if their Gleason score was reported to be 6. The score grading can be subjective and there is room for variation or misinterpretation from one grade to the next, even amongst experienced pathologists. It could be a fine line between a score of 6 and 7. A second opinion may cause the cancer to be upgraded or downgraded.

Although pathologists are becoming more uniform in their approach to grading, individuals may differ slightly in their assessments, causing an inaccurate Gleason score.

How Fast is Fast?

Some people also confuse the Gleason score with PSA level. The two obviously aren't related, and each means something distinctly different.

The PSA level will likely increase over time, with untreated prostate cancer. The Gleason score will likely not change with time. Consider the following analogy:

- A cancer with a Gleason score of 2, very well-differentiated, may be represented as a turtle moving ever so slowly.
- A cancer with a score of 4, well-differentiated, may be represented as a horse and buggy, moving somewhat faster than the turtle.
- A cancer with a score of 6, moderately-differentiated, may be represented as a car travelling at 48 kilometres per hour (30 miles per hour), moving faster than the horse and buggy.
- A cancer with a score of 7, intermediate-differentiated, may be represented as a Formula I race car traveling at 160 kilometres per hour (100 miles per hour).
- A cancer with a score of 8, poorly-differentiated, may be considered as being a 737 jet flying at 640 kilometres per hour (400 miles per hour).
- A cancer with a score of 10, very poorly-differentiated, may be considered as being a supersonic jet flying at 1,600 kilometres per hour (1,000 miles per hour).

Thus, the Gleason score tells us how fast the cancer is capable of moving and spreading. A cancer with a score of 10 will progress from point A to B in a very short period of time, and will reach the critical or dangerous stage very quickly. Similarly, a cancer with a Gleason score of 2 will travel so slowly (like a turtle) that it may never get to the danger zone.

Another important concept is that a car (Gleason 6 cancer) does not transform into a supersonic jet (Gleason 10 cancer), even if we wait for some time.

My Case

> At the time of my diagnosis, my cancer was given a Gleason score of 4 (2+2) from my biopsy samples. After my surgery the pathologist's report indicated that my cancer had a Gleason score 6 (3+3), which was determined from my removed prostate gland. I interpreted that to mean that my cancer really had a Gleason score of 6 (3+3) all along.

Sometimes pathologists interpret the cancer cells abnormalities or differentiations from the biopsy samples as one Gleason score, (2+2 = 4), only to find out later, after surgery, from the final pathology that it was a different score, (3+3=6). This could happen as the biopsy samples are taken only from certain tissues. Of course this can raise concern, because, to some extent, how quickly one seeks treatment could depend largely on this initial biopsy information. As illustrated above, a cancer with a Gleason score of 4 is less aggressive than a cancer with a score of 6. Had I known that I had a score of 6, I probably would have been more proactive in making my decision, and making it sooner.

It's important that this information is accurate, because it's heavily relied upon to make some critical decisions and it does not change throughout the life of cancer.

Score versus Grade

Sometimes confusion arises in a patient's mind regarding the terms Gleason score versus grade, (sometimes referred to Gleason scale or pattern). Since the highest grade is 5, when the number 6 or higher is referred to, you can be assured it means Gleason score. When the number is 3 or 4 or 5, you cannot assume it to be either, so it's best to clarify this with your doctor. Make sure that you understand which one is being referred to. (Remember the grade is 1, 2, 3, 4, or 5. The score is X+Y=Z, and could be anywhere from 2 = (1+1) through to 10 = (5+5).

As mentioned earlier, Gleason score is taken from the two most predominant formation and arrangement or grade in the specimen. Thus grade ranges from 1 to 5, whereas score ranges from 2 to 10.

The higher the Gleason score, the more aggressive the cancer will spread. A Gleason score of 8 to 10 can spread pretty fast and very soon, within weeks or months, can metastasize – escape outside the capsule.

Chapter 18

STAGING THE CANCER

God said "Your task: to build a better world,"
And I answered, "How? The world is such a large place, so complicated now;
And I so small and useless am, there's nothing I can do."
But God in His wisdom said, "Just build a better you."

SUCCESS COMES IN CANS NOT CARROTS
AUTHOR: JOEL H. WALDON

Stage – A Matter of Location

Staging cancer means, determining if it's confined within the prostate or if it has penetrated the wall of the gland or capsule and is spreading (metastasizing) to other areas of the body. Staging indicates how far the cancer has progressed. The finding is referred to as the "stage" or "clinical stage" of the cancer.

The stage is important because it's usually correlated with the PSA for the overall prognosis. The stage may also correlate with the grade – a higher grade cancer, one that grows and spreads fast, is more likely to have reached a more advanced stage by the time it's diagnosed, while a lower grade, which grows more slowly, is more likely to be at an earlier stage.

Staging Methods

There are various systems used for staging. Two will be described here:

    a) The Whitmore-Jewett A-B-C system (where Stage 'A' is the earliest stage) and

b) The more universal T-N-M system (where Stage 'T0' is the earliest stage).

Whitmore-Jewett A-B-C Staging

(This is an older system now used less often, although it's used by the National Cancer Institutes):

Stage A – The cancer is causing no symptoms, and can't be felt during the DRE, nor can it be seen with the naked eye. It's often discovered unexpectedly during a resection for obstructive symptoms with BPH, when the pathologist examines the tissue under a microscope. It's classified A1 or A2.

> **Stage A1** – Stage A with microscopic cancer cells, usually low grade, found in one area of the prostate.
>
> **Stage A2** – Stage A with microscopic cancer cells, possibly a higher grade, found in more areas of the prostate.

Stage B – The cancer, which can be felt during a DRE, is confined to the prostate. It's classified as B1 or B2.

> **Stage B1** – The cancer can be felt during a DRE and is confined to one side of the prostate.
>
> **Stage B2** – The cancer can be felt during a DRE and is felt on both sides of the prostate.

Stage C – The cancer has penetrated the walls of the prostate, and is invading nearby tissues, such as the bladder and/or the seminal vesicles.

Stage D – The cancer has spread to the lymph nodes, organs or tissues. It's classified D1 or D2.

> **Stage D1** – The cancer has spread to the lymph nodes, near the prostate.
>
> **Stage D2** – The cancer has spread to the bones, or other parts of the body.

Recurrent – Cancer, treated and thought to have been eliminated, has returned to the prostate or another area of the body.

T-N-M Staging

Primary Tumour (T)

Stage TX – Primary tumour cannot be assessed.

Stage T0 – No evidence of primary tumour.

Stage T1 – Clinically unapparent tumour not palpable nor visible by imaging.

    T1a – Tumour incidental. Found microscopically in 5 percent, or less, of tissue *resected*.

    T1b – Tumour incidental. Found microscopically in more than 5 percent of tissue resected.

    T1c – Tumour identified by needle biopsy, taken because of elevated PSA.

Stage T2 – Tumour confined within prostate.

    T2a – Tumour involves half of a lobe or less.

    T2b – Tumour involves more than half of a lobe but not both lobes.

    T2c – Tumour involves both lobes.

Note: A tumour found in one or both lobes by needle biopsy, but not palpable nor visible by imaging, is classified as T1c.

Stage T3 – Tumour extends beyond the prostate capsule.

    T3a – Extends beyond the capsule on one side (Unilateral extracapsular extension).

    T3b – Extends beyond the capsule on both sides (*Bilateral* extracapsular extension).

    T3c – Tumour extends to the seminal vesicle(s).

Stage T4 – Tumour is fixed or has invaded adjacent structures other than the seminal vesicles.

    T4a – Tumour extends to any of: bladder neck, urethral sphincter muscle, or rectum.

    T4b – Tumour extends to "levator muscles" and/or is fixed to the pelvis wall.

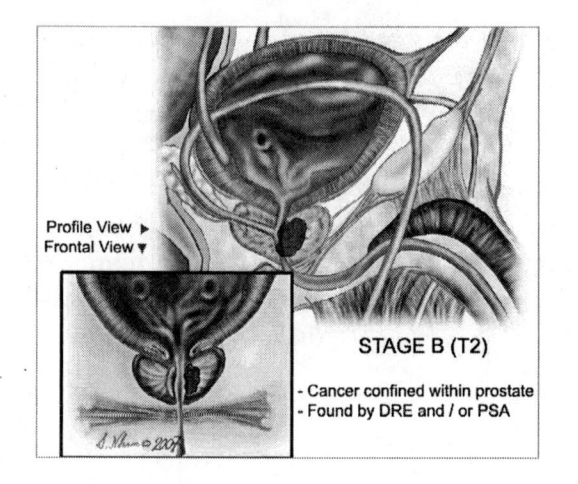

STAGE B (T2)
- Cancer confined within prostate
- Found by DRE and / or PSA

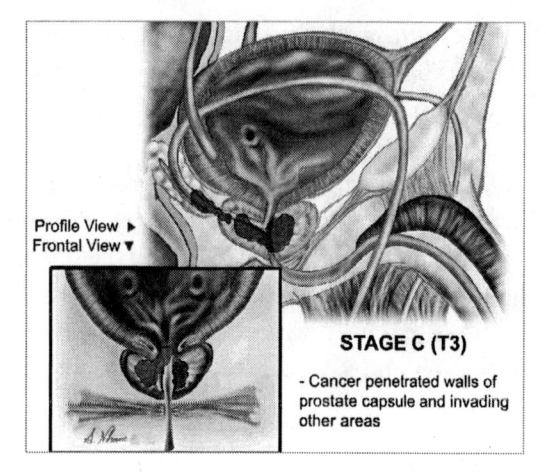

STAGE C (T3)
- Cancer penetrated walls of prostate capsule and invading other areas

Regional Lymph Nodes (N)

Stage NX – Regional lymph nodes cannot or have not been assessed.

Stage N0 – No regional lymph node metastasis.

Stage N1 – Metastasis in a single lymph node, 2 cm or less in greatest dimension.

Stage N2 – Metastasis in a single lymph node, more than 2 cm but not more than 5 cm in greatest dimension, or multiple lymph nodes, metastases, none more than 5 cm in greatest dimension.

Stage N3 – Metastasis in a lymph node more than 5 cm in greatest dimension.

Distant Metastasis (M)

MX – Presence of distant metastasis cannot be assessed.

M0 – No evidence of distant metastasis.

M1 – There is evidence of distant metastasis.

    M1a – Non regional lymph node(s)

    M1b – Bone(s)

    M1c – Other site(s)

Part III   Prostate Cancer Diagnosis

It's important to understand the information regarding the stage of your prostate cancer. It's based on this knowledge presented here, exactly where the cancer is situated in the gland, and whether it has spread (metastasized) – that your urologist can make the best recommendation.

Note: If cancer, resulting from migrated prostate cancer cells, is found in another part of the body, even years later, it's still considered prostate cancer. Often it goes with a certain recognizable pattern of spread. Occasionally, there is uncertainty and a biopsy is needed to confirm its origin. An accelerated PSA will strengthen the suspicion. About a third of men, whose cancerous prostate is removed, will experience recurrence, often years later. See the last chapter for more information on recurrence.

My Case

> Initially, my cancer was staged as T2a (B1). If I was careless in not getting the appropriate treatment, it could easily have progressed to T2b, or T2c, or even beyond.

Most men diagnosed with prostate cancer today fall into stage A, B or T1c, which means that it's confined. Perhaps this is because today, most men are diagnosed while the cancer is at an early stage, due largely to regular (yearly) medical check-up and widespread use of PSA testing.

Chapter 19

BONE SCAN

*One of the most tragic things I know about human nature
is that all of us tend to put off living.
We are all dreaming of some magical rose garden over the horizon –
instead of enjoying the roses blooming outside our windows today.*

DALE CARNEGIE

Preparing to Performing

The bone scan is a radiological process that helps to determine the spread of the cancer.

Your urologist will want to know whether the cancer has spread outside of the prostate gland or capsule to other parts of the body. He gets this knowledge by observing results of a bone scan of your entire body.

Generally, men with low PSA levels or low grade cancers do not need a bone scan, since it's unlikely to be positive and, thus, would not add much information. Your PSA level would have to be about 7 to 10 ng/ml or above, and your Gleason score 7 or above, before a bone scan would be recommended.

In preparing for the bone scan, you will be given an intravenous injection of a radioactive tracer or substance and asked to return in three hours.

During those hours, the radioactive substance will spread through your body and collect in your bone structures, including areas where there may be cancer cells.

On your return, you will remove your clothes, put on a hospital robe, and lie on a table where a radiology technician will guide a massive gamma camera over and around your entire body, slowly and painlessly scanning or taking images of you at various locations and in various positions.

The gamma camera scans your entire body and reveals the whole skeleton, so that areas of increased metabolic activity, called "hot spots" can be seen. These hot spots may be due to an old or new fracture, bone infection, arthritis, or cancer. The scanning is time-consuming and even boring. In fact, I went to sleep during the procedure.

A radiologist later examines the pictures for hot-spots or areas of increased metabolic activity which might suggest the presence of cancer on or in the bones. The radiologist will know which disturbance or activity represents which condition. Occasionally, special X-rays are taken of areas of interest to clarify the situation.

Following the scan, the radioactive substance is automatically eliminated through your urine, so that you do not remain radioactive.

My Case

> My first bone scan was done in August 1995. The only thing that I can remember being told about the images that showed up on the films, was that, "certain signs were indicative of *degenerative disc* disease." That was no surprise to me since I was already aware that I had that condition. Degenerative disc is a deterioration of the disks between the joints of the spinal cord. It has nothing to do with cancer. I've had it for years, but it hardly bothers me at this stage of my life, except sometimes when I am in a tired or depressed state, or when I give up taking my nutritional supplements for a while.
>
> My second bone scan was done in March 1998, soon after I was diagnosed with prostate cancer. The results of that scan were made available to me a few days later. The only thing that I remember about those results was being told, "there was no sign of cancer anywhere outside of my prostate gland." That alone was a relief. If there was any sign of cancer anywhere else, my life would have taken a drastic turn. I really do not know how I would have handled that.

I had a third bone scan in November 1999, at my request, simply because it was so long (almost two years) since I had been diagnosed, and I had taken none of the traditional treatments, except my vitamin and mineral supplements. Again, they found no sign of cancer anywhere else in my body. That does not mean that one or two undetected prostate cancer cells have not migrated to other parts of my body via my blood stream. If they had, then they would probably be stuck somewhere along my spinal cord or on my *pelvic bone*, and will begin to multiply in about seven to eight years after my treatment. It has been known to happen. I hope it does not happen to me.

I did find out from that third scan that I had a minor arthritic problem in my right shoulder and left knee. I did not know of those previously, but I remembered experiencing occasional pains in both areas. I guess my nutritional supplements worked their magic.

Chapter 20

PARTIN PROBABILITY TABLES

Always, that which you most need, is already at hand…
and it's your insistent searching, and belief in its absence, that keeps it from view.
Today you sit on a gold mine … and beneath your feet are acres of diamonds.
Ha! You should see yourself… (as the Universe does).

M. Dooley

Partin Tables – Source for Prediction

Probability tables are models for predicting organ confinement of the prostate cancer, versus the chance of cancer penetration to outside the gland or capsule. These models are designed to help the urologist and other specialists predict the appropriate treatment for specific conditions. We have already identified a simple model in Chapter 13, as utilized by one treatment centre. However, the most popular model among physicians consists of the so-called "Partin Tables," named after one of their developers, Dr. Alan W. Partin, a urologist at Johns Hopkins University in Baltimore, Maryland.

The Partin Tables is a set of probability tables, which, by using their information in correlation with your PSA results, grade (Gleason score) and stage, you and/or your physician can predict the probability of your cancer still being confined within the prostate gland. But let's be clear, it's only a probability.

The Partin Tables consist of coefficients, first developed based on accumulated data from hundreds of patients, by Drs. Partin, J. Yoo, H.B. Carter and others. They were first published in 1993. Four years later they were revised to incorporate data from three major prostate cancer research institutions in the United States, which included treatment of 4,133 patients by radical prostatectomy. The institutions were Johns Hopkins, Baylor School of Medicine in Houston, Texas, and Michigan Prostate Institute in Ann Arbor, Michigan. A revised set of tables was published in May 1997. They are outlined in the succeeding pages of this chapter.

Using the Partin Tables, you and your doctor can make the following predictions about the state of your cancer, and thus reach a reasonable conclusion regarding risks and treatment options:

1. The probability of your cancer being confined (and therefore theoretically *curable*);
2. The probability of your cancer having penetrated the capsule (thus having a somewhat lower chance of a cure);
3. The probability of your cancer having penetrated the walls of the capsule and spread into the seminal vesicles;
4. The probability of your cancer having penetrated and spread into the lymph nodes.

These predictions can have significant impact on what treatment you and your doctor choose.

Example

Let's say you are a 60 year old man who has a PSA level as high as 11.5 ng/ml. There is no family history of prostate cancer, but there is an indication of a problem, based on your DRE. After some discussion, your urologist sends you for an ultrasound-guided prostate biopsy. The biopsy shows indications of malignancy in one lobe of the prostate. The Gleason score is classified by the pathologist as 3 + 3 = 6. The urologist classifies your prostate cancer as clinical stage T2b.

Based on the Partin Tables on the next four pages, particularly the third table, you can make the following predictions about your cancer:

- The probability of you having prostate cancer that's organ-confined (and therefore theoretically curable) condition is 26 percent (actually between 23 percent and 31 percent). In other words, according to this table, there is about 1 chance in 4 that your cancer is confined within the prostate.
- The probability of you having prostate cancer that's established as capsular penetration (therefore a higher risk of positive margins if you were to have surgery, unless the surgeon were to do a wide excision) is 57 percent (actually between 51 percent and 62 percent). In other words, according to this table, there is a 1 chance in 2 that your cancer has already penetrated the wall of the capsule or prostate gland.
- The probability of you having prostate cancer that has spread or invaded into your seminal vesicles is only 7 percent (actually between 5 percent and 10 percent). In other words, there is about 1 chance in 14 that your cancer has spread into your seminal vesicles. **Note:** If it has

Part III   Prostate Cancer Diagnosis

invaded your seminal vesicles, the chance of a cure drops drastically.
- The probability of you having prostate cancer which has spread into your lymph nodes is a mere 10 percent (actually between 7 and 13 percent). In other words, there is a 1 chance in 10 that your cancer has spread through to your lymph nodes and maybe into the rest of your body.

You can conclude that you have a small chance that your prostate cancer is organ-confined, with your greatest risk being that the cancer has established capsular penetration of the gland.

With that information, you are much better armed to decide on an appropriate treatment option that suits your lifestyle.

> Now, review the situation, assuming that you had all the same situation and conditions except that your clinical stage was T1c.
>
> Now, what if your Gleason score was 3+4 = 7?
>
> See the big difference?

Dr. Partin and his colleagues have reported that the use of these tables have resulted in improvements in the number of organ-confined cancers being confirmed at surgery. For example they reported that:
- The number of men who have been diagnosed with organ-confined condition at the time of radical prostatectomy has risen from 33 percent before the tables were used to 55 percent with the use of the tables;
- The number of men diagnosed with positive seminal vesicles or positive lymph nodes decreased from 21 percent before the tables were used to 10 percent with the use of the tables.

Of course, these are based on the fact that, if the Partin tables predict a very high risk of cancer already having spread outside the prostate, that patient is less likely to be undergoing surgery. Thus with improved patient selection, the results are obviously better.

There are other challenges as well. Many people are of the opinion that whereas the tables are very helpful, other factors such as increased use of blood test for PSA level identification, staging, improved technology, have all contributed somewhat to the reported improvements.

Regardless, it appears evident that with the help of the tables, urologists can predict with more confidence, what treatment is more appropriate and what is the likelihood of cure.

Partin Tables (1997 Version)

PSA 0.0-4.0 ng/ml

Gleason Grade	Pathologic Stage	T1a	T1b	T1c	T2a	T2b	T2c	T3a
2-4	Organ-Confined Disease	90 (84-95)	80(72-86)	89 (86-92)	81 (75-86)	72 (65-79)	77(69-83)	-
	Established Capsular Penetration	9(4-15)	19(13-26)	10(7-14)	18(13-23)	25(19-32)	21(14-28)	-
	Seminal Vesicle Involvement	0 (0-2)	1 (0-3)	1 (0-1)	1(0-2)	2(1-5)	2(1-5)	-
	Lymph Node Involvement	0(0-1)	0(0-1)	0(0-1)	0(0-0)	0(0-0)	0(0-1)	-
5	Organ-Confined Disease	82(73-90)	66(57-73)	81(76-84)	68(63-72)	57(50-62)	62(55-69)	40(26-53)
	Established Capsular Penetration	17(9-26)	32(24-40)	18(15-22)	30(26-35)	40(34-46)	34(27-40)	51(38-65)
	Seminal Vesicle Involvement	1(0-3)	2(0-4)	1(1-2)	2(1-3)	3(2-4)	3(2-6)	7(3-14)
	Lymph Node Involvement	0(0-2)	1(0-2)	0(0-0)	1(0-1)	1(0-2)	1(0-2)	2(0-4)
6	Organ-Confined Disease	78(68-88)	61(52-69)	78(74-81)	64(59-68)	52(46-57)	57(51-64)	35(22-48)
	Established Capsular Penetration	19(11-29)	35(27-43)	21(18-25)	34(30-38)	43(38-48)	37(31-43)	53(41-65)
	Seminal Vesicle Involvement	1(0-3)	2(0-4)	1(1-2)	2(1-3)	3(2-4)	4(2-5)	7(4-13)
	Lymph Node Involvement	1(0-7)	2(1-5)	0(0-1)	1(0-1)	2(1-3)	2(1-4)	5(2-9)
7	Organ-Confined Disease	-	43(34-53)	63(58-68)	47(41-52)	34(29-39)	38(32-45)	19(11-29)
	Established Capsular Penetration	-	44(35-54)	31(26-36)	45(40-50)	51(46-57)	45(38-52)	52(40-63)
	Seminal Vesicle Involvement	-	6(1-13)	4(2-7)	6(4-9)	10(6-14)	12(7-17)	19(10-31)
	Lymph Node Involvement	-	6(2-13)	1(1-3)	2(1-4)	5(2-8)	5(2-9)	9(4-17)
8-10	Organ-Confined Disease	-	31(20-43)	52(41-62)	36(27-45)	24(17-32)	27(18-36)	-
	Established Capsular Penetration	-	34(27-44)	34(27-44)	47(38-56)	48(40-57)	42(33-52)	-
	Seminal Vesicle Involvement	-	9(5-16)	9(5-16)	12(7-19)	17(11-25)	21(12-31)	-
	Lymph Node Involvement	-	4(2-7)	4(2-7)	5(2-9)	10(5-17)	10(4-18)	-

Part III Prostate Cancer Diagnosis

PSA 4.1-10.0 ng/ml

Gleason Grade	Pathologic Stage	T1a	T1b	T1c	T2a	T2b	T2c	T3a
2-4	Organ-Confined Disease	84(75-82)	70(60-79)	83(78-88)	71(64-78)	81(52-69)	66(57-74)	43(27-58)
	Established Capsular Penetration	14(7-3)	27(18-37)	15(11-20)	26(19-33)	35(26-43)	29(21-37)	44(30-59)
	Seminal Vesicle Involvement	1(0-4)	2(0-6)	1(0-3)	2(1-5)	4(1-9)	5(1-10)	10(3-23)
	Lymph Node Involvement	0(0-2)	1(0-3)	0(0-1)	0(0-1)	1(0-2)	1(0-2)	1(0-5)
5	Organ-Confined Disease	72(60-85)	53(44-63)	71(67-75)	55(51-60)	43(38-49)	49(42-55)	27(17-39)
	Established Capsular Penetration	25(14-36)	42(32-51)	27(23-30)	41(36-46)	50(45-55)	43(37-50)	57(46-68)
	Seminal Vesicle Involvement	2(0-5)	3(1-7)	2(1-3)	3(2-5)	5(3-8)	6(4-10)	12(6-20)
	Lymph Node Involvement	1(0-5)	2(1-5)	0(0-1)	1(0-1)	2(1-3)	2(1-3)	3(1-7)
6	Organ-Confined Disease	67(55-82)	47(38-57)	67(64-70)	51(47-54)	38(34-43)	43(38-49)	23(14-34)
	Established Capsular Penetration	27(15-39)	44(35-53)	30(27-33)	44(41-48)	52(48-56)	46(40-51)	57(47-67)
	Seminal Vesicle Involvement	2(0-6)	3(1-6)	2(2-3)	3(2-4)	5(4-7)	6(4-9)	11(6-18)
	Lymph Node Involvement	3(0-15)	5(2-11)	1(1-2)	2(1-3)	4(3-6)	4(3-6)	9(5-15)
7	Organ-Confined Disease	49(34-68)	29(21-38)	49(45-54)	33(29-38)	22(18-26)	25(20-30)	11(6-17)
	Established Capsular Penetration	36(20-51)	48(38-60)	40(35-44)	52(48-57)	54(49-59)	48(42-54)	48(37-58)
	Seminal Vesicle Involvement	6(0-19)	9(2-18)	8(5-11)	10(8-13)	15(11-19)	18(13-24)	26(17-36)
	Lymph Node Involvement	8(0-32)	12(5-23)	3(2-5)	4(3-6)	9(6-12)	9(6-13)	15(8-23)
8-10	Organ-Confined Disease	35(18-62)	18(11-28)	37(28-46)	23(16-31)	14(9-19)	15(10-22)	6(3-10)
	Established Capsular Penetration	34(17-58)	42(28-57)	40(33-49)	49(42-57)	46(39-53)	40(31-48)	34(24-46)
	Seminal Vesicle Involvement	10(0-34)	15(4-29)	15(10-22)	19(13-26)	24(17-31)	28(20-37)	35(23-48)
	Lymph Node Involvement	18(0-55)	23(10-43)	8(4-12)	9(5-13)	16(11-24)	17(10-26)	24(13-38)

Clinical Stage

Chapter 20 | Partin Probability Tables

PSA 10.1-20.0 ng/ml

Gleason Grade	Pathologic Stage	T1a	T1b	T1c	T2a	T2b	T2c	T3a
2-4	Organ-Confined Disease	76(65-88)	58(46-69)	75(68-82)	60(52-70)	48(39-58)	53(42-64)	—
	Established Capsular Penetration	20(10-32)	36(26-46)	22(16-29)	35(26-43)	43(34-53)	37(27-47)	—
	Seminal Vesicle Involvement	2(0-7)	4(1-10)	2(1-5)	4(1-8)	7(2-14)	8(2-16)	—
	Lymph Node Involvement	0(0-7)	2(0-8)	0(0-2)	1(0-2)	1(0-5)	1(0-6)	—
5	Organ-Confined Disease	61(47-78)	40(31-50)	60(54-65)	43(38-49)	32(26-37)	36(29-43)	18(10-27)
	Established Capsular Penetration	33(18-47)	50(39-59)	35(30-40)	50(45-56)	57(51-63)	51(43-57)	59(47-69)
	Seminal Vesicle Involvement	3(0-9)	5(1-10)	3(2-5)	5(3-8)	8(5-11)	9(6-15)	15(8-25)
	Lymph Node Involvement	3(0-14)	5(2-11)	1(0-2)	2(1-3)	4(1-7)	4(1-7)	7(3-15)
6	Organ-Confined Disease	—	33(25-42)	55(51-59)	38(34-43)	26(23-31)	31(25-37)	14(8-22)
	Established Capsular Penetration	—	49(38-59)	38(34-42)	52(48-57)	57(51-62)	50(44-57)	54(44-64)
	Seminal Vesicle Involvement	—	4(1-8)	4(3-5)	5(3-7)	7(5-10)	9(6-13)	14(8-21)
	Lymph Node Involvement	—	13(6-24)	3(2-5)	4(3-6)	10(7-13)	10(6-14)	18(10-27)
7	Organ-Confined Disease	33(19-57)	17(11-24)	35(31-40)	22(18-26)	13(11-16)	15(11-19)	6(3-10)
	Established Capsular Penetration	38(18-61)	46(34-60)	45(40-50)	55(50-60)	51(45-57)	45(39-52)	40(30-50)
	Seminal Vesicle Involvement	8(0-28)	11(3-22)	12(8-16)	14(10-19)	14(10-19)	22(16-29)	28(18-39)
	Lymph Node Involvement	18(0-57)	24(10-41)	8(5-11)	9(6-13)	9(6-13)	18(12-25)	26(16-38)
8-10	Organ-Confined Disease	—	9(5-16)	23(16-32)	14(9-19)	7(5-11)	8(5-12)	3(1-5)
	Established Capsular Penetration	—	33(21-51)	40(33-49)	46(38-55)	38(30-47)	33(24-42)	26(17-37)
	Seminal Vesicle Involvement	—	15(4-32)	20(13-28)	22(15-31)	25(18-34)	30(21-40)	34(21-47)
	Lymph Node Involvement	—	40(19-60)	16(10-24)	17(11-25)	29(21-38)	29(19-40)	37(24-52)

Clinical Stage

Part III Prostate Cancer Diagnosis

PSA > 20.0 ng/ml

Gleason Grade	Pathologic Stage	T1a	T1b	T1c	Clinical Stage T2a	T2b	T2c	T3a
2-4	Organ-Confined Disease	-	38(26-52)	58(46-68)	41(31-52)	29(20-40)	-	-
	Established Capsular Penetration	-	47(33-61)	34(24-44)	48(36-56)	52(39-65)	-	-
	Seminal Vesicle Involvement	-	9(1-22)	7(2-15)	10(3-20)	14(4-29)	-	-
	Lymph Node Involvement	-	4(0-17)	1(0-4)	1(0-5)	3(0-11)	-	-
5	Organ-Confined Disease	-	23(15-32)	40(32-49)	26(19-33)	17(12-22)	19(14-26)	8(4-14)
	Established Capsular Penetration	-	57(44-68)	48(40-56)	60(52-68)	61(53-69)	55(46-64)	54(40-67)
	Seminal Vesicle Involvement	-	10(2-21)	9(5-14)	11(6-17)	15(9-23)	19(11-28)	26(14-41)
	Lymph Node Involvement	-	10(3-21)	3(1-6)	3(1-7)	7(3-13)	7(3-13)	11(4-22)
6	Organ-Confined Disease	-	17(11-25)	35(27-42)	22(16-27)	13(10-17)	15(11-20)	6(3-10)
	Established Capsular Penetration	-	51(37-64)	49(43-56)	60(53-66)	57(50-64)	51(43-59)	46(34-58)
	Seminal Vesicle Involvement	-	8(2-17)	8(6-12)	10(7-15)	13(9-19)	17(11-24)	21(13-33)
	Lymph Node Involvement	-	23(10-40)	7(4-11)	8(5-13)	16(11-23)	17(11-25)	26(16-38)
7	Organ-Confined Disease	-	-	18(13-23)	10(7-14)	5(4-8)	6(4-9)	2(1-4)
	Established Capsular Penetration	-	-	46(39-54)	51(44-58)	43(35-50)	37(29-45)	29(19-40)
	Seminal Vesicle Involvement	-	-	22(15-28)	24(17-32)	27(20-34)	32(24-42)	36(25-49)
	Lymph Node Involvement	-	-	14(9-21)	14(9-22)	25(18-33)	25(16-34)	32(20-45)
8-10	Organ-Confined Disease	-	3(2-7)	10(6-16)	5(3-9)	3(2-4)	3(2-5)	1(0-2)
	Established Capsular Penetration	-	24(13-42)	34(27-45)	37(28-48)	28(20-37)	23(16-31)	17(11-26)
	Seminal Vesicle Involvement	-	20(6-43)	31(21-42)	33(22-45)	33(24-45)	38(26-51)	40(25-55)
	Lymph Node Involvement	-	51(25-72)	24(15-36)	24(15-35)	36(25-48)	35(23-48)	42(27-58)

146

Part IV

Managing The Condition

Chapter 21

NO INSTANT DECISION

*What cancer cannot do –
Cancer is so limited, it cannot cripple love, or shatter hope
it cannot corrode faith or kill friendship or stop memories or invade souls.
Cancer cannot silence courage, steal eternal life or conquer the spirit.*

AUTHOR UNKNOWN

Initial Information – May Not Register

After informing me that I had cancer, my urologist outlined various treatment options that are available. He mentioned surgery, external beam radiation, seed implant and watchful waiting. He also told me about some of the after-effects that could result from these treatments.

I confess that very little of that information registered with me at the time. The reasons were three-fold:

1) Having just been informed that I had cancer, I was in no frame of mind to listen to anything else.
2) At that point in time, I really didn't want to think that far ahead – to treatment. I did not even realize what having prostate cancer meant.
3) I was definitely not in an analytic mood to determine what to do next and, truly, everything he was talking about was beyond my comprehension at the time.

The only reason I know my urologist outlined those options, is because, as he spoke, he scribbled some notes and drew some sketches to illustrate what he was talking about. He subsequently gave me those notes and sketches and I kept them.

He also suggested what he considered to be my best option, based on my age (under 70) and general good health. That option was surgery. I subsequently realized that he also suggested, based on the grade, stage and PSA level of my cancer, and the Partin Tables' probability, a successful cure.

Take Time to Understand

As I sat and tried to listen to my urologist, some gnawing doubts came over me. I could not believe I had prostate cancer, that this was happening to me.

I wasn't sure if my urologist expected me to make a decision then and there but, I certainly wasn't ready to do so, partly because I didn't feel that I had the knowledge and understanding I needed and partly because I had no idea what was involved in the treatments, including after-effects.

I knew I needed time to understand. I feel it's important to allow ourselves the time to digest a diagnosis before embarking on serious decision-making, especially of this nature. One should know and understand their options and resulting consequences before making such decisions. However, it's also important to not delay making the decision too long, at the expense of allowing the cancer to grow and spread.

What did I Want?

In my case, I first wanted to understand what this meant to me, how it was going to affect my lifestyle, my future and my family and friends. I wanted to talk to my family and my physician. My urologist encouraged me to return to see him, accompanied by my spouse, for more detailed discussion.

Many family physicians aren't as well informed on these matters as the specialists. That's why they refer us to the specialists in the first place. But I really wanted to chat with someone who could help me find my questions and give me answers, who could afford the time to be patient, empathic and understanding. Yes! I probably wanted to be treated like a child. I wanted to know more about my options. I wanted to fully comprehend the after-effects of potential treatments, to be sure that I was ready to accept and live with them.

I also wanted a second opinion. At that time, my idea of a second opinion was to start all over again, at a different hospital or treatment centre. However, I gathered from my urologist's response that a second opinion was just someone else's interpretation of the same data. He assured me he had the utmost confidence in the radiologist/pathologist who had done my biopsy.

I still wanted to feel more confident – first that I truly had a problem and, second, that I really needed to do something about it. For that I knew I had to research information that was quite foreign to me. The information had to sink into my comprehension. In order for that to happen, I had to read the same material several times, as told by different people in different ways. Only then was I able to comprehend the real seriousness and impact of my condition, and what each of the treatments meant in terms of cure and after-effects.

State of Denial

For a while, I went into what I now consider to be a state of denial. I did not want to deal with the situation. I did not want to believe the diagnosis was true. I did not want to accept the fact that I had to take action, especially regarding treatment choice. After all, of my 13 biopsy samples, only one proved positive, maybe two since one was borderline. Could the diagnosis be wrong? Was it that they were so determined to prove that I had cancer that they found it to be positive? I felt healthy. I had no symptoms. I was therefore in no rush to say "yes," or "do it." I will elaborate on this in a subsequent chapter.

A Gap to Fill

I have spoken to several men, and their spouses, who have been through this experience, and each of them, without exception, admitted that they felt the same way I did. Like me, they felt that a huge gap existed between the initial information offered to them following diagnosis and what they felt they wanted, in order to make an informed treatment decision. That gap, by the way, is not so much a lack of information, as a feeling on the patient's part, that something is missing – that's their understanding of the situation. It stems from the fact that most of us come into this situation not even aware of the location of the prostate or the important role it plays in our reproductive systems. And then, we find out later, that we hardly know or understand the after-effects of the various treatments.

When we become cognizant of their after-effects, our need for additional information increases. It's this that influenced me to write this book, to attempt to fill that gap and help make the decision process easier for others. If I help you, or your partner, become better informed, I have succeeded.

There are people who, understandably, do not care the depth of information I sought. And there are some who seek more. Some just want to have the condition treated. They'll say "Doc, do whatever you think is best." Unfortunately, after the experience, several of them regret acting in such haste.

So, there are many of us who want to understand a little more about what we were dealing with in order to appreciate the decision we had to make about choice of treatment and why we were making those choices.

I believe urologists make an effort to ensure that their patients understand their options and the consequences of their choice. I am not sure all patients understand, or perhaps even care to understand, what they need to know.

Seeking more information is second nature to me. A large part of my work life included researching and collecting information, developing alternatives, then analyzing and evaluating those alternatives, and finally selecting the best choice for implementation. I could not help but feel I should do the same in this situation. After all, when I bought my house I compared it to other houses, and when I bought my car I compared it to other cars, even when I bought my shoes I compared them to other shoes. I felt there had to be more to this prostate cancer treatment decision than met the eyes. There had to be other factors involved, but I had no idea what they were.

This gnawing feeling kept telling me:

"Get more information."
"Get a second opinion."
"Understand what you have."
"Find out what this condition means to you."
"Find out and understand the other available treatments."
"Find out who can best perform those treatments for you."
"Find out what the after-effects are."
"Find out if you can be cured."

I say the same thing to you. If you are uncomfortable with, or uncertain about, the information you've received, seek more. This book may well be all you need, but, if you need more, go find it. There's a wealth of information scattered across the internet, in libraries, and at resource centres. Your doctor can point you in the right direction.

Bear in mind that it may be complicated and confusing. I have summarized it for you, simply, precisely and I hope, in an easy to read format.

Survivors Stories

My training and experience had also taught me that no one person has all the answers. I felt that for a complicated condition like prostate cancer, I needed to hear information and opinion from others. I needed to formulate some questions and get some answers, preferably in layman's terminology. I needed to talk it out with people I could respect, trust, and believe, both experts and those who had been there themselves.

I'd heard of support groups, but I wasn't interested in them. I felt they were based on specific treatments, rather than disease of the prostate in general, and that the members would try to persuade me about the merits of a specific treatment. I was afraid that the support groups would be made up of men who had gone through surgery or radiation, and would try to convince me to do the same. I was wrong. Support groups are made up of men who have experienced various prostate conditions and have gone through treatments, including surgery, radiation and others.

Their experiences, and support in the form of fellowship and understanding, are valuable and helpful.

As word got around that I had prostate cancer, I began to hear from survivors in Canada and the United States, who wanted to share their experiences, although much of what they shared was somewhat negative. What I heard was that many men go through this experience, and even choose a treatment, without fully understanding what they are getting into.

Know the Alternatives

I figured if I was to choose a treatment, I should choose the one which satisfies me best. That had to be done by taking everything into consideration, including my health, quality of life, and desired longevity. First I needed to know the available alternative treatments and their after-effects. My search took me across the continent and I came across a vast array of health care providers and as many approaches to marketing their services.

I discovered that in some U.S. treatment centres specialists might not be open enough to accept a patient's involvement in selecting a treatment. In fact, in many cases American specialists can argue convincingly in favour of their specialty treatment. However, some are still open enough to suggest that another treatment might be just as good or even better.

Understandably, there are biases for one's expertise. After all, these specialists invested years of work to acquire their knowledge. I discovered that many specialists do not really know why another treatment would be better or worse; they only know why theirs is good and possibly best. That made me very uncomfortable.

Despite all this concern, I was determined to look at this in a practical and positive manner and take charge of my situation.

Chapter 21 | No Instant Decision

One doctor I met, each time he diagnoses a prostate condition, particularly cancer, he offers the patient a specific book on the subject to read before he is expected to assist them in making a decision. If your urologist does this, you can assume he wants you to have as much information as you need, to make your decision.

That may be best for some patients, but others may feel overwhelmed with a book, especially when it contains what they perceive as irrelevant information. With that in mind, this book is structured so that readers can bypass areas they prefer to disregard.

I believe it's important that we, the patients, feel comfortable with our treatment choices. For that reason, we may choose to follow one of the following three approaches:

1. Take a very aggressive approach and simply accept our urologist's or radiation oncologist's primary treatment recommendation and have it done quickly; or
2. Take a casual approach, seeking out more information about other options and then make a choice, which may or may not be the recommendation of the specialist; or
3. Do nothing.

People who follow the third approach may die from prostate cancer, or, they may be lucky and die from something else entirely.

Those who take the second, as I did, should not delay too long. I delayed too long. Fortunately, I seem to have been cured, but only time will tell. So far, so good after eight years. But remember my cancer was slow growing.

I was tempted to follow the third approach. I was thinking that I preferred to live a good quality lifestyle, even if life was shortened. I reasoned that treatment would take something away from my manhood and quality of life. I thought that after treatment I would never be enthusiastic, vibrant and full of life again. I believed that I would lose my charm and sex appeal, that I would be reduced to a sad, grouchy, old man, just sitting around, waiting to die. And as I looked at the alternative, I realized the "do nothing approach" could very well take other things from my life, perhaps many years of being a husband, father and grandfather, and inspiration to others.

When I considered my family, I felt that I owed it to them to live as long as possible. It was then that I opted for the second approach, so that I could understand more and make an informed decision.

Subsequently, I went on my search and after almost two years, I became very concerned about the time that had elapsed since my diagnosis. I then did my analysis and evaluation based on my knowledge and information, and opted for my urologist's original recommendation, which was surgery.

Part IV   Managing The Condition

I close this chapter by saying that part of the equation for choosing a treatment is consideration of the after-effects. You must understand clearly what you will be left with or without, what, if any, shortcomings you will have after treatment. I doubt there is a doctor in practice who can explain everything to you, especially the after-effects. I believe that this book comes close to doing so.

Remember, after you are cured, you still have to live with the after-effects. If you aren't aware of those potential limitations, and aren't prepared to accept them, you could be left feeling devastated. At least ensure that you get basic appreciation of what are the potential effects of your treatment. Everyone is different.

Chapter 22

BEHAVIOUR TENDENCIES – "DISC"

We feel our behaviour and adjust it according to our circumstances and environment.

Dr. Robert A. Rohm, Ph.D.
Author of "Positive Personality Profiles"

Why We Behave the Way We Do

One of the personal development workshops offered within my portfolio as a Life Enrichment Coach and Trainer is entitled "Understanding Your Behaviour." In that workshop participants learn to "know themselves better than others know them" and "understand others better than those others understand themselves."

Research in human behaviour shows us that we have predictable patterns of behaviour that we exhibit. According to this premise, every human being exhibits tendencies based on four sets of characteristics. In a given environment, we tend to exercise one of these sets of characteristics more predominantly, although not necessarily consistently, than we exercise the other three. The environment consists of "the people, place, processes and practices." A specific environment forms a portion of the characteristics that influence the behaviour tendencies, which could differ depending on whether you are at work, home, socializing or somewhere else. For example we may behave differently at work than at home, or in a social setting.

Some other characteristics, which influence the behaviour tendencies are whether you are a naturally 'slow-paced laid-back' type of person or 'fast-paced go-getter' type, as well as whether you are 'task-oriented' or 'people-oriented.' Other conditions of influence are how comfortable or intimidated you feel at home, work, or in a social setting. Lastly, ones 'values' or 'standards' also influence the behaviour.

Part IV Managing The Condition

The Four Characteristics

Based on the characteristics mentioned above, each of us tends to behave in a Dominant (D), Influential (I), Steady (S), or Conscientious (C) manner. This is called the DISC system of behaviour tendencies.

In any given environment we exhibit behaviour, to some extent, in each of these four tendencies, but we predominate in one more than the others. We are then considered a 'high' in that tendency.

When the environment changes, such as when something snaps inside of us, maybe because of some stressful news we received, or we have a new arrogant boss, we could change that behaviour instantly.

* **Dominant Characteristics (High 'D'):**

    High 'D' people like to be in charge. They are direct, demanding, determined, decisive, fast-paced, task-oriented and fearless. They thrive on challenges and changes and do not like to waste time with details or facts. They are 'what is the bottom line?' oriented, and 'let us get this over with' types.

    When you **speak** to a 'High D,' you should get straight to the point, and speak assertively and with confidence.

    When you **listen** to them, you should be prepared to hear the bottom line quickly, because they will give you very little details. They expect you to do your own analysis later. You should listen to them with your ears, eyes and mind.

    High 'D' people are marked by a fast-paced approach to work that's task-oriented. Their goal is to shape the environment by overcoming opposition to accomplish results.

    15 percent of the people in the world are High Ds.

* **Influential Characteristics (High 'I'):**

    High 'I' people like to be liked, to influence people to do things. They like challenges and engage in small talk before breaking news or asking favours. They are enthusiastic, influential, inspirational, interactive, fast-paced and people-oriented. They are disorganized, active and positive.

    When you **speak** to a 'High I,' you should be prepared to first establish a positive, friendly relationship, using some small talk.

    When you **listen** to them, you should be prepared to listen to some personal things or current events, before they get to the point. You should listen to them with your heart.

High 'I' people are marked by a fast-paced approach to work that's people-oriented. Their goal is to shape the environment by influencing and persuading others to achieve results.

15 percent of the people in the world are High Is.

* Steadiness Characteristics (High 'S'):

High 'S' people are reliable and predictable. They are slow-paced, people-oriented, submissive, steady, status-quo specialists, shy, composed, fearful, and indecisive. They do not like change. When change is to take place they prefer it in small increments. They listen well then get to work to accomplish a task.

When you **speak** to a 'High S,' you should be empathic, gentle and slow, without giving a massive amount of new information or changes all at once.

When you **listen** to them, you should be empathic, patient and polite.

High 'S' people are marked by a slow-paced and reserved approach to work that's people-oriented and cooperative. Their goal is to shape the environment by cooperating with others to accomplish tasks.

35 percent of the people in the world are High Ss.

* Conscientiousness Characteristics (High 'C')

High 'C' people are methodical. They are cautious, careful, concerned, calculating, slow-paced, task-oriented, fearful, analytical, critical and sensitive. Their approach is opposite to the quick and dirty approach and therefore they always want more information.

When you **speak** to a 'High C,' you should be prepared to give lots of details and reasons.

When you **listen** to them, you should be patient, because they will want to give you a lot of details and reasons.

High 'C' people are marked by a slow-paced approach to work, and a natural desire for perfection that's task-oriented and predictable. Their goal is to shape the environment by working to ensure quality and accuracy in their output.

35 percent of the people in the world are High Cs.

It's important to understand that none of the above characteristics, D, I, S or C, is bad. In all environments, we need different people who predominate in each of these, in order for the world to move on and be a better place. We cannot have everyone predominating in the same set. What is important is that we understand them and recognize them in ourselves and others, so that we can relate to each other better and react appropriately.

Another element that integrates with these characteristics to form our behaviour tendencies is our "**values**" such as, quality of life, life versus death, crime, integrity, morals, and so on.

My Behaviour Tendency

Generally, my predominant characteristics is 'influential' or 'High I,' but during the early days, when I was with my urologist, I felt that I exhibited a 'steady' or 'High S' set of characteristics. I felt that I clammed up, more out of respect for him and, perhaps, due to concerns about taking up his time. However, as soon as I left his environment, I felt that my behaviour immediately switched to being 'conscientious' or 'High C.' I wanted more information, answers to questions such as, "What am I dealing with? What are the treatment options? What are the after-effects? How will any treatment affect my quality of life?" I was not satisfied with what I had heard during the short visit with my urologist and I was not about to make a decision based on what I felt was limited information and understanding on my part. Frankly, I did not really know what else I wanted to know. I think what I needed was a conversation where I could hear the pros and cons. That's where some support groups are quite effective.

My Urologist's Behaviour

On the other hand, I felt that my urologist's behaviour tendency in his doctor/patient environment, or at least with me, could be characterized as Dominant or 'High D.' I suspect that because of my values of humility and respect for his specialist status and tight schedule, I perceived this as 'High D' and shifted my behaviour to one characterized as Steady or 'High S.' I clammed up, became concerned about using too much of his time or irritating him by wanting more understanding or of what he might have considered enough information. So I held back. For example, I once asked him a question that he claimed, to my embarrassment, that he had already addressed. Later, on referencing my notes, I realized that he was right. The problem is that his explanation was given immediately after telling me that I had a malignant tumour. I was hardly hearing him at that time and, in addition, the vocabulary was foreign to me. So each time, immediately after leaving his clinic, I jumped out of a 'High S' into a 'High C' seeking information elsewhere.

Interestingly, based on what other patients have told me, it appears to be a common trait in patient/specialist relationships. I suspect, however, that it's largely a matter of perception on the patient's part. Out of respect for the specialist, and because of their status, the patient probably becomes humble and reluctant to ask questions fearing they may be seen, mistakenly, as questioning.

As time passed, I became more comfortable with my urologist and was pleasantly surprised to find him to be a warm, sensitive, and caring individual.

Words of Advice

To doctors, I assure you, that if I feel this way, more than half of your patients feel the same or worse. Do not misunderstand us. We respect you. We just want you to treat us with empathy, be more patient with us and respect our circumstances. We understand that you're busy, but we would still like you to steer us in a direction that will lead to greater understanding of the condition. Perhaps urologists/radiation oncologists, medical oncologists and other treatment specialists, might consider setting up educational sessions within their clinics for such purpose.

To patients, I hope that this information will help you to be more bold and assertive, and less reluctant to ask questions. When you are in your doctor's office, tell yourself that you need to understand and you are just as important as anyone else and have every right to answers.

Some hospitals and health care centres use a multi-disciplinary team approach, with treatment discussions for unusual or difficult cases. That's good, but what I am referring to here is an educational service for patients.

Above all, go to your doctor with prepared questions, and write down the answers. Your doctor/urologist will not object or deny you the answers. Some of these answers take on new meaning with time, more knowledge and deeper understanding.

Chapter 23

STATE OF DENIAL

By not choosing, you have chosen;
by not deciding, you have decided;
by not acting, you have acted!

HAROLD USHER, P. ENG., DTM
LIFE ENRICHMENT COACH

Did I Really Have Cancer?

Some people say there is a fine line between, 'holding out for hope' and 'being in denial.'

From my perspective, I initially went into a state of denial for about six months. I say that because I was not thinking much about my prostate condition, nor treatment for it. Instead, I occupied my mind with other things. I intentionally chose to be busy doing those things that were part of my busy life. Somewhere in the back of my mind, I found it difficult to admit this was truly happening to me.

Did I really have cancer? I did not feel that I did. I was not feeling any of the symptoms that I expected to experience. That's not unusual for prostate cancer patients. Most do not have troubling symptoms.

This delay – occupying myself with work rather than considering what treatment I would pursue – was bad judgment. I guess I was expecting that one day, I would wake up and find it was just a dream. I was lucky in that I had a slow growing cancer. Most men have a higher grade or faster growing cancer and therefore do not have the luxury of spending time in denial. Frankly, as I look back, I can only think that being in denial was just another cowardly way of deferring a critical health decision.

Based on conversation I've had with several prostate cancer survivors, many who encouraged me to write this book, it's apparent that denial is a common phase. Fortunately, it can be avoided or the time can be shortened. It results from a lack of understanding and knowledge of the prostate, prostate cancer, and the various treatment options. If I were to advise you on it, I would say, "snap out of it."

Need for Assurance

As I mentioned earlier, I had no troubling symptoms nor did I in any way feel unhealthy. So I tried to convince myself that my situation was not critical, that there was no urgency to deal with it, that I had time on my side. That was so dangerously wrong, especially when you consider that my PSA level had risen to 11 ng/ml, my stage was considered a T2a (or B1), and my grade was a Gleason score of 2+2 = 4, which I was ignorant of at the time. That's why I believe we need to understand this information. It's not difficult to understand, it's simply new and somewhat foreign. We need someone to patiently and empathically explain it.

I visited and talked to my family doctor, who was truly patient and empathic. He assured me that I had cancer. I asked him how could he tell and, for the first time, he told me he could feel the lump and hardness.

But I knew I wanted more understanding before I made a treatment decision. My concern began to change. I wondered whether I could afford to delay making the decision while I conducted the necessary research for information that would make me understand. If I could delay the decision, then the question becomes, for how long? That was something I was reluctant to ask my urologist, because I thought he would say "No! you cannot delay." I was not ready to accept that.

Woman Power

Were it not for my wife, who kept pressing me to go to the library and get some information about prostate cancer, I would probably still be walking around with a cancerous prostate inside me. Perhaps by now it would have metastasized.

I went to the cancer treatment centre's library and borrowed books and videos and brought them home. Fortunately for me, my wife viewed the videos and told me about them, because even though I had brought them home, and it was my illness, I made no effort to look at or read them. In fact, she practically sat me down and forced me to look at them.

Part IV   Managing The Condition

What I saw and heard on those videos helped me to begin to think about my life, my children and the consequences of dying unnecessarily and leaving my family behind. I realized that I could avoid that by simply taking some action toward my healing.

Chapter 24

BREAKING THE NEWS

To think too long about doing a thing often becomes its undoing.

EVA YOUNG

I am a member of large family – nine brothers and eight sisters, and thus, of a large extended family. I also have a network of friends and acquaintances throughout North and Central America, the Caribbean and Europe.

Initially I confined the news of my prostate cancer to only a few close friends and family members. In most cases, they had the distinct disadvantage of not having seen me for a while. When I informed them by telephone, some of them thought that I was dying. If they received the news second-hand, it was even worse.

None of the people with whom I associated daily knew of my condition. I never gave them a hint. To them, I was always upbeat and on top of the world and I wanted it kept that way until I decided what treatment I would pursue.

You must decide who you want to tell, and how, when, and where you will break the news. Then do it! Having a prostate problem, and in particular prostate cancer, is nothing to be ashamed of. In fact, I firmly believe that the more I spread the word that I am a prostate cancer survivor the more I am helping people.

My Immediate Family

My first concern was how I would break this information to my wife and three daughters, who were scattered across the country. I wanted to do that gently and, at the same time, assure them I was not dying. I have always made them understand that some day we all die and the chances are that we, the parents, are likely to precede our children. So they ought to be prepared to accept it bravely when it happens. That's the way it's supposed to be.

I think the best decision I made was to keep them informed from the beginning, when I started to visit my urologist. I believe the best time to bring your children into the picture is when you are referred to a specialist. I had also kept them apprised of my condition and test results.

I decided to break the news to my wife in the same casual manner in which my urologist had broken it to me. That was the gentlest way I could think of. It was done while I was driving her home one afternoon. It was done with a simple statement, "One of the samples of my biopsy came back positive."

I did the same in making the announcement to my daughters. My youngest was visiting us from her home in Victoria, British Columbia and while we were sitting around the dining room table one day, I casually broke the news to her. With the other two, I simply said to each of them separately, on the telephone: "I have prostate cancer and I have to make a decision as to the treatment I want to pursue. I will let you know how that decision develops." They accepted it the same way, with empathy and concern, but nobody went berserk.

I convinced each of them that I was alright, and would be thinking about the alternatives before making any treatment decision. I invited their input, questions and expressions of concern at any time. I also advised them that I had some time to think and do some research, and it was not an emergency. Perhaps I also convinced myself of that too much, because I did not jump to action as I now believe I should have done.

Self-Education First

I did not make another appointment with my urologist for three months. In fact, I went to see my family doctor first. He convinced me to go back to the urologist, because he was the best.

Three months after I was diagnosed with the cancer, my wife accompanied me on a visit to my urologist. We agreed it would be best for her to personally hear what he had to say. My wife remembers things much better than I do and she asks more relevant questions about health, than me.

We were so ignorant on this subject that we really did not know what questions to ask. Moreover, we felt the questions we could think of were not those that the urologist wanted to hear. Hindsight tells me we should never make such assumptions. We wanted to know of all alternatives, including the good, bad or indifferent, and their after-effects. Should we seek an alternate approach other than my urologist's recommended surgery?

There is a saying that "a little knowledge is too much." Well, I wanted all the knowledge I could get.

So off I went on a journey of educating myself. Did I learn enough to understand? I certainly did! Most of what I learned is in this book.

The Rest of the Family

With time, I gradually and casually broke the news to other members of my family around the world, as if I was telling them what I had for dinner the previous night. Their reactions were amazingly varied. Despite that, many worried, thinking that I might be dying slowly.

Later that year, I visited my native country of Belize for a family reunion. No one knew that I had been diagnosed with prostate cancer. A few days into my visit, after all the celebrations and parties, I was sitting around a table with some relatives having dinner, when I calmly announced that I had prostate cancer. Everyone immediately looked up in shock with open mouths and eyes for a moment, as if they were gasping for breath. Then they expressed disbelief. They expected that if I had prostate cancer, I would be bed-ridden and dying.

Spreading the Word

Be prepared to hear the news spread and become exaggerated. I told one of my brothers who lives in New Jersey about my condition, and he told a friend. That friend told an acquaintance in California who dropped the word "prostate" as he told others just that I had cancer. People began to tell others across the United States, and some of those people began to believe that I was dying. That rumour spread until someone decided that I was dead. So someone told someone else that I had died of cancer. The rumour spread to Belize that I was dead. You can imagine how my family and in-laws there felt when they heard that I had died. Fortunately, I had kept them informed, so they knew I was actually alive and well.

Part IV   Managing The Condition

Touching Lives

In the process of breaking the news, I convinced several people to go and get medical check-ups. Some of them did. In fact, a couple of them even found that they had prostate cancer themselves, but caught it in time to act on treatment, before it spread.

That, my friend, is what I call "touching lives." I hope to touch many more through this book, and if I touch your life, it would be nice to know.

Chapter 25

CHANGE YOUR LIFESTYLE

Simple choices in one's diet and lifestyle can make a powerful difference in personal health.

DEAN ORMISH, M.D.
CREATOR OF THE BEST-SELLING ORMISH DIET

Attitude Check

One of the more important things to consider doing when you find out you have prostate cancer, or any cancer for that matter, is to have an attitude check-up, and if necessary, an attitude adjustment. Most of us need to do one or the other, or both.

Develop a Positive Mental Attitude

It's definitely advisable that, you develop a positive mental attitude. Read this book from cover to cover, then obtain a copy of the books, **"The Magic of Thinking Big,"** by David Schwartz, Ph.D. and **"Don't Sweat The Small Stuff . . ."** by Richard Carlson, Ph.D. Also, read **"Renewal"** by Timothy J. Smith, M.D. or a similar one on nutrition. Acquire a copy of the audio cassette tapes, **"Psychology of Living LEAN"** by Dr. Denis Waitley, or something similar. These will begin to put you in a better frame of mind to accept what you are experiencing.

In "The Magic of Thinking Big," Dr. David Schwartz helps you develop the power of belief and cure you of "excusitis." You will stop finding excuses for everything.

In "Do not Sweat The Small Stuff…" Dr. Richard Carlson teaches simple ways to keep "little things" from taking over your life, and that everything is "little," when compared to your life.

In "Renewal," Dr. Tim Smith discusses how to rejuvenate your cells, by eating right, taking nutritional supplements and exercising.

In "Psychology of Living LEAN" Dr. Denis Waitley offers you inspiration to help you believe in yourself and realize that "you" can take care of "you."

Together these material will help you realize that nothing in the world is as important as you. It's up to you to take care of you. And you can do it! I call it "self-care."

You may also want to supplement these with regular readings from your guiding religious book.

The Change Starts Now

You need to change and discipline your lifestyle, starting right now. This means drastic changes to attitude, diet, physical activities and lifestyle. However, it's important to understand that meaningful changes come slowly and they must be woven into the fabric of your life.

If you smoke or drink alcohol, give it up. If you love sweets and fats, cut down on the amount you consume. If you love sex, increase doing it. You need to prepare your body and your mind and soul for what is to come. You cannot afford to continue dumping junk into your mental or physical system if you are to fight this condition, regardless of your chosen treatment. You have to change your lifestyle, starting now.

My Case

Like most people it was difficult in the beginning for me to do what I am suggesting. However, when my daughter explained to me how my life and body could change by making some lifestyle changes, I accepted her idea.

When I gave up smoking in 1979, did I find it easy to do? No! But I knew that I wanted to be healthy, and smoking is definitely unhealthy. Based on what I've heard, today's cigarettes are even more unhealthy and addictive than those I used to smoke in the 1970's.

Soon after my prostate cancer diagnosis, I chose to change other aspects of my lifestyle. I had already started taking a more balanced and complete spectrum of nutritional supplements. I simultaneously started reducing my consumption of junk food. That meant less munchies and chips, fewer cookies, less soda, and so on. It was not long before I began to feel the toxins being cleansed from my body. And whereas I used to feel fatigue early in the evenings, I began to feel more energetic longer into the evenings and slept better at nights. My body weight dropped by six pounds in six months.

Later that year, I started on a more formal fitness program with the objective of burning some of the accumulated fat from around my waist and flatten my stomach. The program I chose is a video series directed by Dr. Michael Colgan, internationally recognized for his cutting-edge research on fitness, nutrition and aging, in partnership with Nancy Popp, ESPN's Fitness Pros and Buns of Steel PLATINUM 2000 trainer. It includes exercising regularly, controlling my food intake and taking supplements. Within 13 weeks I lost another 20 pounds and my waist went from a 34 to 31 inches. Each of my weight, waist and stomach have been pretty well the same since.

I met both Dr. Colgan and Nancy Popp personally during my initial introduction to the program, the weight-bearing exercises are done, by following their instructions on the videos, using dumb-bells four days per week, half an hour each time in the privacy of my home. These exercises involve two days on one day off, two days on and two days off. All are done first thing in the mornings, before any food is consumed, in order to burn the fat from my body, rather than burning the energy from consumed food. On day one the exercise is to the chest back and lower abdomen, day two is to the legs and oblique abdomen, day three is to the shoulders and upper abdomen, and day four is to the arms and complete abdomen.

I complement these exercise with occasional walking and aerobics (also directed by Nancy Popp on video) on the off days.

My daily food intake, consists of a balance between high and low glycemic food:

- 180 grams of carbohydrates,
- 108 grams of protein, and
- 36 grams of fat spread over five servings. This is considered a 5:3:1 ratio by weight.

This change in lifestyle worked, and continues to work, for me. However, that does not mean it will work for everyone. There are other plans available. The important message is to eat healthy and be active.

One of the things I did was to reduce and control the amount of sugar, white flour, white rice, fat, red meat and dairy products that I consumed, daily.

I love oatmeal porridge. But I love it only when I can mix it with a substantial amount of condensed milk. Condensed milk is concentrated sugar. When I decided to cut down on my sugar,

Part IV   Managing The Condition

that's where I started. Did I like it? No! But I knew that it was the way I had to go to become healthier. So I learned to live with it and now I enjoy it. I could have chosen to give up oatmeal, but to replace it with what? Something less healthy? After all, I also needed the fibre.

I like rice, especially white rice. Do you know what white rice is? It's simply sugar with all the natural nutrients removed, and no fibre. Is that good for me, or you? Absolutely not! So I decided to switch to whole grain rice which has more fibre. Did I like it? Not at first. But I became accustomed to it over time.

I became especially conscious of fats, and the amount and type I consume, particularly hydrogenated fat, and saturated fat, when I was made aware of what they can do to your body. I like bread, but commercial breads are made of enriched white flour and shortening. Is that good for me, or you? Absolutely not! Ask any diabetic. Do you know what is? Do you know what shortening is?

Enriched white flour is simply sugar with very few nutrients and no fibre. That does tremendous damage, particularly to the colon.

Shortening is hydrogenated fat, oil cooked at a high temperature to chemically alter its structural composition, thereby changing it from a liquid to a more solid state. Hydrogenated fat requires a much higher temperature to melt or liquefy. That's the fat that's assumed to cause cellulite, especially in the legs, and maybe even cancer.

So I changed my bread to those made of whole wheat flour and *unsaturated oil*, or canola oil. Did I like it? Not at first, but it was healthier, and I grew accustomed to it slowly.

I began to incorporated essential Fatty Acids (EFA) – Omega-3 and Omega-6 – plus coenzyme Q10, garlic, more Vitamin E (to a total of 850 IUs daily), as well as grape seed extract with pro-anthocyanadin, into my diet and nutritional supplement program.

If you decide to have surgery and are taking Omega-3, check with your surgeon to find out if you should discontinue since Omega-3 fats may increase bleeding time. In fact, it's advisable to disclose to your urologist everything you are consuming, including vitamin and mineral supplements.

I added saw palmetto, lycopene, and pumpkin seed (for extra zinc) to my spectrum of supplements, in addition to my regular supplements, specifically to help shrink my prostate. Remember I said that these aren't drugs or medicine, they are food supplements!

Note: If you are diagnosed with prostate cancer, check with your urologist before you start taking saw palmetto and zinc (pumpkin seed).

The consumption of liquor was also something I chose to quickly reduce from my bad habits, although I was never a big consumer.

I reduced consumption of dairy foods, as they contain an enormous amount of fat.

I tried to add more fruits and vegetables to my daily diet, although I must admit that I do not do a very good job of it.

I still practice this lifestyle and am still relatively lean. I must admit though, that age is catching up on me, even though people think I am under 50. Most of my exercises, except walking, are done in the confines of my own home with my personal trainer, on video. Now I feel good. I am healthy and never feel bloated or tired.

So, to me and to many others with whom I have spoken, lifestyle changes are essential as a starting point. No matter what treatment choice you opt for, even if you choose to do nothing, you will still need those changes. They will make you feel better, live longer and reduce potential complications. You will also be a happier man with a positive mental attitude. That alone will make a world of difference in tackling the challenges ahead.

Chapter 26

MY SEARCH FOR MORE UNDERSTANDING

Men don't die because of prostate cancer.
They die, rather, because of ignorance –
a lack of knowledge and the ability to
apply that knowledge to their specific disease.

James Lewis, Jr., Ph.D. – Co-Director,
The Education Centre for Prostate Cancer Research
Westbury, New York

Understanding is the Key

Was I ready to go the surgery route and have a piece of my anatomy sliced out and thrown away? Such an important piece? Definitely not! Would you be ready? Probably not!

I decided that I needed to focus on what it is I was looking for in terms of more understanding and available alternatives.

From the beginning, I made a conscious decision that I was not going to let my prostate condition control my life. I had things I wanted to do and I was not going to let this condition stop me. In fact, I was in no hurry to make a decision about treatment. Nor was I ready to take just any treatment without knowing all the options available, and how they would ultimately affect my quality of life.

Chapter 26 | My Search for More Understanding

Unfortunately, information that I needed to provide a clearer understanding was not readily forthcoming. Nobody was voluntarily offering it. Part of the reason was because I did not really know what I wanted, but I also felt that the doctors do not use enough time to communicate with the patients and they did not want their patients to have too much detailed information that might confuse them. If that was the case, perhaps they were of the opinion that we the patients would not understand, having not been trained in the anatomy of the body. Or perhaps they thought too much information was not good for us. Or maybe I just did not ask enough of the right questions in the right tone of voice.

That's one of the concerns that some patients have with the process. I would have liked a process whereby the doctor might diagnose you and refer you to a team of counselors. These would be people with knowledge, patience and empathy, to explain, in detail, what he doesn't have time to explain — the various options that were available, as well as their benefits and after-effects. Little did I know that not all the experts really understand those benefits and after-effects. Fortunately, my urologist does. As I said earlier, he gave me some information, although I did not feel that I had a clear enough understanding to make an informed decision. I was also not ready to take the first recommendation that came my way without first having a better understanding, even if it was from my trusted urologist. I took his recommendation seriously, but as recommendation only. I believe doctors offer their recommendations to help their patients make the appropriate choice. However, in the final analysis, their recommendation carries a significant of weight.

Some people might perceive my concern as my inability to accept, or be satisfied with, a little bit of information. I am not blaming anyone for my concern and insufficient understanding. But, as long as I am not comfortable with my level of understanding, then I do not have enough to base a decision on. And I fully appreciated the information initially given by the urologist is enough for some people. Unfortunately, it was not enough for me.

As I said earlier, I am an analytical person who was trained to consider alternatives and, fortunately, I have a concerned wife who kept encouraging me to go to the library and get more information. So I embarked on this mission. I was not totally absorbed in this adventure at first, but my wife kept reminding me. She helped me realize there were many options for treatment, and I needed to find the one I wanted and choose it.

I decided to examine, in more detail, the various options that came to my attention. I researched, read and analyzed a wealth of information. You can always find additional information, if you are tenacious and look in the right places. But it takes time and patience and, of course, depending on the grade of your cancer, you may not have those luxuries. So be cognizant of the grade of your cancer before you embark on anything that will cause a delay in treatment. It could ultimately cost you your life.

Part IV   Managing The Condition

Don't Procrastinate – Get On With It!

It's worthwhile to spend time weighing options, but it's dangerous to procrastinate, because your cancer might be growing and spreading. If you are going to do research, do it expeditiously. You can also be inundated with reams of information, much of which could be worthless to you and could also be outdated. You need to know how to decipher the information to determine what is appropriate, valuable and current.

Taking time to do research caused me to delay my treatment decision. That was a dangerous risk. I did it and I have seen others do it. I was lucky, but some others were not so lucky. Their cancer spread in the interim. That's one of the reasons I am telling you what I learned, in order to save you some time.

I started my search by visiting the library at the cancer centre here in my home city of London, Ontario, Canada, where I live. The people there were very empathic and helpful. Even though I never told them of my condition, I could hear the empathy in their voices. I borrowed several videos and books on prostate cancer. The videos consisted of mostly interviews and offered some valuable insights.

An inspiring video entitled, "Two Men and Prostate Cancer," tells the story of U.S. General, Norman Schwartzkoph, and Canadian broadcaster, David Crichton. One took the bull by the horn and opted for prostate cancer surgery immediately, while the other initially went into a state of denial, then opted for surgery.

I learned of various prominent public and political figures and entertainment personalities who had experienced prostate cancer, had surgery and went on to enjoy a healthy life, people such as comedian Jerry Lewis, Senator Bob Dole (it impressed me that he had his surgery before he campaigned for the U.S. Presidency in 1996 – he looked so healthy), CNN Crossfire's Robert Novak, actor Sidney Poiter, U.S. Secretary of State Colin Powell, former leader of the Canadian Alliance party, Preston Manning, former Canadian federal health minister, Allan Rock, to name a few.

I also learned that prostate cancer killed Nobel Peace Prize recipient and scientist Linus Pauling at age 93, actor Telly Savalas and musician Frank Zappa.

Then, while I was doing my research, several prominently people died as a result of prostate cancer. For example, 1960's Black activist Stokely Carmichael, died at age 57 in 1998; Idi Amin, former President of Uganda, died at age 82 in 1999; a former Premier of The Bahamas, Sir Lyndon Pindling, died at the age of 70 in 2000; former Canadian Prime Minister, Pierre Elliot Trudeau, died at the age of 82 in 2000; the originator of TV game shows and famous entrepreneur, Merv Griffin, dies at age 82 in 2007. We also heard of others who suffered from the condition but died from other causes, such as singer (Godfather of Soul) James Brown, who died of pneumonia at the end of 2006.

I read an account of extensive research carried out by the CEO of Intel Corporation, Andrew Grove, which led to his decision to opt for *high dose rate radiation* treatment (a form of seed-implant therapy or *brachytherapy*, which I will explain in chapter 32), at a medical centre in Seattle, Washington.

I spoke with other people who had the same treatment as Andrew Grove and discovered this was an increasingly popular treatment in the United States. It has since become an established treatment in Canada.

When I investigated the possibility of brachytherapy – using the radioactive substance "Iodine125" – for myself, I was informed that the qualification is based on general health, age, PSA, the grade and stage of the cancer, and the size of the prostate gland. You must also be able to medically withstand an anaesthetic. Your PSA level must be under 10 ng/ml, Gleason score no greater than 6, and your stage a T1 or T2. You should also check to ensure that insurance will cover this treatment, or any treatment for that matter, as they are very expensive.

I read of several cancer survivors who had sought non-traditional methods of treatment. Chief among them is Larry Clapp, author, attorney, corporate CEO and co-founder of the Bank of Honolulu, and more than 20 years prostate cancer survivor. His extraordinary adventure in treating himself, using his own personal healing plan consisted of cleansing, nutritional healing, pH balancing and other intriguing approaches to rid himself of his prostate cancer in 90 days without drugs or surgery. I do not doubt his story, although it obviously took a tremendous amount of faith and discipline. I am confident that with the right state of mind, anything can be accomplished and no doubt about it, Larry Clapp had the right state of mind. However, this was a single person's account, and as plausible as it appears, it may not be widely applicable to others, although he is teaching it to others. He has authored several books on the subject.

I read material by Dr. Michael Colgan of The Colgan Institute, including his nutritional supplementation recommendations. Dr. Colgan believes strongly in nutrition for prostate treatment and has developed a specific formula to nurture the prostate. His formula contains a large quantity of vitamins and minerals. I do not get the feeling that he advocates that he can cure prostate cancer, but I do believe that his formula can nurture the prostate, rid the body of free radicals, and help with BPH. My only concerned would be related to the uncertainty, given the many months required for the formula to take effect, and the financial cost.

A booklet entitled "Prostate Cancer: A Booklet for Patients," developed by the Canadian Prostate Cancer Network in 2003, provides some really good educational introductory information.

Part IV   Managing The Condition

The Naturopathic Route

Soon I was being introduced to a few alternative treatments. Unfortunately, they were costly, some in the vicinity of thousands of dollars, just for consultation. For example, I started one consultation that was costing $250 U.S. per half hour monthly. Another required extremely expensive products and analysis that I could not envision curing me, as was promised by the supplier. Not to mention that I could not afford them, and they were not covered by my insurance. Cost and insurance coverage are factors that certainly form a part of the equation. For some people, money is not an issue, but for many, it is. More importantly, I could not find any positive evidence to support the effectiveness of any of these treatments.

I was gaining knowledge, but I was not hearing what I really needed to make me understand more.

I decided to try the services of a naturopathic doctor. The one I chose was very reputable, judging by references I received of him. He undoubtedly knew his work and could probably cure me as he said he would, but it appeared to be a long process and I soon lost faith in it. Part of the reason for my loss of faith, was that I did not understand what he was doing to me and giving me to consume. I also understand very well that you have to allow an appropriate time for a therapy to take its course – perhaps I didn't. But time spent fiddling around with what I ultimately began to believe was a lengthy and uncertain procedure, when I had cancer eating away at my prostate, could cost me my life.

When I first visited the naturopathic doctor, I told him my medical diagnosis was prostate cancer. Surprisingly, he did not examine me. I was not asked about my PSA level, my stage, grade or Gleason score, if the tumour was contained, or any such information. From my perspective, he had no idea of the state of my condition. It's almost as if he did not consider this to be cancer. He chatted with me and then told me that he was going to recommend some nutritional supplements and shark cartilage. I asked him about the supplements, since I did not want to abandon or change the vitamin and mineral supplements I was already taking. He suggested that I bring in my supplements so that he could test them and satisfy himself that they were of sufficient standard and quality. I took them in, and they were tested, and in fact, surpassed his set standards. Neither he nor his staff, ever mentioned taking nutritional supplements to me again.

I visited this doctor office once per month for five months. Each time, I paid a hefty fee and bought a large jar of very expensive shark cartilage and other products that he prescribed, some which were unfamiliar. Some of the products were like supposedly medicinal, provided in small dark bottles with a dropper insert to take by the drops. All the prescribed products were purchased from his supply. When I suggested that I could purchase the products at the health food store, his staff informed me that they were not of the same quality. Their selling price was about

Chapter 26 | My Search for More Understanding

20 percent more expensive than what I would have paid at the health food stores. He justified that difference by saying that their products were of superior quality.

My concern began to materialize when the doctor insisted that I purchase all his prescribed products from his supply. I wondered how ethical that was. I consoled myself with the consideration that he purchased the best so that his patients could have the best. But considering that none of these costs were covered by my insurance, I could hardly afford them. And I had no idea how long this would continue. When I sought an answer to that question, I was told, "until you are cured."

My concern was increased later when I realized that the doctor never personally attended to me after my initial visit. After the initial consultation, I was seen by therapist, which I suspected was the normal routine. On each of these visits, the therapist conducted tests on me, using, a "Electrodermal Screening" (EDS) device. This is an instrument that produces a tiny electrical current – too small to be detected by the human sense.

The EDS device (instrument) was made up of:

- A computer with a terminal and a printer.
- An electronic board, with various mechanisms to adjust different requirements, connected to the computer.
- A pen-like probe (sensor rod) which was a thin metal rod with a cone-shaped rounded tip at one end, and the other end inserted into a plastic bar similar to that of a screw driver handle. This was connected to the electronic board, by a long, flexible, plastic covered wire.
- A hand-held conductor (short cylindrical, heavy metal weight) covered with a canvas cloth. This was connected to the opposite end of the electronic board, by wire.

When the hand-held conductor, which was covered by the wet canvas material is held in the palm of the patient's hand and the pen-like probe touches the body, a complete electrical circuit was created. It's designed to produce an energetic blueprint of the patient's body/organ system and environmental sensitivities in order to supposedly help establish wellness and balance for a healthy quality of life.

The therapist conducted tests on me by pressing the rounded tip of the pen-like probe to the inner edge of each of my fingers and toes just above the first joints. These were the parts of my fingers and toes that had no flesh or fat but rather just skin and bones. She told me that by doing this, she was observing various "feelings" or "energy levels." In doing this she would moisten the canvas cloth on the hand-held conductor and ask me to hold firmly in the palm of one hand. I would squeeze it tightly while she applied the pressure of the probe against the side of my fingers and toes. Each time she applied the pressure, it hurt and simultaneously a beeping sound would go off on the electronic board and a new graph and reading would appear on the computer screen and print out on the printer. She said that these graphs and readings were indi-

Part IV   Managing The Condition

cating levels of various feelings or energy inside me. When I looked on the print out, there were numbers related to various organs, tissues and systems, such as the lymphatic, intestines, heart, joints and others, plus conditions such as allergies, and others that I could not comprehend.

I assumed she was accumulating information to create a health profile so that appropriate treatment can be determined. I was never told.

The therapist would review these readings, tore the printed paper off the printer, then disappeared for a few minutes. I believe that she went to consult with the naturopathic doctor. She would then return with a prescription for a special medication to be filled from their own supply.

Generally, the prescription consisted of the liquid (what I understand to be special Naturopathic medicine) in the small dark bottle, which I mentioned before and which would indicate that it was sensitive to light. The recommended dose would be anywhere from one drop, up to 25 drops, three times per day, depending on which medicine and for what purpose. I asked how these medications were linked to curing my prostate cancer, but never received a clear explanation. They did tell me that I would be cured and that I had to believe that I would be cured. These medicines were in addition to the shark cartilage and other items prescribed by the naturopathic doctor on a regular basis, including psyllium powder, capriol oil, and bentonite to cleanse my intestines, and of course my vitamin and mineral supplements. None of these were covered by my insurance.

My decision to terminate my visits to the naturopathic doctor came five months after I started visiting him. At that time, there was an apparent abnormal reading registering on the terminal, resulting from one of the applied pressures. The technician became concerned about the reading and asked me if I was worried about something. I was not initially aware that I was worried about anything, then it dawned on me that I did have some concerns. It was a day after I had visited my urologist who had chastised me for not taking some positive steps regarding treatment. He was not aware that I was seeing the naturopathic doctor, although he was aware that I was taking vitamin and mineral supplements.

I mentioned to the assistant that I had been to see my urologist the previous day, and that he was very concerned that I was not taking action regarding treatment. I told her that I felt badly that he was concerned about this. For some reason beyond my comprehension, the technician appeared to act in a strange, confused and nervous manner. She did not set up another appointment as she usually did, which I found unusual. Instead, she told me that when I felt that I wanted another appointment I should call. I sensed some kind of paranoia in her behaviour. I left that office trying to figure out the reason for her behaviour, but could not. I never returned, and they never contacted me. Needless to say, I was disappointed.

Alternative Medicine Options

There are several other non-traditional alternative options for the treatment of prostate cancer; however, few, if any, traditional health care professionals from the Western world will tell you about them. In fact, most of them do not know and do not want to know much about them. That may be simply because they do not believe in non-traditional options, and do not want to waste their time hearing about them. For them the traditional options are the only proven way to treat a patient.

Well, I found out that there are many other ways. However, they are expensive, require discipline, and aren't well publicized, recognized or accepted by the medical profession in North America, mostly because they aren't scientifically proven. If you decide on using any of them, you will have to be prepared to take the risk on your own, and probably drastically alter your lifestyle.

I also believe that what will work for one person may not necessarily work for another. No two people do exactly the same thing when they are using non-traditional treatments, unless they are under the care of a specialist in that treatment. And no two prostate cancer conditions are the same.

Decision Time

You can make the experience much more economical and far less frustrating by just dealing with your urologist or radiation oncologist and accepting their advice. They are well trained and I firmly believe that, by and large, they make recommendations in the best interests of the patient. The big consideration is that in the Canadian medical system, which does not operate on a free enterprise system, specialists do not jockey for business, whereas in the more free enterprise system as exists in the United States, they apparently do so. So, one has to be aware of this in their quest for information. Read the literature (sales pitch) with this in mind.

When I was introduced to Dr. S. Larry Goldenberg's book, "Prostate Cancer," and read it, I knew that it was time to make a decision. I made an appointment with my urologist who had expressed concern that I was delaying action. But before I get there, let me tell you in the next few chapters about the various available options for treatment that I encountered.

If your urologist/radiation oncologist expresses concern that you aren't taking action regarding therapy, be grateful that he does so. He is probably concerned because of your lack of treatment, and/or that you may be following a treatment that has no sound scientific basis. His concern would stem from the belief that you may be doing more harm than good to yourself. He has a right to be so concerned, because after all, you are his patient, and to an extent his responsibility.

Chapter 27

WHAT THE WOMAN IN YOUR LIFE CAN DO TO HELP

*"When we learn to say a deep, passionate yes to the things that really matter...
then peace begins to settle onto our lives like golden sunlight sifting to a forest floor."*

THOMAS KINKADE

At the beginning of this book, I stated that it's written for men, and women who have men in their lives. There are several reasons for this, but most significant is that, in our society, women tend to be more concerned about personal and family health than do men, including that of their children, parents and partners. Women do not see their bodies as invincible, as men often do, and women aren't as reluctant to admit to health problems.

Women become involved in men's health for several reasons, including the fact that they are:

- Accustomed to making the healthcare decisions for family members;
- Committed to reading, learning and knowing more about health and the healthcare system;
- Affected by their men's health, sexual pleasures and displeasures, and ultimately their quality of life.

When it comes to prostate disorders, women are faced with their own challenges, arising from the fact that they care for their men and know they are suffering – physically, mentally, socially and emotionally.

The partners of men, suffering from erectile dysfunction, incontinence, or reduced erection size, suffer too, losing not only intimacy but, sometimes, self-esteem. In some cases, those partners may even assume that they have become unappealing.

Women generally want to help their men live longer and better quality lives. Following are some recommendations of things they can do to help accomplish this. These recommendations adapted from several sources, particularly the Male Health Centre in Dallas, Texas, are sprinkled with some of my personal experiences, as well as those of other families of prostate cancer survivors.

Understand your man's mentality regarding health, and check-ups!

Before you can help your partner, you need to learn about his particular health concerns, his feelings of fear and embarrassment regarding the condition and particularly his manhood, as well as his attitude. Educate yourself about his health problems. This book can be a start in that direction.

Create an atmosphere for your man to want to share his feelings!

From an early age, males are taught to "take it like a man." The messages from society and the media are strong, but you can help to change that mentality. Tell him that it's okay to show emotion, to cry, to touch, and to talk about his problems.

Talk about it together! Encourage him to talk!

Many men have trouble telling a doctor or their female partner about a health symptom or problem.

For example, one day I went outside and shoveled the snow off my driveway. It was fresh, wet, soggy and therefore heavy. In the process I dislodged my spine. I was out of commission for several days. I even felt sick. When my wife asked me where it hurt, I was hard pressed to tell her exactly where it hurt. To me it felt as if "it was hurting all over my body." I could not express what was happening with my own body.

When a man with whom I am acquainted, recognized that there was a relatively long delay before his urine began to flow, he chalked it up to "old age." By the time his wife learned of his dilemma his bladder was already damaged. He required major surgery to correct the situation.

Talk to your man about how he is doing and help him to talk to you. Remember as he passes the age of 50 he becomes vulnerable to prostate disorders.

Share your understanding of male health problems!

As his partner, you can talk with your man about his health, share printed information or the telephone number of a health or support group hot line. In many instances your man may need to be encouraged, or prodded, to pay attention to his health and to take action, even for a regular medical check-up – you can do that.

Recognize symptoms that indicate the need for medical attention!

When a red light signal appears in a man's car, he will probably quickly take it in for service. However, when a similar warning sign goes off in his body, he may well ignore it. You, the woman in his life, may better recognize what those warning signs are and can encourage him to have them checked out immediately.

A man used to get up at nights to urinate. According to his wife, he would spend more than 15 minutes each time. When she asked him why he took so long in the bathroom, his response was: "Old age is catching up on me." His wife took him to the doctor where he was diagnosed with BPH.

Chapter 6 of this book identifies several symptoms associated with an abnormal prostate gland. Observe your man's actions and behaviour and question him. Remember however that prostate cancer may not present any symptoms.

Know when your man is due to have his medical check-up!

While most men know the maintenance schedule for their cars, or when to cut the grass, few know how often they should visit the doctor for a check-up. Many men do not even know where their prostate is located, or what's its function. Many men I encountered were not aware of these functions until I told them. One likened removing his prostate to removing his appendix – he was so wrong. Some men don't even know about the DRE, and many who do, refuse to have their doctor perform it as part of their check-up. Know that your man should have a medical check-up yearly after he turns 40. Insist that a Digital Rectal Examination is performed each time.

Encourage your man to write a list of questions for the doctor!

It's said that the average woman asks four questions during a doctor's visit, whereas the average man asks one. Most doctors can tell when a woman has helped a man prepare for a visit, because he comes prepared with a list of questions. I recently helped an acquaintance prepare some questions before he visited his urologist to receive the result of a biopsy. His urologist was very impressed that he came prepared with those questions. Men, or women for that matter, should not be reluctant to prepare for a visit to the doctor.

Men tell me that when they arrive in their urologist's office they totally forget the questions they wanted to ask. Write them down in advance. They don't have to be many – three to six are sufficient.

When it comes to prostate disorders, check Chapter 6 to determine if you can relate to any of those symptoms and report them to your doctor. Turn to Chapter 10 for examples of some questions you may want to ask your doctor during the testing and diagnostic process.

Accompany your man to the doctor and help him prepare questions!

Most men prefer to handle daily chores, such as dealing with the carpenter, the furnace maintenance man or even the service man at the garage; however, when it comes to dealing with the family physician or any health specialist, they are more reluctant to take charge. Women, on the other hand, deal with physicians as if it's second nature to them. Women visit doctors far more frequently than men do, if not for themselves, for their children or parents. They develop a much closer affinity with doctors. So they can help their man get the most from visits to the doctor. They can especially help with those special visits when something is wrong and treatment is required.

Today's brief office visits, multiple treatment options, and improved diagnostic procedures, have made it crucial that patients ask questions, identify symptoms, ask for tests, be able to answer their doctors' questions, and offer insight that can help with diagnosis and treatment. Men tend to be very passive in these areas. Women are more proactive. These passive approaches to healthcare by men create one-way communication, and sometimes result in incomplete or wrong diagnoses, or misunderstanding by patient and physician. Women can help their men to be more proactive by taking the bull by the horn and helping the men prepare for that visit to the doctor.

Part IV   Managing The Condition

Encourage your man to keep track of his visits to the doctor!

Encourage your man to keep a health diary for tracking check-ups, doctor's recommendations, tests and results. In the case of urological or prostate problems, he may want to record his length of time of incontinence, erections or dysfunction and how long the erections last and length of the erected penis. While he is in the record keeping state of mind, it would not hurt for him to keep records of his medications, treatments, appointments, new or troubling symptoms, side-effects, and questions and concerns that may materialize. Women are more conscientious about this, but be assured these records are very useful. Remember, you both have to live with the condition. I used to review my information many times when I was sitting alone at home, particularly my PSA readings. You can help your man start and maintain his health diary. Some health centres give patients passport type books for this purpose. Ask for one!

Encourage your man to compile his family health history!

In addition to keeping track of visits, a compilation of family health history can be helpful. Encourage your man to do this. Get him to record his parents health experiences and don't hesitate to ask the parents about this yourself, especially if he is reluctant to do so. Researchers are discovering many links between genetics and disease. They are urging people to compile a history of the diseases that run in the family so that preventative measures can be taken.

Most people aren't aware of how old their grandparents were when they died, or what caused the death of other family members. Did your man's dad have prostate problems? I found out that my father died from an aneurysm, as did my eldest brother. I found out that my mother's brother, his two sons and daughter each had diabetes, all discovered late in life. I found out that one of my older brothers and two of my older sisters suffered from angina and later other heart problems, and so did I.

Compiling a family health history will help your man and his doctor identify his health priorities. Do not wait until it's too late. Do it now. If his brother or father had prostate cancer, he is twice as likely to have it himself. If both his brother and his father had prostate cancer, he is four times more likely to have it.

Talk with other women whose men have similar problems!

If your man has a certain problem, help him find others with the same problem, with whom he will talk. Talking with another man, and his spouse, who share the same problem, has a positive impact. Find out how male problems affect other women, and what they have done or not done about them. Possible sources for such contacts are support groups, often found through health organizations. The physician or urologist may also be able to contact other male patients to see if they and their partner might be willing to help out. Give your man this book to read.

Partner with your man to work on a shared solution!

Most man's problems aren't just the man's problems. Many spill over to the woman in their lives. Most urological problems do spill over, so they are dual problems. For example, erectile dysfunction, or other sexual dysfunctions, or incontinence are male problems that can be most effectively dealt with when the man and his partner talk about them, experiment together, or visit the urologist together.

Talking together can be of great benefit. This is especially so when cancer is involved. It has been observed that men whose partners are actively involved with their healthcare tend to be more optimistic and confident, develop a sense of balance and well-being and recover more rapidly. I believe that I am living proof of that. My discussions with other couples have led me to believe that this is more widely the case than we may want to recognize. The woman is stronger in times like these.

Be your man's caregiver without becoming stressed out yourself!

If your man develops a serious, long-term illness, you, may become the primary caregiver. You need to know how you can help him, and also how to take care of yourself during this stressful time. Men are like babies when they become ill and sometimes all they need is your presence and assurance that you won't leave them alone. Seek help as you need it, from family, friends, professionals and support groups.

Lifestyle changes in diet, nutrition and exercise are often longer lasting when a couple adopts them together. That's the way it happened in my household. I had to depend on the inspiration and persuasion from my wife and daughter to eat right, add nutritional supplementation, exercise and to eliminate or reduce the harmful items from my diet, such as sugar and fat. They became my partners. If you do most of the shopping and cooking, you can change and manage what your man eats at home; however, be cognizant of the fact that it may take some time for him to become accustomed to new tastes. Read the first section of this book to learn more about nutritional suggestions.

Be creative in love-making and proactive in seeking help!

After submitting to prostate cancer treatment, your man is not exactly the same – neither mentally, physically or emotionally. He may not want to admit it, but it's a fact. How he copes will depend on his attitude and yours. If he had surgery, his penis and his stomach have gone through considerable abuse, as a result of the treatment and perhaps the anaesthetic. He may even be experiencing some level of incontinence. He may have difficulty developing an erection. In fact he may not be able to have an erection at all. It's not because he lost his love or desire for you. He has a lot of that. However, he may be incapable of penetration during sexual intercourse, although, he can still give and have an orgasm. In fact, his libido may be stronger than ever. He may discover that his erected penis is smaller than it used to be. He needs every assurance and encouragement to make the best of these situations and to give whatever he can give, and receive whatever he can receive from you.

The one person who can help him most is you, the woman in his life. Be creative for both of you. A close personal relationship, including a sexual relationship, can be maintained without having an erection. You can learn to stimulate each other with hugging and petting techniques, as you did when you first fell in love. Oral sex is a common technique that's sometimes conducted very successfully with good effect and enjoyment, sometimes culminating in a bursting orgasm or climax for each party, even if not simultaneously.

Ultimately, both of you may be quite satisfied to give up this aspect of life and live a life of celibacy.

Listen to your man!

Above all, listen! The following simple rules for good listening will help you to do that just right:

- Talk less and listen more – you cannot listen if you are talking.
- Put him at ease – help him feel that he's free to talk.
- Show him that you want to listen by giving him your full attention and listening to understand, rather than to reply.
- Remove distractions. Do not doodle or fiddle around with things when you should be listening.
- Empathize. Try to put yourself in his situation, so you can see his point of view.
- Be patient, allow plenty of time and do not interrupt.
- Control your emotions. An emotional or angry person gets the wrong meaning from words.
- Go easy on argument and criticism. He may clam up or get angry.

- Ask questions. This is encouraging and shows that you are listening.
- Talk less and listen more – you just cannot do a good listening job, while you are talking.

Accept the final breath – Death!

The chances are that one day you will be left alone. Statistics shows that women outlive their spouses, on average by about seven years. Many men, as do many women, practice unhealthy living in their younger days that affect them adversely as they grow older. For example smoking, unhealthy eating, poor diet, consuming large amounts of saturated and hydrogenated fat, inhaling of pesticides and dioxins, lack of exercise, and no regular medical check-ups. The result may be early death, or long drawn out suffering – or as Dr. Walter Bortz II and Dr. Myron Wentz put it, "they live short and die long." Be prepared to accept his shorter life, if it happens, and move on with yours.

Part V

Treatment Options

Chapter 28

OPTIONS FOR PROSTATE CANCER TREATMENT

"All men and their families must be informed of all of their treatment options, not just those that special interest groups may want them to know about, and to understand their respective expected risks and benefits."

RICHARD J. ABLIN, PH.D.

No Easy Answer

There are several treatment options available for prostate cancer. They include non-invasive watchful waiting, surgery, radiation, hormone therapy, freezing and heat. Others are being created as you read this. There is no easy answer when it comes to selecting an option. No one has been able to say definitively which treatment is best for anyone. Even the experts cannot agree. Perhaps that's why so many people accept the treatment that their urologists or oncologists suggest and never seek another opinion, or even ask any questions. That in itself is not such a bad thing, if you can accept it.

What I find surprising is that some people accept a suggestion for treatment without understanding:

- the risks involved,
- the real situation with their condition,
- the probability of the cancer being totally confined versus having penetrated beyond the capsule,
- the chance of a complete cure versus the chance of recurrence,

- the potential after-effects, particularly,
  - incontinence,
  - erectile dysfunction,
  - shortened erected penis,
  - never experiencing an ejaculation again even though you may have an orgasm,
  - infertility

Of course it's up to you, if you want to go blindly into a treatment without knowing the effects it may have on your future lifestyle. But is that really what you want?

Making the choice of treatment is difficult partly because of the limitations of the current scientific data. There have been no studies completed in which large, comparable groups of patients are randomly assigned treatments and then followed for a significant period of time. There are some studies ongoing, but they are still inconclusive. The majority of today's published information is based on observation after the fact. In fact, many of them are biased and are gauged by their apparent success rate.

Many prostate cancer patients delay choosing a treatment, not because they are practicing watchful waiting or observation therapy, but because they see this decision to choose a treatment as potentially life-altering and theywant to:

- be made more aware of the condition and the after-effects that accompany each treatment.
- assure themselves, once they make the choice, it's the best choice, based on current understanding and technology.

This level of awareness and assurance is difficult to achieve since the marketing and publicity surrounding the more common treatments are on the rise and can be overwhelming. This is particularly true in the free enterprise health care system. Little of the marketing and publicity seems to offer the full story. They probably try, or feel that they do, but they really do not. Granted, some patients do not want to know the full story.

In reviewing information, one must be mindful of the health care system's method of operation, particularly if you reside in Canada and are reviewing material from the United States. Many of the health care centres in the United States operate on the free enterprise system, meaning they may be private and for-profit. Thus, "profit," "turf," "and marketing" are important elements of survival. Health care centres in Canada are primarily government-sponsored, so profit and turf are immaterial for them.

In the free enterprise system, specialists tend to recommend a treatment based on their own specialty. If more than one option is equally viable, surgeons will recommend surgery, radiation oncologists will recommend radiation, brachytherapists will recommend brachytherapy, cryosurgeons will recommend cryotherapy, and so on. That's analogous to purchasing a car – the Ford

Part V   Treatment Options

dealer will talk about Ford, the Chrysler dealer will talk about Chrysler, even the SUV dealer will try to sell you only an SUV. In the Canadian medical system, specialists strive to provide a balanced view. In many centres, teams of specialists will discuss options, based on the patient's age and general health, the cancer's characteristics, and the potential side/after-effects. The multidisciplinary approach is what most Canadian centres strive for.

In this era when prostate cancer is being diagnosed earlier and more frequently, it's imperative that patients understand the risks of traditional treatments and the more experimental ones. Every treatment carries certain risks and potential after-effects and quality of life degradations. Patients should understand what those are, for each specific treatment.

Partnering

I believe it should be the responsibility of the specialist, or at least the health centre, to ensure that the patient has a clear understanding of the downside of a particular treatment. It's usually not a pretty picture, so do not expect the specialists to make it sound so. Accept the facts. In the same context, it's not that gloomy, either. Hopefully, the specialists will make it clear so the risks not only are 'not' buried or omitted, but that they do not 'appear' to be buried or omitted either. It should be up front in bold prints of the patient's contract.

Based on my experience, I believe the patient should be a partner in the decision making process. Not everyone is alike, especially in terms of values and lifestyle needs. Neither is every prostate cancer the same. Some men want to get rid of all cancerous cells at any cost. Others prefer to hold out on any invasive treatment and preserve their potency, erectile function, and accept the risk of dying earlier. Ultimately, it's the patient who should decide how much risk he is prepared to take, and the consequences he is prepared to live with.

The American Prostate Society states:

> "As a man with prostate cancer faces a decision, the question before him is not the decision itself, but HOW he arrived at it. The decision, no matter what it is, is not reversible. There is no guarantee it will turn out to be the right one. This means the man, and his family, must not have to second guess the decision if it turns out to be wrong. It's critical for all concerned to be able to say the decision was based on weighing ALL knowledge available, plus the recommendation of trusted medical experts.
>
> An essential rule in deciding which, if any, therapy to accept is NEVER to accept just one doctor's judgment. The point is that by gathering opinions from more than one source, preferably three sources, a man can be reasonably confident he has weighed all positives and negatives of each therapy.

Do not be rushed into anything. Prostate cancer generally grows so slowly it takes about four years for an average tumour to double in size. To take a few more weeks to gain full knowledge of your condition, and alternative therapies, is the right thing to do.

Only then can you say with confidence, I made the best decision using every bit of information I could find."

Even with this advice, some men aren't in the right state of mind, to make a decision. It's difficult to make these decisions if you're not aware of, or don't understand, what will be done to you and therefore exactly what are the risks. Think also about family members who are involved or concerned about you?

And patients should be cognizant that not all prostate cancers grow slowly. We really may not have years to wait and therefore should make a decision expeditiously.

It appears to me that there's a link missing in the process. Perhaps, as was suggested earlier in Chapter 26, there should be a group of specially-trained health care counsellors who understand the psychology of human behaviours, as well as the various treatments available and their implications. These counsellors should be empathic and possess the skill as well as have the welfare of the patient at heart. They should be able to help the patient arrive at a decision, that's best suited for him and his family, quicker. They would fill the information gap and help the patient understand what he wants to understand. Knowledge of the level of information presented in this book should be a pre-requisite for these counsellors.

Traditional Treatments

Current western traditional treatments for prostate cancer include:
- Watchful waiting
- Surgery (removal of the prostate gland)
- External beam radiation therapy (EBRT)
- Internal radiation treatment
  - (including brachytherapy or seed implant, high dose rate radiation, etc.)
- *Hormone therapy* (including *orchiectomy* or *castration*)
- Cryosurgery (freezing cells to death)
- HIFU
- Chemotherapy

Doctors generally recommend one or more of these as the most appropriate treatment, after they have determined the grade and stage of the cancer, and considering your age, PSA and health condition. I will address each of these traditional treatments separately, in the next few chapters,

Part V   Treatment Options

in order to give you an appreciation for each.

Be reminded that these are being offering to you as information that I learned, while I was trying to understand more on each treatment so that I could ask questions and analyze the situation more effectively, in order to make my decision. I have also added what I learned since then, as developments occurred. It's more than you will get in most places or books. If you feel that this is not enough for you, I urge you to explore further until you are satisfied.

Non-Traditional Treatments

There are also many alternative or non-traditional forms of treatment that aren't recognized by the western medical establishment, primarily because each lacks sufficient scientific study to fully document it as viable treatment. Some of these can go under the general heading of:

- Nutritional (diet, supplementation and exercise)
- Herbal
- Cleansing
- Vegetarian
- Homeopathic
- Others

Some, particularly diet and life-style modification, may be helpful in conjunction with recognized western treatments.

Some other interesting alternate non-traditional approaches that may have worked for some, but which aren't officially endorsed in the West, are:

- Antineoplastin therapy (developed by Dr. Stanislaw Burzynski)
- Ayurveda (Deepak Chopra is one of the practitioners of this method)
- Bovine cartilage (said to have been used successfully by its discoverer Dr. John Prudden – Columbia-Presbyterian Medical Centre)
- Burton's Immuno-augmentative therapy (developed by Dr. Lawrence Burton while serving as an oncologist at New York's St. Vincent's Hospital)
- Essiac tea (inherited by Rene Caisse, a Canadian nurse, from an Indian healer, by way of a patient they both treated)
- Gerson therapy (one of the oldest, devised by Germany's Dr. Max Gerson)
- Kelly's nutritional-metabolic therapy (developed by a dentist named William Kelly)
- Live-cell therapy (developed by Dr. Paul Niehans of Switzerland in the 1930s)
- Livingston therapy (created by the late Virginia Livingston-Wheeler, M.D.)
- Macrobiotics (based on the oriental concept of yin and yang)

- Moerman anti-cancer diet (based on a diet of fresh, organically grown fruits and vegetables, whole grains, buttermilk, and natural seasoning)
- Revici therapy (developed by Dr. Emanuel Revici)
- Shark cartilage (utilized by several naturopathic practitioners)
- Urea therapy (based on a 1950s report by a Greek doctor that urea, a substance found in the urine, can kill cancer cells)
- Wheat grass therapy (developed and promoted in the U.S. by Ann Wigmore and based on drinking juice made from wheat grass)

These and many other therapies, are intriguing, and have been said to help individuals, in various countries. Whereas they should not be considered as "quackery," they should not necessarily be considered as successful or permanent treatments in all cases for all people. Although they may work positively for Joe, they may not necessarily work as positively for John. If you can believe strongly in any of them and commit to their program completely, it may work for you. Remember that everything takes time, and time is precious, because during any delayed period, your tumour could be growing in a ravaging, or a mild way, or perhaps not be growing at all.

Standards for Cure

For some time, many treatment specialists simply assume they were curing or eliminating the cancer, without any formal acceptable standardized measure or specification for cure. In 1996, American urologist Dr. Frank Critz, Medical Director of the Radiotherapy Clinics of the state of Georgia, in the United States, suggested that the cure rate for prostate cancer treatment, regardless of the treatment used, should be standardized. He recommended a standard specification for cure across the nation. He suggested the establishment of a PSA *nadir*, the lowest PSA level measured after any type of treatment. He suggested a PSA nadir of no more than 0.5 ng/ml. He even suggested that we might consider using a PSA level as low as 0.2 ng/ml or less. In addition, he suggested that for men to be considered cured of their prostate cancer, by any treatment, they must not only achieve the PSA nadir, but must maintain it for at least 10 years after treatment. Such qualification across the board places each treatment on the same basis, something that was lacking at the time, but apparently improving today.

Surgeons in Canada advised they use an "undetectable" PSA level that is to be sustained forever, as the proof of cure after surgery. Unfortunately, they cannot use that with other forms of treatment, such as radiation or others. My PSA level has been practically zero or "undetectable" since my radical prostatectomy in March of 2000.

Perhaps some consideration should also be given to standards for after-effects, such as erectile dysfunction and incontinence, as part of the total cure success picture. At the least, such after-effects standards or expectations could help to assess the quality of the cure.

Part V   Treatment Options

In order for these measurements or specifications to be credible, they would have to be collected and analyzed to ensure that they meet standard guidelines and benchmarks. These would have to be recorded and tracked by a neutral group. The problem today is that most, if not all, of the work in this area is being recorded and tracked by the individual therapist in the individual treatment centres or hospitals. That opens the potential for bias.

There is also a wide variation in the surgical skills of doctors who perform treatments. The data quoted in published literature regarding cure rate and success rate may not necessarily be that of your local urologist, oncologist or radiation therapist, but possibly of top experts in the field. It has been shown that specialists who perform their procedure regularly, whether it's surgery or radiation, have better outcomes and fewer complications than those who perform the procedure only occasionally. That's so in any profession – practice makes perfect, as the saying goes. In fact in some cases, the more expertise one has, the more they are inclined to get patients seeking them out.

Fortunately, many experienced specialists report observations and results in peer review journals and invite criticism and feedback from colleagues.

More Questions to Ask

Some other good questions to ask your doctor – understanding that answers could depend on the surgical skill and experience of the surgeon, the patient's pre-surgery conditions and other factors – are:

1. "Approximately, what percentage of patients, overall, achieved and maintained an undetectable PSA after surgery, or a PSA nadir of 0.2 ng/ml or less for 10 years after their treatment?"

2. "How many patients have YOU personally performed this treatment on?"

3. "What percentage of YOUR patients have achieved this undetectable PSA if it's surgery, or a PSA nadir of 0.2 ng/ml or less, for 10 years after this recommended treatment?"

4. "What is your record of winning the battle of erectile dysfunction and incontinence?"

5. "Assuming that I will be capable of having an erection, will my erection be of the same strength and length as I experience today (before treatment)?"

6. "What are my chances of achieving normal ejaculation (versus retrograde ejaculation or no ejaculation) during orgasm?"

You think that these are harsh questions? What is far more harsh or shocking is when you end up with an after-effect situation that you can't handle emotionally.

When you ask the questions, you might find that the treatment you first considered is not necessarily your best choice. Even if it is, can you prepare yourself mentally to live with the degradation?

Conclusion

Every therapy, including watchful waiting, has a certain positive outcome attached to it; however, it appears that much depends on the PSA level, the stage and grade of the cancer, your age and general health. If the stage indicates that your cancer has progressed too far, and the PSA levels and grade are high, you will have a lower probability of being cured, regardless of the treatment you choose. If the cancer has not progressed too far and the levels are low, you might have a higher probability of a cure. Those are reasons your specialist will be recommending different options. You still have to choose.

After carefully weighing all the consequences, I opted for surgery from the list of options presented to me. Did I make the best choice? I honestly do not know, but I was satisfied with it. It seemed like the best choice at the time. My consideration was influenced by several circumstances, including finances, close proximity to the treatment centre (hospital) relative to my home, the limited availability of choices locally at the time, the standard of cure that I was promised, the quality lifestyle I was promised and a surgeon in whom I had confidence, who presented it as the best choice for me at that time. Only time will tell if I made the best choice.

I might add that at that point in time, residents of Canada did not have as many treatment choices as did residents of the United States. That's changing. So unless I was prepared to come up with a substantial amount of money, to pay for other choices that were available south of the border, I had to choose from what was offered in Canada. Canadian health care plan will also not cover treatments abroad that are similarly available in Canada (meaning if they can get the same results in terms of cure). I was fortunate in that the treatment I selected (surgery) was available in Canada, with the same levels of expertise as in the U. S.

Chapter 29

WATCHFUL WAITING

The key to your universe is that you can choose.

CARL FREDERICK

To Treat or Observe – That is the Question

It's said that if a man lives long enough, he will experience prostate cancer. At the very least, he will likely have some cancer cells in his prostate. Some of those cancers are aggressive, fast growing and deadly; however, many are slow growing or even dormant and for those, no treatment is recommended. This is called "watchful waiting" and sometimes "active surveillance" or "observation." It's simply managing or monitoring the condition for stability versus aggressiveness, without undergoing invasive treatment.

Who is Best Suited?

This treatment (or non-treatment) is based on the theory that since this type of prostate cancer grows slowly, many older men with the condition will never need treatment. They will probably die from some other cause, long before their prostate cancer becomes critical or chronic. In fact, it's reported that some men with prostate cancer die from other causes, without even knowing that they had the condition. Can you imagine that?

It's wise to bear in mind though, that some prostate cancers do require urgent treatment.

Thus watchful waiting is particularly suited for older men with early-stage slow-growing cancer, and/or those with other serious health problems from which they may die before the cancer becomes a real threat.

Watchful waiting may also be recommended to others, if their cancer is:

- Expected to grow slowly,
- Small,
- Contained within one area of the gland, and
- Not causing any symptoms.

Some younger men with a borderline PSA level and low Gleason score may choose this strategy, although most of the time they do so at a high risk. In most cases, they suffer the consequences, especially if this is against the recommendation of a specialist who has analyzed the condition and suggested a treatment.

Studies have shown that, in general, a 70 year old prostate cancer patient who accepts treatment, will survive approximately three years or more longer than a 70 year old patient who accept only watchful waiting.

Some men may also practice watchful waiting out of fear, or because they think that faith will heal them.

Watchful waiting is not for everybody, and those who embark on that strategy may want to get the full agreement of their urologist or oncologist. Below are some guidelines established by some urologists to qualify patients for watchful waiting. Any one of these can qualify you, if you:

- Are 75 years of age or older.
- Have some sort of significant other health problem.
- Have a low volume and low grade tumour.

How it is Monitored

The monitoring process for watchful waiting includes a DRE and a PSA blood test every six months. Occasionally, a scan or a TRUS is warranted. Sometimes this might be accompanied by repeating TRUS-guided biopsies. Action is taken only if bothersome symptoms begin to emerge or if growth begins to accelerate. The danger for younger men is that the cancer is still growing and you certainly do not want even one of those cells to escape via the blood stream and become attached to your pelvis bone or spinal cord or somewhere else, only to grow and spread later in life.

A young man, has a longer life expectancy and thus stands to lose more by succumbing to the cancer. For an older person, this may be less of a consideration.

If the cancer continues at the same safe level of activity, the monitoring continues with no treatment. Many men live this out and die from other causes, such as heart failure, diabetes, stroke, Alzheimer's, and so on. If the cancer should show signs of progressing, then another treatment or therapy is recommended.

Study Aims to Answer The Big Question

In September 2007 the Canadian Cancer Society and the National Cancer Institute of Canada announced jointly that they are launching a large, multi-year international study to try to find a way to help men who are diagnosed with prostate cancer to decide whether to opt for a "watch-and-wait" approach or "choose a supposedly curative treatment." Researchers from the two institutes said they are hopeful that the trial, named "Surveillance Therapy Against Radical Treatment" (START), will resolve the dilemma in prostate cancer care. Unfortunately, it will take 20 years to have an answer.

Hopefully the trial will provide answer to the question, "does active treatment make a difference in terms of long-term survival from prostate cancer?" The study is designed to follow 2,100 newly diagnosed volunteers in Canada, the United States and Britain who will be randomly assigned to receive either "treatment" or "to undergo active surveillance (watchful waiting)." It will take about four to five years to enroll all the patients, then they will be followed for 10 to 15 years, thus the 20 years wait for the answer that so many men and their physicians would like to have. Men in the surveillance group whose cancer progresses or who later decide they want to have treatment can do so.

The principal investigator, Dr. Laurence Klotz, chief urologist at Toronto's Sunnybrook Health Sciences Centre, had this to say: "Choosing to take no immediate action is a particularly difficult one, running counter to what he calls society's "cancer hysteria" – the equivalent of a cancer diagnosis with a death sentence. By having treatment, you elect to avoid risk of prostate cancer death, but you also incur very major risk of erectile dysfunction, urinary incontinence, rectal problems, if you have radiation, surgery and so on. The idea is we're trying to kind of drive a middle road between treating everybody, which will result in over-treatment, and treating nobody, which will result in under-treatment and just identify the ones who look like the bad actors."

Every prostate cancer patient had to make that tough choice. I did, eight years ago, when my DRE, PSA and subsequent biopsy revealed I had prostate cancer, even though I waited two years to do so.

Chapter 29 | Watchful Waiting

Many men with prostate cancer need to undergo treatment to stop the advance of the disease. But in many others – perhaps as many as half the cases that come to light – doctors know the cancer is unlikely to break out of the prostate and spread to other parts of the body. The question is, are they brave enough to suggest watchful waiting?

Since the advent of PSA testing, large numbers of men who were seemingly healthy have been told they have cancer cells in their prostates and have faced this difficult choice. Experts say a significant portion of these men will die from other causes and would never require any prostate cancer care, if the screening test hadn't signaled the presence of malignant cells.

"With a disease like this, which typically is diagnosed in either late middle age or more, death from other causes is by far the commonest cause of death in men with prostate cancer. Heart disease is the commonest cause of death in men with prostate cancer," Klotz said. He noted that at age 50, about one out of every two men will have some cancer cells in their prostate. By age 80, the number is 80 per cent.

The problem is, doctors don't know how to determine with certainty, which are the cancers that will progress (and therefore should be treated) and which are the types that won't. As a result, many men receive treatment they would never have needed if their cancer hadn't been picked up by a PSA test.

"I think there's a strong consensus, not only in the United States but around the world, that there is over-treatment," said Dr. Barnett Kramer, associate director for disease prevention at the U.S. National Institutes of Health in Bethesda, Md. "The magnitude of over-treatment is probably debated, but not the fact that some men are over-treated. Finding a way to be able to determine at the time of diagnosis which is which would be a valuable contribution to the field of cancer care, Kramer suggested. "Day in and day out the decision is being made with regard to therapy of screen-detected prostate cancer whether to treat or how aggressively to treat," he said. "And it affects over 100,000 men a year just in the United States, and around the world it affects that many more, so it's not an unusual question that a patient and his physicians face."

General Comments

If you are recommended for watchful waiting, you should not lose sleep over it. However, you should expect that, at some point in time, the condition might require you to take a different action, or a more aggressive treatment or even a more invasive one.

Watchful waiting is practiced in the United Kingdom and Europe more than in North America. It's not an option you should choose on your own, or without understanding your condition. If you do, you may die earlier than you would otherwise.

Part V   Treatment Options

Of course watchful waiting is not a strategy that's controlled and monitored by you. That's done by a urologist, with your cooperation, which is essential. You need to be conscientious, as it's important to keep all appointments with your urologist/oncologist.

There are people who profess to be watching and waiting and at the same time trying other treatments, such as seeing another practitioner, or taking certain medications. It's important that your urologist be made aware of everything you do during watchful waiting. Otherwise, it's not watchful waiting; it's a treatment.

Watchful waiting is not something that you decide upon and then do it. It's something that's recommended and monitored by your urologist. It's to be practiced with his full co-operation and instructions. It might also do you good to re-read "Part I" of this book to get some appreciation for taking control of your health.

One might say that delaying a decision is practicing watchful waiting. That's a false notion. Only with co-operation and active monitoring by a urologist, can you consider it watchful waiting.

Examples

Here are a couple of examples or first-hand stories:

> A man who was undergoing watchful waiting for his prostate cancer, decided to take saw palmetto. He was boasting that his PSA level was going down, as a result. Finally, he decided to go for surgery in an effort to get on with his life. He was surprised to find that the cancer had grown. It appears, as some medical experts suggest, that the saw palmetto contains some enzymes that lowered the PSA activity and show a false indication of the decreasing PSA level. This made it appeared that the cancer might have been regressing. That wasn't the case. So if you have cancer, you should avoid taking saw palmetto, unless you are instructed to do so by your urologist.

There are thousands of men who are practicing watchful waiting and are happy doing so. I have met a few of them personally.

Chapter 29 | Watchful Waiting

> On one occasion, upon entering a restaurant in Miami Beach, I encountered four men sitting at a table eating what appeared to be health food and drinking bottled water. Each had some vitamins laid out on the table in front of them. These men were dressed in shorts, polo shirts and walking shoes. As the vitamins looked familiar to me, like the ones I was taking, I stopped to chat with them, and found out that all of them had been diagnosed with prostate cancer. Two had prostatectomy (surgery), one had brachytherapy, and the other was practicing watchful waiting with full consent of his urologist who was monitoring his condition. They were all happy and jovial, although the one who was practicing watchful waiting appeared to be a lot happier and younger, even though he was the oldest! I did not ask for his exact age or his general medical condition. Nor did I ask for his cancer's stage/grade/PSA. Since he had the consent of his urologist to practice watchful waiting, I assumed that he fit the criteria mentioned earlier.
>
> In our conversation, he attributed his happiness, as he put it to me, whispering in my ear, "to his exceptional sex life," meaning his capability of having an erection and ejaculation during orgasm. His colleagues were not able to enjoy their sex to the same extent, since their erection capability were severely limited and ejaculation was impossible for them, as a result of their surgery and brachytherapy.

Note: In the watchful waiting approach, the patient and his urologist agree upon what is to be watched, monitored or observed (PSA, PSA change, DRE, bone scans, or anything else) and what is being waited for (development of a proven therapy capable of improving the condition, or development of numerical values of parameters being watched, progression to symptoms, and any others), with the intention of taking the next step after the occurrence of any of those events.

It should also be noted that watchful waiting, like many other treatments, will become obsolete after a cure for prostate cancer is found. However, until we can convince the Government that a drastic increase in research funding is in order, that discovery may be in the very distant future.

Chapter 30

SURGERY

Make visible what, without you, might perhaps never have been seen.

Robert Bresson

The Sure Way for the Right Man

The technical word for prostate surgery is prostatectomy. It's an invasive procedure that can be performed in any of three ways, classified according to the type of incision, namely: *retropubic* – a single open incision to the lower abdomen; *perineal* – a single open incision to the perineum; and *laparoscopic* – a series of small keyhole like incisions to the lower abdomen. Each type involves the surgical removal (radical) of the entire prostate gland including the prostatic urethra, as well as the seminal vesicles and vas deferens tubes to avoid spread of the cancer. The premise is: "remove the cancerous organ to treat the condition." Thus, it will only help those patients with confined or early stage prostate cancer.

Surgery also includes sparing or preserving the *neurovascular (nerve) bundles* or more specifically the cavernous nerves, that are responsible for erection, and the external sphincter muscle to help control urine flow.

History has shown that most men with prostate cancer choose surgery as their preferred treatment. Many of them did not consider any other option. This proportion can be expected to decline slightly as newer treatments are developed and these prove more successful. However, it appears that more prostate cancers are being detected earlier today, when the cancer is still contained, which means most patients do qualify for surgery.

Because of the risks involved – side-effects and after-effects – surgery is generally recommended more often for men 75 years of age and younger, with a PSA level under 15 ng/ml, a clinical stage T1C or T2, and a Gleason score of 7 or less. Patients with a Gleason score of 8 or higher would likely require additional treatments. The 75 age limit's chosen as a benchmark because it's assumed that the average male, who is in good health at age 75, has a life expectancy of about 10 years. So unless a patient can reasonably expect to benefit for another 10 years, doctors will not generally recommend prostatectomy.

Notwithstanding the above statement, surgery is still the most common choice for men in their 50s and early 60s since urologists and oncologists generally agree that younger patients have more to gain by going for a one-time definitive procedure.

Before surgery is undertaken, the surgeon would determine, based on the DRE finding, PSA, ultrasound, Gleason score, and possibly a bone scan, and CT scan, that, to the best of his knowledge, the cancer has not metastasized, or spread.

Retropubic Radical Prostatectomy

Retropubic radical prostatectomy is a major invasive procedure in which an open incision, approximately six to 10 centimetres long, is made down the centre of the lower abdomen, from the navel toward the pubic bone.

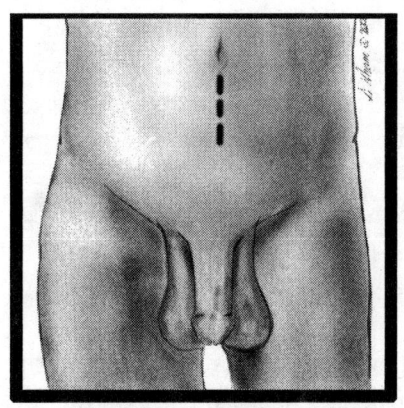

Incision for Retropubic Radical Prostatectomy

Retropubic means the prostate gland is located behind the pubic arch, which is made up of the pubic bones. This surgery, in use since the 1940s, is designed to take the gland out from behind the arch. Some high grade cancers need a longer incision to ensure that all the cancer is removed. After the operation is completed, the incision requires 10 to 20 staples to close it.

Part V   Treatment Options

In performing retropubic prostatectomy, the patient is first put under general anaesthesia. The surgeon then pushes past the pool of tissues – fat, blood, nerves, arteries, and muscles – to get to the prostate gland. Think about this when you set that date for surgery because any excess fat you can burn away beforehand, will help you and the surgeon.

Sometimes, early in the surgery, depending on the PSA level and Gleason score, the surgeon may take biopsy samples of the lymph nodes or may remove the entire lymph nodes, and have them examined by a pathologist. Removing the lymph nodes is referred to as "pelvic lymph node dissection (PLND)" or "pelvic lymphadenectomy." Once he is assured that there is no evidence of cancer metastasis to the lymph nodes, he will continue with the surgery. If the nodes have been invaded, the surgery would be terminated, the incision closed and another form of treatment chosen.

The surgeon carefully separates the nerve bundles from both sides of the gland and leaves them intact and, it's hoped, specifically the cavernous nerves, undamaged. This is referred to a "*sparing the nerve bundles,*" and is necessary to preserve erectile function. This will be addressed in more detail further on in this chapter.

The surgeon detaches the gland, along with the prostatic urethra, from the rest of the tube, just above the membranous urethra. This is done in such a way that the urinary sphincter muscle (external sphincter muscle) that surrounds the membrane urethra is preserved, as this alone will henceforth control urine flow, or "continence." He then separates the prostate gland from the surrounding tissues and the rectal wall, leaving it attached only to the bladder. Finally he dismembers the gland by slicing it off from the bladder, taking with it the two attached seminal vesicles and a piece of the neck of the bladder. This leaves an opening at the bottom of the bladder about the diameter of a 25 cent coin. The freed prostate gland, along with the prostatic urethra, the seminal vesicles and portions of the two vas deferens tubes, are then removed.

The remains of the two vas deferens tubes are tied, as is done for *vasectomy*, thereby rendering the man infertile. The removal of the prostate gland and seminal vesicles, also render you unable to father children, since they provide fluid nutrients for your sperm.

The surgeon then pulls the urethra and connects what's left of it to the bladder. He first sews up the opening of the bladder to make it smaller, then takes the urethra at the membranous end, pulls and attaches it to the new opening of the bladder and sutures (attaches) them together. This may contribute to a shortening of the penis. Subsequently, nature takes its course in healing and sealing the attachment.

The internal tissues are put back as best as possible. The incision on the abdomen is sealed like a zipper, with staples, and the healing process begins. A urinary *catheter*, is inserted through the head of the penis, up through the urethras to the bladder. This remains for about three weeks until it's extracted by the surgeon. Often, another tube is inserted through the lower abdomen to drain any excess fluid. That remains for about five days.

The prostate gland is sent to the pathologist for examination. The pathologist slices it into sections and examines each under a microscope to determine the extent of the cancer and reconfirm its stage and grade.

After surgery, the patient is taken to the *recovery room*, where he is closely monitored by a nurse for about one and a half hours. Later, he is taken to the ward to recuperate, for one to three days.

The entire surgical procedure takes about two to three hours, plus recovery time. To the patient, it feels like two minutes, because one minute he is awake in an operating room and the next, he is lying in the recovery room in a daze. To the family, especially the spouse, it feels like eternity.

Retropubic radical prostatectomy has a cure rate of 75 to 80 percent after five years.

A 1997 report from Johns Hopkins University, provides statistics for cures five and 10 years after surgery performed by Dr. Patrick Walsh, using a PSA level of <0.2 ng/ml as a PSA nadir benchmark, as follows:

PSA Before Treatment	cure 5 years after percent	cure 10 years after percent
0—4 ng/ml	94	87
>4—10 ng/ml	82	75
>10 -20 ng/ml	72	30
>20 ng/ml	54	28
Overall	80	68

Dr. Walsh is the world's expert on radical prostatectomy procedure and nerve-sparing technique.

Some recent reports indicate up to an 85 percent survival rate after 10 years. Unfortunately, they do not state any specific range of PSA prior to treatment.

It can be assumed that with more early diagnosis and improved technology for treatment these records will improve with time.

Perineal Radical Prostatectomy

Perineal radical prostatectomy is a major invasive procedure, in use since the early 20th century, in which an approximately six centimetre long curved incision is made across the perineum – the space between the scrotum and anus, which comprises of mainly skin and muscle.

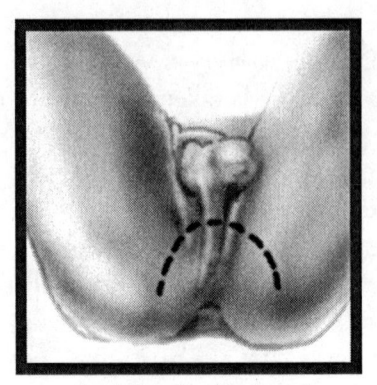

Incision for Perineal Radical Prostatectomy

In performing this procedure, the patient is positioned in the high *dorsal lithotomy* position, with the legs extending up in the air and elevated above the head while supported by stirrups behind the knees. This position gives the surgeon a clear view of the incision site as the operation is performed from a different angle than for the retropubic approach. A self-retaining perineal retractor is used to hold the incision open.

In general, the procedure is similar to the retropubic, except for the sparing of the nerve bundles and reaching the lymph nodes. If the lymph nodes must be worked on, a separate incision would have to be made in the abdomen in order to access them. Some patients exhibit what is called "pubic arch interference" which also inhibits access to the nerves. Thus, if the nerve bundles are to be spared, it would be wise not to choose this approach.

Because of the earlier detection of prostate cancer, most patients today do not experience the cancer spread to the lymph nodes. The surgeon relies on the PSA, DRE findings and Gleason score as sufficient indication of nymph node metastasis when performing this procedure.

It's said that patients who suffer from significant obesity are generally candidates for perineal prostatectomy over retropubic.

It's strongly advised that patients who are interested in saving the nerves in hopes of preserving their erectile function should speak frankly with their surgeon about his previous success with this technique.

After the operation is completed, the catheter and drain are put in place and recovery follows the same process as with the retropubic approach. The incision requires 8 to 12 staples to close it.

The patient may begin to walk within a few hours and may be released from the hospital within one to three days. He would, however, be cautioned to not lift any heavy items for six weeks.

Laparoscopic Radical Prostatectomy (LRP)

Laparoscopic radical prostatectomy is a minimally invasive procedure. It requires a few small keyhole-type incisions, each approximately five to 10 millimetres long, in the abdomen, around the navel.

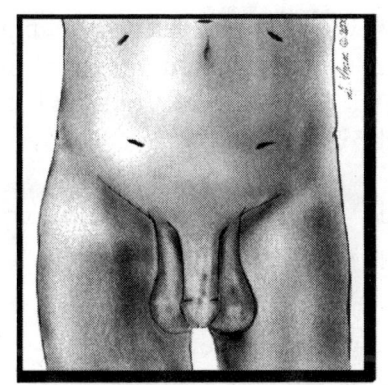

Incisions for Laparoscopic Radical Prostatectomy

One incision is made first just above the navel and a laparoscope, a slim tube with a tiny video camera on the end, is inserted into the abdomen. The camera projects the image to a monitor, placed where it can be seen by the surgeon.

The surgeon inserts a small needle into the abdominal cavity just above the navel. It's connected to a tube that passes carbon dioxide gas into the cavity, lifting the abdominal wall to provide a view of the cavity and ensure the *laparoscopy* procedure is safe. If the surgeon sees significant scar tissue, infection, or abdominal disease, he will discontinue the procedure. If he decides that the surgery can be performed safely, he will make four additional small incisions, two on each side of the navel with two in line with, and two lower than, the navel in the lower abdomen. These incisions provide further access to the abdominal cavity.

Guided by the laparoscopic images, the surgeon, using long thin instruments which he inserts through the incisions, manually separates the nerve bundles from the gland and dislodges, disconnects and removes the gland, seminal vesicles and vas deferens tubes through the incisions, protecting the external sphincter muscle in the process. He then *sutures*, or reconnects, the urethra to the bladder.

The procedure is very similar to the retropubic method, except that here everything is done through the small incisions, using long thin instruments that are controlled manually by the surgeon's hands.

This technique is still evolving, although it's gaining popularity as it shows promise for worldwide acceptance. It's a standard procedure in the U.S.

Robotic-Assisted Laparoscopic Radical Prostatectomy

This variation of laparoscopic surgery, sometimes referred to simply as robotic surgery for prostate cancer or robotic-assisted laparoscopic radical prostatectomy, is performed, as the name implies, with the assistance of a "robot," or "robotic arm." It's still in clinical studies in Canada, although commonly utilized in the U.S.

The robot (most commonly the da Vinci Surgical System) is a computer-enhanced minimally invasive surgical system, which allows 3-dimensional greatly magnified vision during laparoscopic surgery. The system consists of three main components:

- The InSite 3-D Vision System, which provides the surgeon with a 3-D view of the operative field with both high magnification and resolution,

- The Surgical Cart, which provides the robotic arms that control the articulating EndoWrist instruments. These instruments move in all directions giving the surgeon greater control and manipulation for performing delicate maneuvers inside the patient. The movement of the instruments are precise and are done only at the command of the surgeon.

- The Surgical Console where the surgeon sits, and views the operative site while controlling the movement of the instruments through their range of motions.

This da Vinci Surgical System has been used successfully in the U.S., Canada and some centres in Europe and has been deemed safe and effective by the U.S. Food and Drug Administration for use in urologic, abdominal and thoracic (chest) surgical procedures.

The surgical procedure is the same as the LRP except in this case the instruments or robots are controlled and augmented by computer. The first keyhole incision is made, the laparoscope is inserted and the carbon dioxide gas is injected. This is followed by the other four small keyhole incisions in the abdomen around the navel, as with the LRP.

The surgeon inserts robotic instruments (arms) through the incisions and maneuvers them by use of the computer and the monitor. The entire procedure is then performed using the robotic arms, controlled remotely by the surgeon.

The surgeon controls the EndoWrist instruments, allowing him greater control with delicate maneuvering of the robotic arms. The movements of the arms are precise and allow laparoscopic removal of the cancerous gland, as well as the delicate preservation of the urinary sphincter muscles and vital nerve bundles.

According to several reports, the use of the robots enables the surgeon to work less invasively and with more precision than the manual LRP procedure. The 3-dimensional camera allows excellent visibility.

According to Dr. Joseph Chin, co-author and editor of these medical chapters, who is leading research in this area at the London Health Sciences Centre in London, Ontario, Canada through a program called CSTAR (Canadian Surgical Technologies and Advanced Robotics), "the robot provides much better visualization, magnification, and improved dexterity, which translates into greater surgical accuracy overall." Dr. Chin and several of his colleagues, along with CSTAR, are utilizing the "da Vinci" robot's 3-dimensional images. They performed the first robotic assisted laparoscopic prostatectomy in Canada in 2004 and have come a long way with very satisfactory and encouraging results.

CSTAR is a collaborative research program of London Health Sciences Centre and the Lawson Health Research Institute and is affiliated with The University of Western Ontario, all located within an arm's reach of each other in London.

Although it's too early to categorically state that the robotic procedure provides a better cure rate, it's reasonable to say that it aids the surgeon in identifying vital anatomy such as the delicate nerve and blood vessels surrounding the prostate and also provides him with increased dexterity, not available using other methods. It also lends itself to the performance of a delicate and precise surgical dissection and reconstruction of the bladder and urethra.

According to preliminary research, the robotic system enhances the surgery as follows:

- Nerve sparing thus improved erectile function
- Possibly more rapid regaining of urinary control
- Very few transfusions required
- Small incisions
- Less pain
- Shorter hospital stay
- Faster return to normal activities
- Faster recuperation

Risks and After-Effects

The risks associated with radical prostatectomy are similar to those of any major surgery, including potential for heart attack or heart failure, stroke, blood clots in the legs that could travel to the lungs, infections at the incision, and potential for recurrence of the cancer.

Some possible after-effects are:

- Erectile dysfunction (which is of a greater concern than you might think),
- Incontinence (some more problematic than others),
- Penile shortening (reduced length of erected penis),
- Shrinkage of the penis (reduced girth of the penis),
- Loss of ejaculatory capability during orgasm,
- Soreness in the urethra, and
- Stress pains in the bladder.

Fear of recurrence is a major stress factor in this or any treatment, but what is far more stressful, as I have learned from survivors, is dealing with the following three after-effects:

- Erectile dysfunction.
- Incontinence, and
- Reduced size penis.

These are major factors to be reckoned with socially, emotionally and psychologically.

Erectile Dysfunction (ED)

Erectile dysfunction (ED), sometimes referred to as "impotence," is the inability to achieve or maintain an erection sufficient to satisfy the sexual needs of the man or his partner, or the ability to achieve only brief erections.

There is a high likelihood that following radical prostatectomy, regardless of age, you will experience a decrease in your ability to have an erection. This could range from a mild problem to total erectile dysfunction. At any level, it's a frustrating experience. All patients should prepare to experience this to some degree.

Chapter 30 | Surgery

A Case of Nerves – or Erection

The primary objective of prostatectomy is the removal of early stage prostate cancer which is accomplished by the complete removal of the prostate gland. A secondary objective is to ensure retention of urinary continence and a third is to *spare* or preserve the neurovascular nerve bundles, particularly the cavernous nerves which are the nerves responsible for stimulating penile erection (see chapter 6).

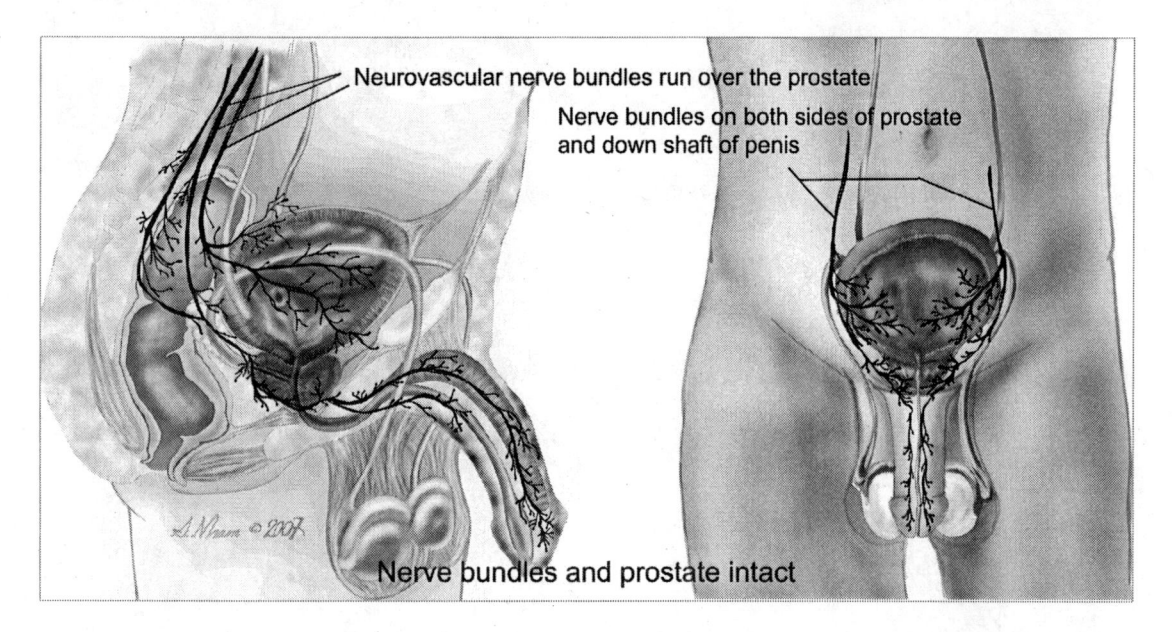

Neurovascular nerve bundles run over the prostate
Nerve bundles on both sides of prostate and down shaft of penis
Nerve bundles and prostate intact

Sometimes, achieving those secondary objectives may result in some undesirable after-effects. No surgeon, with whom I am familiar, will sacrifice that primary objective simply to accomplish the others.

To spare or preserve the nerves from damage, the surgeon must separate the nerve bundles from the surface of the prostate gland on both sides, a task more difficult, at least more delicate, than it might seem. He does this by skillfully lifting them from the gland as one would lift a wet tissue, undamaged, from a surface. This should only be done if the cancer has not extended to the surface of the gland.

Part V Treatment Options

Nerve bundles continuous down to shaft of penis after prostatectomy - nerve spared

Prostate removed - nerve bundles intact

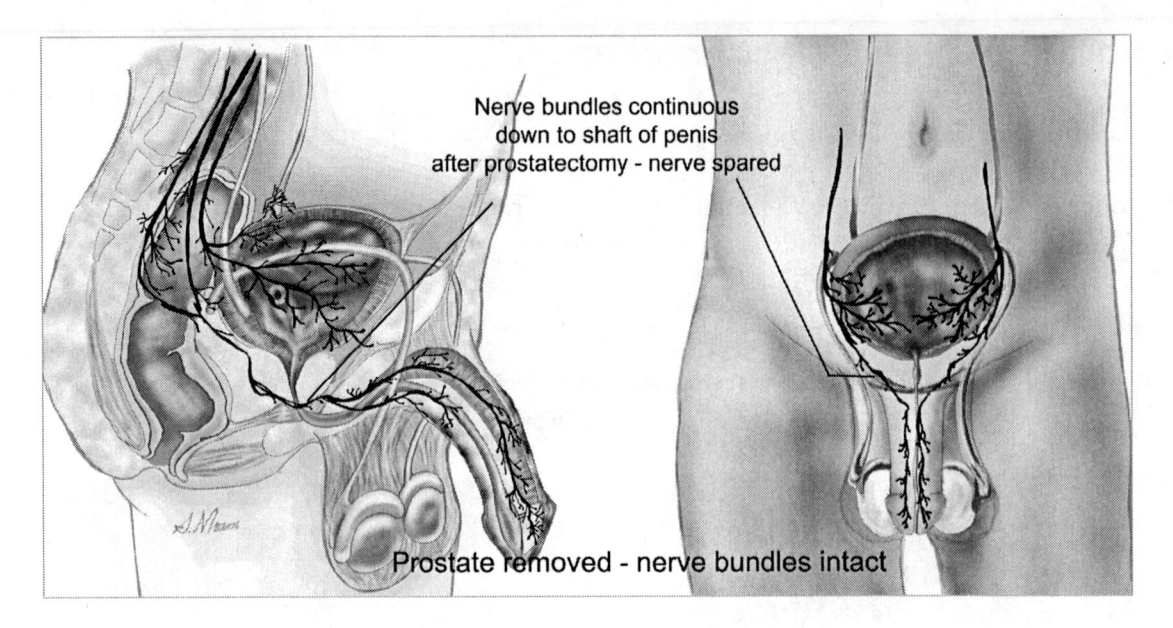

When both sets of nerves bundles are spared, the procedure is called "bilateral nerve-sparing radical prostatectomy." If only one set of nerve bundles is spared, it's called "unilateral nerve-sparing radical prostatectomy." If none of the nerve bundles are spared, the procedure is called a "non-nerve-sparing radical prostatectomy."

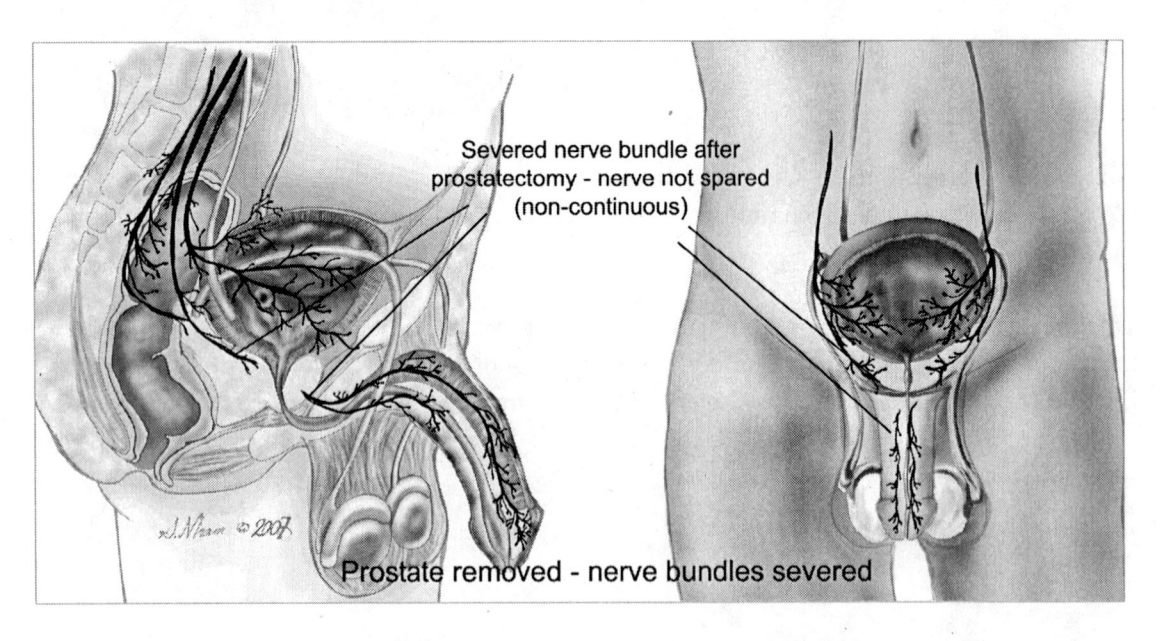

Severed nerve bundle after prostatectomy - nerve not spared (non-continuous)

Prostate removed - nerve bundles severed

Being informed by the surgeon that the nerve bundles were successfully spared always bring a sigh of relief to the patient, although it would be immaterial if accomplished at the cost of a shortened life span due to not getting all the cancer.

Many surgeons have successfully performed nerve-sparing surgery. However, not all of their patients subsequently succeed in achieving a quality erection. The question you might ask your surgeon, is: "How many of your patients subsequently succeed in having an erection that's hard enough for a sustainable period of time and that can penetrate the vagina for enjoyable sexual intercourse until climax or orgasm is achieved?" Ask the surgeon how long after the surgery did it take for those men to accomplish that quality of erection. Remember you are asking this simply to decide if surgery is for you.

As you read further in this chapter you will understand the importance of this and why it's so important for you to ask the questions. It's not to question your surgeon's ability, but rather for you to understand what you are getting yourself into. It's also important for you to understand that sparing the nerve is no guarantee that you will continue to be capable of having that quality erection. The nerve could be physically preserved but some damage may have occurred in the process that would affect the quality of the erection. This is not to scare you, just to inform you.

Damage to the nerve tissue usually result from the surgeon's inability to distinguish between the prostate's tissue and the nerve tissue. The requirement to be able to identify and avoid the cavernous nerves as they adhere to the prostate.

Theoretically, if the cavernous nerve are preserved undamaged, the capability of achieving an erection should be retained, or at least returned within six to twelve months. That is, of course, if you had that capability prior to having radical prostatectomy and you have no other physical or psychological challenges.

Erectile function depends on several physical and psychological factors including preoperative functions and the absence of conditions such as hypertension, diabetes, obesity, artherosclerosis, anxiety and history of smoking, among others.

Sometimes some unavoidable damage is done to the nerve bundles through handling and these may take three to twelve months to heal, sometimes even longer. On occasions, patients have had to be encouraged to be patient (no pun intended) with a new proviso that it could take up to three years for normal erection capability to return.

Studies suggest that upwards of 50 percent of men who have undergone radical prostatectomy subsequently have almost no erection capability. Another 30 percent have reduced erection capability.

None of the many men with whom I have spoken on this subject have ever been able to say, categorically, that they have full erection capability, equal to what they had prior to surgery. That would be an erection capable of successful or direct penetration of the vagina, without wobbling, bending or softening. Many men complain, for example, that the head of their penis does not become as hard as it once did.

Some reports suggest that even in cases where the nerves are supposedly properly spared, there could be about 25 to 30 percent of men under 60 years, and 70 to 75 percent 60 and over, who will experience erectile dysfunction.

In his book entitled, *The Prostate: A Guide for Men and the Women Who Love Them*, published in 1995, Dr. Walsh wrote: "for patients who had both neurovascular (nerve) bundles left intact, potency was preserved in 91 percent of the men younger than 50 years of age, 75 percent of the men between 50 and 60 years of age, and 25 percent of the men over 70 years of age."

My surgeon in London, Ontario, (co-author of this book) has very acceptable success rates, as he too performs several radical prostatectomies each week. Ask your surgeon about his success rate. Review the questions in chapters 10, 16 and 28. Understand that you may not get fully comprehensive answers to all these questions, but you will get some. And know that every person's condition and situation is different and every surgeon's experience is different.

It is important to note that the surgeon's success rates of preserving erectile function, partly depends on the stage and grade of the cancers he operates on.

Sparing the nerves is not always possible. Neither does sparing them necessarily guarantee satisfactory erection after surgery; but, if they are severed, achieving erection will definitely not be possible.

Some men already suffered from erectile dysfunction before the cancer. In such cases it's useless to make the effort to save the nerves and run the risk of leaving some cancer cells behind. Such malignant cells can ultimately spread into the nerve bundles and other areas. It's better to focus on removing all the cancer.

Today, when more younger men are being diagnosed with prostate cancer, or when prostate cancer is being detected earlier than previously, it can be expected that fewer and fewer men who choose prostatectomy will experience erectile dysfunction as a result.

Nerve Graft Procedure

Sometimes a wide margin of surrounding tissue (wide resection) must be removed with the prostate in order to ensure that no cancer is left behind. Likewise, sometimes it becomes necessary to remove a portion of the nerve bundles (wide-excision) with the gland. An innovative procedure, called the *"nerve graft,"* is used by some surgeons, to repair the nerve bundles and regain erectile capability. Nerve grafting was developed in 1998, by physicians at Baylor College of

Medicine and The Methodist Hospital in Houston, Texas and reported in the Journal of Urology in January 1999.

The surgeon extracts a small nerve, called the *sural nerve*, from near the ankle. This nerve provides sensation to the side of the foot and ankle. Extracting, or *harvesting*, this nerve can be done during the prostatectomy. The harvested sural nerve is then *grafted* onto the two cut ends of the nerve bundle around the prostate. The nerve graft *bridges* the cut ends of the nerve bundle, serving as a *scaffolding* for the nerves to heal. Thus the electrical pathways necessary for an erection are regained. This may be performed on one side (unilateral sural nerve graft) or on both sides (bilateral sural nerve graft).

Recovery takes about 12 to 18 months with 35 to 50 percent success in regaining erectile function. This technique is suitable for selected patients only.

Another nerve that is occasionally used by some surgeons for grafting is called the *"genitofemoral nerve,"* taken from inside the pelvis. Results are relatively comparable to those achieved with the sural nerve grafting.

You should ask your surgeon if you are a candidate for any of these in the event your nerve-sparing fails to accomplish what you hope for. But do so before surgery, because after surgery would be too late.

Treatment for Erectile Dysfunction

Current treatment options for erectile dysfunction in men who have received treatment for prostate cancer include:

- Oral medications, such as Viagra, Cialis or Levitra
- Injections of medicine into the penis before intercourse (called intracavernous injection therapy)
- Use of a vacuum constriction device to draw blood into the penis to cause an erection
- Medicine taken as a suppository placed in the penis prior to intercourse
- Penile implants

Sometimes you have to try a number of these until you find one that you can best live with. Consult your doctor to find out which of these, if any, would be suitable for you.

Part V   Treatment Options

Down-Sized Penis

Regardless of the stature of your erection capability, don't expect the penis to return to its original hardness, length or girth. Many men have expressed anger and disdain at their reduced penis size after surgery. This reduction is either a general shrinkage, shortened erection, or both. Unfortunately, most men who experience this are reluctant to speak about it, as it brings with it major emotional and psychological stress.

The penis is essentially muscles, muscles and more muscles, and muscles shrink when they aren't exercised or used. They may also shrink when they experience severe trauma. Having a catheter inserted through the urethra for three weeks could be a severe trauma. Also, not using the penis for sexual intercourse or even to have an erection for an extended period of time after surgery, up to a year or more in some instances, could cause the muscles to shrink. Unfortunately, there is very little research or written material on this subject, except by those who have experienced it and even they are reluctant to address it openly. However, it's undoubtedly an after-effect that must be accepted, understood, reckoned with and treated. Perhaps, as some literature have advocated, counselling might be offered to handle this potential emotional situation. We cannot be in denial about it forever.

Some people also believe that scar tissue resulting from handling the nerve bundles could prevent sufficient blood from flowing to the penis to create the engorgement. This is certainly an area that warrants research and if necessary, correction.

In case you might think this is irrelevant, read the following three sample articles on the subject:

"Changes in Penile Morphometrics in Men with Erectile Dysfunction after Nerve-Sparing Radical Retropubic Prostatectomy," by M.C. Fraiman, H. Lapor and A.R. McCullough (Department of Urology, New York University), printed in Molecular Urology, 1999; 3(2):109 – 115. This thesis, based on a sexual inventory of 124 men ages 47 to 74 in the flaccid and erect states all who underwent nerve-sparing retropubic radical prostectomy (NSRRP) by the same surgeon, supports the view that there is a significant decrease in penile size in men who experience erectile dysfunction after NSRRP. It suggests that the reason may be denervation smooth muscle atrophy, apoptosis, or hypoxia-induced damage to the corpora. It calls for further research to clarify the nature of these postoperative changes.

"A prospective study measuring penile length in men treated with radical prostatectomy for prostate cancer," by M. Savoie, S.S. Kim and M.S. Soloway (Department of Urology, University of Miami School of Medicine), printed in Journal of Urology, April 2003; 169(4): 1462 – 4. This article is based on a study which measured penile size of 124 men before radical prostectomy performed by the same surgeon with repeat measurements at three months following surgery – including flaccid length, stretched length, depth of prepubic fat pad and circumference. They found that the size of the penis was significantly smaller after prostectomy. It supports observations of decrease penile length after radical prostatectomy and suggests that men should be counselled before radical prostatectomy, that penile shortening may occur.

"New insights into the pathogenesis of penile shortening after radical prostactomy and the role of postoperative sexual function," by P. Gontero, M. Galzerano, R. Bartoletti, C. Magnani, A. Tizzani, B. Frea, N. Mondaini (Universita degli Studi di Torino, Torino, Italy), printed in Journal of Urology, August 2007; 178(2): 602 – 7. This article is based on assessment of penile changes on 126 patients after radical prostatectomy, by performing serial penile measurements on them at catheter removal, three months, six months and 12 months postoperatively. It concluded that penile shortening occurs after radical prostatectomy and peaks at catheter removal and continues to a lesser but significant degree for at least a year. It suggests that age, nerve sparing surgery and the recovery of erectile function were independent predictors of the final changes in penile size and that these figures should be taken into consideration when counselling patients for radical prostatectomy.

My Experience

> In case you are wondering, and I'll bet you are, my erection capability began to surface within six months after surgery, although I did not recognize the limited erection I was experiencing as evidence of it. The reason I did not initially recognize it was because when my libido stepped in and sent warmth through my head and body I became aroused and my penis felt expanded, extended, and hardened, but it was only minimally so, compared with the same conditions prior to surgery. In addition, the little more than flaccid hardness never seemed to last very long. In fact, my mind was telling me that everything was working, based on my libido, through my brain and body, until I looked down and noticed that it was not translating into much physical result.
>
> The limited erection capability that I was experiencing was far from the level it was prior to the surgery. It was inconceivable to me that I should consider this as an erection. However, according to my urologist, the fact that limited capability occurred was evidence that the nerve bundles were spared and working, at least to some extent. I was therefore convinced that it would improve.

> By about a year after my surgery, my erection had improved somewhat. I was still concerned that it was not near its old self. I began to convince myself that this was the extent of erection that I could expect to achieve. At the same time, I was beginning to hear from specialists that it could take up to three years to return to its old self.
>
> Although the condition continued to improve with time, it took me awhile to accept that the once monstrous 'beast' of a penis would get harder and stay harder only with the aid of drugs. It took me even longer to accept that the erection I was achieving, still a fraction of its previous self, was as enormous as it would get. It seemed to have lost its ability to become as hard as a rock, stout and long. It looked so small in comparison to the monster it used to be.
>
> One might assume that this limitation could be due to a not-so-successful sparing of the nerve bundles, or that the penis, which is a spongy tissue, may have sustained some changes in the period it was not in use, and/or the *tethering* or new connection of the urethra to the bladder may have contributed to a small reduction in penis length, or perhaps a combination of some or all of these. Or maybe it's something entirely different.
>
> It became clear to me, a couple of years after my surgery, that the mediocre erection capability would probably be the best that I would achieve without some form of aid. So, as reality finally struck home, I have chosen to supplement my libido with the aid of prescribed drugs.
>
> One final note on this subject: you have to share your feelings, findings, understanding and decision-making with your spouse. This is not just your problem, or just your decision; it's your joint problem and decision.

Reality

Here is what I found out through my research, from talking to other survivors and from my own experience:

1. The fact that the penis could become firmer rather than just flaccid is a good indication to the surgeon that the nerve-sparing was successful. That's how the surgeon will consider it, even though it may be far from being really hard. This is a major concern for survivors. Most men assume that it's only a matter of a time before full erection capability returns to normal, meaning that it will be able to stand erect, tall and firm, as it did before the surgery. Don't count on that!
2. The penis, when erected, may not be able to stretch to the length that it once did. Some men experience an erected penis that's shortened in length and/or reduced in girth. The

removal of a portion of the urethra within the prostate gland and the tethering of the new connection of the urethra to the bladder may contribute to this shortening to an extent, but there must be other underlying factors such as scar tissue, trauma, lack of use and other unknowns.

3. Some of the small blood vessels or nerve bundles, or parts thereof, could get damaged and form scar tissue, which could prevent the blood from flowing with the same pressure to all parts of the penis. That, in turn, could prevent the erected penis from enlarging, expanding, hardening and reaching the full length, diameter, volume and shape. The beauty of the beast, as it was, would then never return. As one man described it: "It looks uglier and only a dwarf of its former self."
4. Because of possible scar tissue and perhaps other damages, the hardened penis may look bent, ill-shaped, asymmetrical and to some extent, out of proportion. Some of these conditions may also be attributed to Peyronie's Disease, caused by scar tissue in the penis. It happens in men who have not had surgery, and can occur or be exposed in some men after surgery.
5. There are several methods to achieve a firmer or harder erection, although not necessarily a physically longer erected penis, and more than likely not as satisfactory to the man and his spouse. These methods are:

- use of drugs,
- suction pump,
- injection, and/or
- *penile implant.*

To try any of these, one should consult a qualified and experienced urologist, who will refer you to the appropriate specialist. You shouldn't take anyone's word for preference of these – you have to try them yourself and decide which is the one you prefer. Everybody has a different taste and preference for each of these on a different scale.

Incontinence

Incontinence is the inability to control the flow of urine. This can range from an occasional leakage of urine to a complete inability to hold any urine.

The loss of bladder control, known as urinary incontinence, is a common occurrence after treatment for prostate cancer, especially prostatectomy, often causing embarrassment and frustration for most men.

Before surgery, the patient relies on the internal sphincter muscle, the prostate or the muscles around the prostatic urethra and to a smaller extent, the external sphincter muscle, to control urine. Surgery removes the prostate, the prostatic urethra, and bladder neck, which accommodates the internal sphincter muscle, leaving only the external sphincter muscle to control the flow of urine. The external sphincter muscle surrounds the membranous urethra. This is a major shift in urine control and this muscle requires training through exercise to function effectively. Therefore, for a while after surgery, you can expect to experience some level of incontinence.

The three types of incontinence that are likely to occur after surgery, are: urge, stress and overflow, although the most common is the urge. More than 50 percent of men will quickly regain complete control of their urination; however, approximately 20 percent will develop short-term urinary incontinence, and one to two percent will experience long-term, severe incontinence.

Urge incontinence occurs when there is a sudden intense need to pass urine because the bladder becomes irritated and goes into a "spasm," expelling urine involuntarily. Wetting oneself because of not getting to a restroom quickly enough is a sign of urge incontinence. Because the bladder cannot hold the normal amount of urine, patients may feel the urge to urinate every few hours, or that they have a very weak bladder. Wetting the bed at night is not uncommon.

Stress incontinence is caused when the sphincter muscle around the urethra is weak. In such cases, lifting heavy weights, getting up from a chair, coughing, laughing, sneezing, sitting cross-legged or exercising may cause urine to leak. It's caused by the excess load that is suddenly thrust upon the weak external sphincter muscle. You need to exercise that muscle regularly by doing Kegel exercises (see Chapter 42 of this book for methodology), walking, sit-ups or a combination of all. These need to be life-long activities. Many men can control the leaking during the night, but may leak when they get up in the morning. Going to the bathroom more often is a good way to avoid accidents.

Overflow incontinence occurs when the bladder fills up and is not emptied, so it overflows, causing a constant dribble. It's caused by scar tissue or blockage. Signs of overflow incontinence include getting up often during the night to urinate, taking a long time to urinate, urinating small amounts and not feeling empty, the need to urinate but being unable to, leaking urine throughout the day, and having a weak, dribbling stream with no force. If you experience these symptoms, you should immediately consult your urologist. He can help you.

Treatment of incontinence depends on the type, severity, and cause of the problem. Health care professionals can recommend exercises to strengthen the external sphincter muscle and medication if necessary.

Generally, with proper exercises, stress incontinence can be conquered within six weeks to six months. Other types may need to be treated with drugs, such as anti-spasmodics for urgency or with some other corrective procedures.

According to Dr. Walsh, the nerve-sparing technique expert, "In the hands of a skilled surgeon, the likelihood of long-term urinary control problems is less than two percent." Dr. Walsh is probably the most skilled surgeon in this field. However, other urologists, also highly skilled, back up this theory by achieving this success rate.

Almost all the men with whom I have spoken, who had radical prostatectomy, confessed that their incontinence never really left them completely. A sudden laugh, cough, shout, jerk, jump, bend or even sitting cross-legged, can cause a quick spurt of urine. For long periods everything will seem great, then suddenly the spurt happens and they do not feel completely continent. These are experienced in different situations and occasions, such as after consuming a glass or two of wine or a few slices of watermelon. These seem to act as muscle relaxants or provide lighter urine.

The important message here is to know yourself and exercise, exercise, exercise, otherwise always know where the washroom is located.

PSA Level After Surgery

After surgery, theoretically the patient's PSA level should be zero, because the prostate is completely removed and it's the prostate cells that produce PSA. However, many laboratories report the PSA level after surgery as less than (<) 0.01 or 0.05 depending on the measurement method. This means essentially "zero" or "undetectable," but it's important to take note of the "less than" or "<" symbol and not misinterpret the laboratory's report. The <0.05 is what we want, but 0.05 may be significant.

Sometimes, in order to spare the nerve bundles, a minute amount of prostate tissue may, inadvertently, be left behind; or the cancer may have been too advanced to be completely removed; or a cell or two may have escaped via the blood stream before the prostate was removed. Any of these can cause live prostate cells to still produce the antigen.

It's estimated that it takes a few days after the prostate is removed for the blood to rid itself of the PSA. If, after six months, the PSA level is much higher than 0.2 ng/ml, you may want to start considering some other therapy. Some surgeons consider a level of 0.05 ng/ml or higher after surgery to be an indication that somewhere in the body, some prostate cancer cells may be manufacturing PSA. If these cells are cancerous, they could grow and cause recurrence. Most specialists will say that if the PSA level is not moving up (accelerating) over time, there's nothing to worry about. However, if the PSA level rises, it's time to start considering further treatment.

Sometimes, if the pathologist finds that the cancer was extensive and the resection margins (edge of the specimen) show presence of cancer, or if the seminal vesicles were diseased, the surgeon may consult with a radiation oncologist to include radiation as an additional precautionary treatment. The surgeon may also suggest radiation after surgery even if the PSA remains under 0.2 ng/ml.

Recurrence

Recurrence may result from one or more cells being left behind in the *prostatic bed*, or from cells that had already escaped and set up micro-colonies elsewhere prior to surgery, or perhaps from cells left behind that were not removed or destroyed. The best way to avoid recurrence is by early detection and very quick action.

In 20 to 25 percent of cases, recurrence takes place within five years of surgery.

See the last chapter in this book (chapter 45) for an in-depth discussion on this important subject of recurrence.

How Much is Enough Experience

A friend of mine who lives in New York City visited a urologist – at my insistence – who diagnosed him with prostate cancer. The urologist offered to perform a bilateral nerve-sparing radical prostatectomy, admitting, as a result of my friend's questions, that he performs an average of one of these operations per week, and about 100 in total to date.

According to my urologist, who does three to five radical prostatectomies each week, this one per week and a total of 100 to one's credit's good credentials. He says that one such surgery per week is what most urologists would do.

In my opinion, for a surgery as delicate as radical prostatectomy, 100 performances is not that many. Nevertheless, I would want to know his record of success as it relates to risks and after-effects. That's one of the reasons why you must ask questions.

Bear this in mind – a surgeon performing LRP would have to be first very experienced in radical prostatectomy procedure. Likewise, a surgeon performing robotic-assisted laparoscopic would have to be pretty well experienced in LRP procedures. Both of these have a long learning curve, not to mention the excessive cost of the equipment. Thus it's understandable that these would only be conducted in centres where the equipment is affordable and the experience exists.

Conclusion

In conclusion, surgery is an option to be considered by any relatively healthy man with *localized* prostate cancer, whose aim is to achieve cure. If you decide to opt for surgery, you would be wise to understand your diagnosis, know the difference between each variation of surgery that's available to you, which variation you prefer and the experience and track record of your surgeon. Some people will travel a long way to have the surgeon of their choice perform the surgery. In such cases, if you are a Canadian resident it may cost you practically nothing if the surgery variation is standard and offered in your province. If you choose to have it done in the U.S., make sure you know if it's covered by your insurance or that you have sufficient money to pay for it. The same is true if you live in the U.S. or another country.

Cost

The cost of prostatetectomy in the year 2008 is between $20,000 and $45,000 U.S. depending on which procedure you choose and where you have it done. Your health care plan may cover this expense, particularly if it's done in your own state or province.

Chapter 31

EXTERNAL BEAM RADIATION

Challenges make you discover things about yourself that you never really knew.
They are what make the instrument stretch – what makes you go beyond the norm.

CICELY TYSON
ACTOR

Energy to Kill

Radiation treatment is the delivery of beams of high-energy particles or waves, such as x-rays, gamma rays, electrons, or protons, to the location of a patient's tumour. In the case of the prostate, it may be delivered from outside the body, referred to as **External Beam Radiation Therapy (EBRT),** or from within the body, referred to as **Internal Radiation Therapy (IRT).** This chapter will address EBRT and the next chapter will address IRT.

Radiation affects cells which are actively reproducing or multiplying, by damaging their genetic material or *DNA*. The radiation does not of itself kill the cells; however, since cancer cells multiply constantly and quickly, they are the ones that get damaged, whereas normal tissues, or cells that do not multiply, are spared.

The goal of EBRT is to direct radiation through the body to damage the cancer cells, or at least control their growth in the prostate. It accomplishes this by killing, or inactivating, the cells that the radiation comes in contact with. It's applied in such a way that damage to the surrounding skin and tissue is minimized. In the process, some surrounding normal cells are unavoidably damaged, and one may experience *radiation burns*. Fortunately, those damaged tissues will eventually heal.

Despite its penetration ability (like that of a beam of light from a flashlight), EBRT is painless, non-invasive, and one of the more popular therapies used to treat prostate cancer.

An estimated 20 percent of prostate cancer patients choose EBRT annually. This is attributable to several factors, such as, health condition, age, available expertise, stage of the cancer and others. The proportion is expected to remain the same, or rise slightly, in future years as the techniques continue to improved, even in the face of strong competition from other developing treatments.

History of EBRT

For many years EBRT was considered an alternative to prostatectomy, particularly for:

- men with advanced cancer,
- older men with other serious health problems, and
- men with large bulky tumours that were difficult to remove.

The early technology suffered many complications, including:

- radiation injury to the rectum (mainly bleeding),
- bladder irritation,
- urethra burning, and
- problems with control of the bladder and bowel.

As more precise state-of-the-art technologies emerged, EBRT became less damaging and, thus, gained increasing acceptance.

Current EBRT is safer and more efficient than its predecessors, thanks to advances in technology, technique, types of radiation and precision in delivery to the target, thus avoiding collateral damage to surrounding tissues or *organs*.

Most EBRT uses "high-energy linear accelerator machines," which emit the radiation in small packets of energy called *photons*. These machines, combined with state-of-the-art techniques, enable radiation oncologists and therapists to aim and deliver the radiation, in high doses, safely and precisely to the targeted organ, while sparing the healthy tissue and significantly reducing side effects.

Three of the more popular and recognized state-of-the-art techniques are the:

- Three-dimensional conformal radiation therapy (3D-CRT),
- Conformal proton beam radiation therapy (CPBRT) and
- Intensity modulated radiation therapy (IMRT).

Research is also being conducted on other techniques.

Three-dimensional conformal radiation therapy (3D-CRT) is an advanced form of EBRT where the tumour is mapped with imaging equipment and then treated with multiple beams of radiation from different directions. It takes a 3-D image of the tumour and surrounding organs, using a computed tomography (CT) scan, magnetic resonance imaging (MRI) and/or positron emission tomography (PET) and a targeting computer, so that the radiation oncology team can plan multiple radiation x-ray beams targeted to a shape that conforms exactly to that of the treatment area. 3D-CRT thus delivers the radiation, not as a box with fixed dimensions, but as a dosage conforming to a target the shape and size of the prostate. This technology allows the oncologist to aim high doses of radiation precisely at the target from different angles.

Conformal proton beam radiation therapy (CPBRT), uses a similar approach as the 3D-CRT, except that it utilizes proton beams instead of x-rays to kill the cancer. Protons are positive parts of atoms that cause little damage to tissues they pass through, but are good at killing cells at the end of their path. The protons travel through non-cancerous tissue and come to rest in the targeted area, where they deposit their radiation dose. This means that the proton beam radiation may be able to deliver more radiation to the prostate and do less damage to normal neighbouring tissue. This technique has a very limited offering as there are only a few of these expensive machines available. Also medical insurance may not cover this, as it's not yet widely accepted.

Intensity Modulated Radiation Therapy (IMRT), an advanced form of 3-D conformal radiation therapy, allows radiation oncologists to customize the dose by modulating, or varying, the amount of radiation given to different parts of the treatment area. The radiation intensity is adjusted with the use of computer-controlled moveable "leaves," which either block or allow the passage of radiation from certain selected beams that are aimed at the area. The leaves are carefully adjusted to the shape, size and location of the tumour. As a result, with IMRT, more intense or higher doses of radiation can be delivered to the tumour cells directly while less or lower doses are directed at adjacent sensitive areas such as the rectum, bladder and urethra, minimizing damage in these areas.

An analogy for IMRT is a shower nozzle that shoots several streams of water in different directions. Imagine each hole in the nozzle being able to shut off or on, or be set to adjust to different intensity and quantity, rather than a constant flow of equal intensity from each hole.

Administering EBRT

EBRT is administered by a *radiation therapist*, under the direction of a radiation oncologist. It's done in two stages: simulation (planning) and treatment.

Simulation, or the planning process, takes place on the first visit for treatment. In this process, the therapist "customizes" or prepares the area to receive the radiation. This is a process to map out the precise area of your body that needs to receive radiation and is similar with all forms of EBRT. You are asked to arrive at the treatment centre with a full bladder, so that it can be pushed out of the radiation path. The therapist will place you in the treatment position on the linear accelerator x-ray machine and strap you down with a body supporter to keep you from moving. He will then determine specifically what area is to be treated, and mark it. He may even make a mold of the area to be treated and put marks on the mold. These marks are small red lines or crosses, drawn on your skin, or the mold, using special ink, or tattooed dots that are permanent pin pricks in the skin. They will be used to position you precisely, during treatment, thus you will be required to protect those placed on your skin from washing off until you have received all your treatments.

After you are marked, you will be positioned in a specific manner and prepared for x-ray. For better visibility on the x-rays, a special dye may be squeezed into your urethra and barium into your rectum. You will be asked to breathe normally and stay very still. You will be x-rayed to locate the prostate, tumour, seminal vesicles and perhaps other areas, as well as to take measurements of some areas so that they can line up the radiation beam accurately.

Prostate cancer requires a high dosage of radiation in order to be lethal. To lighten the radiation toxicity and minimize potential damage to other organs and tissue, the dosage is divided into a number of uniform portions delivered regularly over about six to eight weeks, with the radiation being delivered for up to five minutes each day, five days each week for a total of up to 35 doses. A two-day rest period each weekend, allows normal body cells to recover from the effects of the radiation.

The radiation oncologist and his team use a special program to calculate the dose of radiation that will be delivered to the tumour and the surrounding tissue. They calculate how long the treatment beam must be left on to deliver the prescribed dose each time.

Treatment begins, on the second visit. Again you are asked to arrive with a full bladder for the same reason as above. You are placed in the treatment position on the linear accelerator x-ray machine in the same position as was used for the simulation, using the same immobilization devices. You are then positioned, using the marks that were made during simulation and alignment lasers. This can take considerable time and effort to get it right. It's important so be patient and cooperate. The therapist then goes outside the room to turn on the x-ray or radiation machine, which delivers the dose of radiation across the pelvic area. This is done daily for two weeks to destroy any cancer cells that may have escaped from the tumour inside the prostate, via the blood stream, and perhaps stuck to the pelvic bone and possibly the lymph nodes. For the subsequent two weeks, the focus of the treatment shifts to the tumour itself, then during the fifth week, pelvic radiation is administered again. The focus is returned to the tumour for the sixth and seventh weeks. The treatment is then considered complete.

The treatment may take 10 to 30 minutes each day, with most of the time used to position the patient.

Current EBRT techniques allow the therapist to deliver radiation beyond the prostate gland to the seminal vesicles and the side-walls surrounding the gland. Thus it reaches cancerous cells outside the prostate gland, as necessary.

The radiation beams travel through healthy skin, muscles and tissue to attack and kill the cancerous cells. They leave the prostate gland intact but damaged and shrunken. They also unavoidably kill or damage some normal cells in their path and unavoidably damage some other important tissues, nerve bundles and blood vessels, including tissues of the bladder, anus, rectum, urethra, intestines and overlying structures, despite protection.

During treatment, you will see your radiation therapist every visit, but you will see your oncologist only occasionally, perhaps once weekly to review your progress and respond to any questions that you might have. It would be a good idea for you to write down any questions that you might think of and take them with you to those visits.

When is EBRT Applied?

Any man, whose cancer is confined within his prostate gland, qualifies for EBRT, even if he is over 75 and especially if his PSA level is 10 or lower, Gleason score of six or lower and no extensive abdominal scar tissue from another situation. Those with significant chronic health problems who aren't suitable candidates for surgery may also qualify. It's also suitable for cancers that may have a limited spread beyond the capsule.

EBRT may be delivered:

   i) As an isolated treatment, or
   ii) Combined with other treatments, such as:

      a. *interstitial radiation,* (internal radiation or brachytherapy)
      b. radical prostatectomy or surgery (this first and then EBRT after), or
      c. hormonal therapy.

EBRT is generally delivered as an isolated treatment when:

   i) The patient has opted for radiation as his choice of treatment;
   ii) The patient is not a candidate for surgery, because of other health reasons and/or age;

iii) The cancer has not spread beyond the pelvic area; or
   iv) The cancer has not metastasized.

EBRT is delivered in combination with interstitial radiation (High dose rate), when

   i) The cancer is a high grade and may have spread and the interstitial radiation alone would not be sufficient to get the cancer cells outside the capsule.
   ii) The oncologist, in performing interstitial radiation, wants to ensure that in the event of any potential spread of the cancer cells they would be caught by the EBRT and killed.
   iii) It's the partner treatment that the specific cancer treatment centre offers.

EBRT is delivered in combination with, but subsequent to, surgery when there is evidence or likelihood that the cancer had extended beyond the prostate and surgery alone may not be sufficient to remove all the cells.

EBRT is delivered in combination with hormonal therapy:

   i) To have the hormone shrink the prostate prior to EBRT, or
   ii) When there is positive evidence or suspicion that the cancer has spread to other parts of the body. This is a relatively late stage cancer where EBRT is used to control the growth of the cancer, but is not working as a cure. The hormones are used in hope of controlling the cancer cells that have already spread elsewhere, or
   iii) For high grade cancer, where the hormone therapy is used to eliminate the male hormones in addition to radiation therapy. This is further explained in the Chapter entitled Hormone Therapy.

Side-Effects

Side-effects of EBRT during treatment, may include some or all of the following:

- loose bowels
- diarrhea
- fatigue
- urination urgency
- irritated intestines
- red dry tender skin
- some hair loss in the pelvic area

If these side-effects become too severe, treatment may be postponed or discontinued.

After-Effects

As treatment proceeds, the prostate may swell. At first, this may cause a narrowing of the urethra passage, resulting in a slow urine stream. Your radiation oncologist may prescribe a medication to relieve this problem. Later, scar tissue may form along the urethra causing further narrowing and affecting the passage of urine from the bladder. This is called urethral stricture. If it occurs at the neck of the bladder, it's called a bladder neck contracture. If you experience any of these, inform your radiation oncologist immediately. They can be treated.

Some short-term after-effects, experienced up to two months after treatment is completed, are:

- burning during urination
- frequency of urination
- the need or urge to urinate regularly at nights
- loose bowels or diarrhea
- skin irritation
- discomfort in the bladder, rectum, and urethra (commonly referred to as sunburn effect)
- rectal spasm or unawareness of losing bowel control (resulting in soiled underwear).

Some long-term after-effects that may not appear immediately, but may follow as long as a year after treatment is completed, may include:

- erectile dysfunction
- urinary obstruction or incontinence.

Another serious potential after effect is severe rectal damage, requiring corrective surgery, such as temporary colostomy, to allow the area to heal. Fortunately, this occurs in less than one percent of cases.

Erectile Dysfunction

Since the nerve around the prostate are in the path of the radiation beam, they are subject to radiation damage, which might result in shrinking, scarring and repairing, and could affect the functioning of the penile erection. More than 50 percent of men who choose EBRT experience delayed erectile dysfunction which slowly develops over a year after their EBRT. About 75 percent of men experience it within five years of treatment. The erectile dysfunction may improve with the aid of drugs prescribed by your physician.

The older the man is, the more likely it is that he will experience erectile dysfunction.

Incontinence

Incontinence may be experienced early, as the radiation begins to irritate the bladder muscles, causing frequent spasm and challenges in controlling urination. Later you may experience seepage, leakage, or sudden spurts. You might discover this when you suddenly laugh, cough, sneeze, or strain, or even when you sit in a meditating position with legs crossed, rise from sitting, run, or following any sudden jerk of the body.

Although this is less common than after surgery, sometimes it does not surface until years after treatment, leading some to suggest that the rate after six years is almost as high as that of surgery.

Most people will recover from incontinence eventually. The radiation oncologist can prescribe some anti-spasm medications to help relieve the problem, if it's severe.

About three percent of men who chose EBRT experience long-term incontinence.

PSA Level After EBRT

Prostate cancer treatment outcomes are generally predicted by PSA nadir levels in the years following the treatment.

Radiation therapy generally results in a gradual declining PSA level over a year to get to below 1.0 ng/ml. Thus it takes awhile to know if you are cured by EBRT, although, it's claimed that the 10-year success rate is virtually equal to surgery.

Generally, damaged DNA molecules in a cell are repairable, but sometimes they produce fatal damage, so when those cells divide into two cells (mitosis), the off-springs cells have fatally flawed genetic information and aren't viable cells. They either die at mitosis or peter out after a few generations. Hence, the life span of prostate cells may range from a few months up to a year or so. The cells with damaged DNA will continue to produce PSA until they die, so the PSA level after EBRT will decline gradually instead of instantly.

EBRT administered in conjunction with other treatment, such as hormone therapy, may speed the drop of the PSA level to 0.1 ng/ml or less to within a few weeks following treatment. However, this would be a result of the other treatment. Recognize that it will never go to zero, or undetectable, because with EBRT, the prostate is not entirely destroyed or removed.

Generally, one's concern is not whether they are responding to the treatment, but rather its long-term effects. That may take up to five years to realize. During that time, the doctor will continue to monitor the PSA levels periodically, but only after the entire treatment is completed and some time passes.

It's imperative that you track your PSA levels continuously after treatment. A temporary rise, or bounce (rise and subsequent fall) in PSA level should not be cause for concern, as it may be intermittent "bounce," occurring anywhere between one to three years after treatment. The magnitude of the bounce lies in the range of about 0.5 ng/ml to 2 ng/ml and may last for a few months to about a year. Having said that, monitoring PSA at intervals is necessary and if a consistent rise continues to occur, that should be cause for concern, because it likely means a recurrence is in process. Your oncologist will take care of this for you, but you should be aware of the consequences.

Recurrence

There is no guarantee that the radiation will get every single cancer cell in and/or around your prostate. If even one cancer cell remains alive, that single cell can trigger a re-birth or recurrence of the tumour. Unfortunately, if it recurs, you cannot return to radiation, since the tissue in the area cannot withstand additional radiation without causing serious damage or burn to the rectum, bladder, overlying skin and other tissues. If recurrence happens, other treatments, such as salvage prostatectomy, hormone therapy, and possibly salvage cryotherapy, are the treatment options.

Unlike all the statistics of successes for other treatments, the statistical successes of EBRT would probably not be comparable with those, since many of the patients treated with EBRT are older (73 years and up) or troubled by other health problems.

For a more in-depth discussion on recurrence, see chapter 45 of this book.

Advantages of EBRT

The major advantages of EBRT are:
- no incision
- no anesthesia
- no bleeding (no blood transfusion)
- less chance of immediate erectile dysfunction
- less chance of immediate incontinence
- no hospital stay
- not much discomfort

Disadvantages of EBRT

Disadvantages of EBRT include:

- fatigue
- long period of treatment
- risk of early bladder irritation
- risk of early bowel problem
- risk of rectal irritation (can be relieved by medication and/or enemas)
- possibility of blood in the urine
- diarrhea
- possibility of delayed erectile dysfunction
- possibility of urinary incontinence years later
- injury to rectal wall
- PSA falls too slowly over too long a period of time
- possibility of damage to healthy tissue near the prostate
- possibility of recurrence – if all cells not killed
- success cannot be determined until long after treatment

Conclusion

EBRT is an option to be considered by any relatively healthy man, with a localized (contained within the capsule) cancer, or cancer with limited spread, whose aim is to achieve cure. If you opt for EBRT you would be wise to ensure that your radiologist is using the most state-of-the-art tools and techniques and that he has the experience to utilize them.

Cost

The cost of EBRT in 2008 is approximately $30,000 to $40,000 U.S., depending on the technique used and the number of treatments received. Your health care plan should cover this expense, particularly if it's done in your own state or province.

Chapter 32

INTERNAL RADIATION TREATMENT

*"The road to happiness lies in two simple principles:
Find what it is that interests you and that you can do well,
and when you find it, put your whole soul into it –
every bit of energy and ambition and natural ability you have."*

JOHN D. ROCKEFELLER III

It's All in the Inside

Internal radiation treatment (IRT) is a minimally invasive procedure that's an alternative to EBRT. It's sometimes referred to as *interstitial* (within the tissue) radiotherapy which is the placement of radioactive sources or material directly into the cancerous area, and more commonly as brachytherapy (pronounced break–ee–therapy) which is interstitial, in that treatment is administered from within the tissue by an application of radioactive material that's delivered in or near the tumour. This method of treatment allows *radioactive* material to be placed in the part of the body to be treated. It puts the radiation right where the cancer is located.

The advantage of IRT over EBRT is that with IRT, the radiation is spread over a small area; the volume of tissue treated is limited; and surrounding normal tissue receives little radiation.

History of IRT

Internal Radiation Treatment dates back to the early 1900s, but because of problems encountered it was dropped from use until the 1970s when new methods were developed to overcome those. Initially it was not successful in curing prostate cancer, largely because the doctors were not able to see the internal areas of the prostate gland, making precise placement of the radioactive material difficult.

Advances in ultrasound imaging, particularly transrectal ultrasound (TRUS) and computerized tomography (CT), coupled with more innovative methods of implanting the radioactive material, non-surgically and uniformly, emerged in the 1980s. Their combined use has positioned IRT as a promising treatment. However, it was not until the early 1990s that it became widely accepted. Information on treatment effectiveness has now surfaced. Today, there are variations in the seeds and radioactive sources that make the treatments even more effective.

Currently, there are two major methods of IRT, namely:

- Seed implant (SI) which provides "permanent low-dose radiation (LRD)," and
- High dose rate (HDR) which provides "temporary high dose rate radiation."

1) **Seed Implant (SI),** or brachytherapy, utilizes 60 to 120 high energy radioactive seeds (tiny metal pellets) placed permanently into the prostate gland, each continuously emitting radiation at a low-dose-rate over an extended period of time.

2) **High Dose-Rate (HDR),** or rapid interstitial therapy utilizes five to 32 implantations of high-energy radioactive sources, transferred into the prostate gland, each emitting radiation at a high dose rate for short periods of time. These radioactive sources are withdrawn, initially, after a planned fraction of the treatment is completed, then after a specific period another fraction is applied.

Both methods work by emitting a specific amount of radioactivity to its immediate area. Ideally, when they are placed inside the prostate gland the radiation kills the adjacent cancer cells.

SI brachytherapy, has dominated non-surgical prostate cancer therapy in the U.S. since the mid 1980s. Its effectiveness for low-risk prostate cancer is widely accepted; however, because of limitations in delivering sufficient radiation to areas outside of the prostate capsule it's considered optimal treatment only for low-risk disease. With the invention of the *"remote afterloading"* machine (used to store radioactive material) in the late 1980s, treatment centres began to offer an alternate protocol utilizing HDR radiation temporary implants for higher risk patients.

In 1995 Andy Grove, the then CEO of Intel Corporation, selected HDR as his treatment choice after extensively researching available options.

> "Who is Andy Grove, you ask? He is one of three people most responsible for putting computers on our desks and in your home. (The other two are Bill Gates and Steve Jobs.) Without Intel's chips, the computer revolution wouldn't have happened, and without Grove,

Intel never would have managed the chip revolution as masterfully as it has. It was Grove who made Intel realize that "the PC is it," and it was his combination of managerial and technical expertise that put Intel inside so many PCs around the world."

Grove's prostate treatment story, printed in the March 13, 1996 Fortune Magazine, gained wide publicity, popularizing brachytherapy, especially HDR, as a good potential treatment. Today HDR is offered in many combinations of modalities.

How is IRT Applied?

IRT application varies from centre to centre; however, in general, SI is applied primarily as a stand-alone treatment (monotherapy), whereas HDR, although occasionally applied as monotherapy, is more commonly applied in combination with other treatments, as follows:

- Hormone therapy followed by HDR
- HDR followed by EBRT (combined radiation therapy)
- EBRT followed by HDR (combined radiation therapy)
- Hormone therapy followed by HDR followed by EBRT (triple *modality* therapy)
- Hormone therapy followed by EBRT followed by HDR (triple modality therapy)

Hormone therapy is generally administered prior to IRT to shrink the prostate.

The term "combined radiation therapy" has different meanings depending on how it's used. It may refer to combined radiation therapies, or combined hormonal and radiation (*neoadjuvant*) therapy. The same can be said for the term "triple modality therapy." Combined radiation therapy is based on the fact that the therapies give a more homogeneous treatment to the tumour, while delivering some radiation to the surrounding areas. Recent research suggests that they may improve survival. Triple modality therapy gives the added advantage of shrinking larger glands down to a manageable size before the prime treatment.

IRT, in one form or another, has become an attractive treatment to men with prostate cancer. It has been suggested that, in Canada and the U.S. alone, the number of men seeking IRT as their treatment is nearing or surpassing the number seeking surgery. Unfortunately, they don't all qualify.

How does a Person Qualify for IRT?

IRT is not for every prostate cancer patient. However, with the current trend towards early detection, more could become candidates. In fact, most patients who qualify for stand-alone IRT (IS and HDR monotherapy) have *low-risk* prostate cancer. They are generally younger men, under

75 years of age, with a low PSA (under 10 ng/ml), a slow-growing grade cancer (Gleason of six or less), an early stage confined tumour (T2b or better), and a prostate smaller than 40 cubic centimetres. These criteria vary depending on the treatment centre. A patient whose cancer does not satisfy all these criteria, or whose pelvis interferes with access to the prostate, will not be considered a suitable candidate.

Intermediate (PSA 10 to 19.9 ng/ml, or Gleason score of 7, or tumour stage of T2c) or high-risk (PSA 20 ng/ml or higher, or Gleason score of 8 to 10, or tumour stage of T3a or worse) prostate cancers are better treated with the more comprehensive strategies, such as combined radiation or triple modality therapy. These are conditions that have a higher likelihood that the cancer has spread.

Seed Implant (SI)

Seed implant (SI) brachytherapy provides for safe delivery of a higher dose of radiation to the prostate than EBRT, but at a low-dose rate. This is possible because it's delivered over an extended period of time – approximately 12 months.

There are three phases to SI treatment: planning, implantation and post implantation. Generally, the planning phase precedes implantation by about two weeks. The process, however, may vary somewhat from centre to centre.

The planning phase involves a series of preparatory tests, including blood tests, EKG, X-rays, and ultrasound volume study, to determine the exact shape, size, and location of the prostate, the tumour, and the position of the prostate gland with respect to the pelvis.

If you are having your SI done outside your home community, such as another or country, you may have to travel back and forth a few times, to get these tests done, or you may be allowed to have them done in your home area and the results forwarded to your radiation oncologist in advance of the implantation.

The ultrasound volume study is performed in the same way as ultrasound imaging for the biopsy, as is explained in "Chapter 14" entitled "Biopsy." However, in this case, it's being done mainly to:

- Get a picture of the shape and size of the prostate gland;
- Visualize the prostate and tumour;
- Calculate how many radioactive seeds are required, and where they should be placed;
- Determine if the implant is feasible, as occasionally the pelvis interferes with direct access to the prostate from the outside, rendering implantation of seeds impossible.

Part V Treatment Options

The results of the ultrasound volume study are transferred to a computerized treatment program, which determines the optimal number of seeds and their distribution, to achieve the proper dose.

With this knowledge, your medical team will be in a position to prepare an implantation map.

This implantation map is prepared to assist the medical team to select the appropriate radioactive seeds and lay out the optimal position of each seed within the prostate gland. It will also help ensure that virtually no radiation reaches adjacent organs, such as the rectum, bladder and urethra.

The implantation phase is conducted in the hospital or treatment centre. It takes about an hour. In some centres, a radiation oncologist and a urologist perform the procedure together. However, in other centres, the radiation oncologist may perform it without the urologist. Like most procedures, you will take a bowel-cleansing drink and subsequently refrain from consuming anything.

The procedure starts with either a local or a general anaesthetic. You will lie on your back in the dorsal lithotomy position. Your perineum will be shaved and cleansed with an antiseptic solution.

Your urologist may perform a cystoscopy to visually examine your bladder, prostate and urethra. A urinary catheter is then inserted into your bladder through your penis to keep it drained during the procedure. An ultrasound probe, connected to a computer, will be inserted into your rectum. Sometimes, a non-radioactive seed is initially injected into the lowest part of the prostate to serve as a reference marker for future CT Scans, or any EBRT planning that might follow.

Your radiation oncologist or urologist will then insert some hollow needles through the skin at your perineum to be used as conduits for implantation of the seeds. Up to 120 or more seeds may be implanted. Usually, three to five are delivered through each needle, requiring, on average, insertion of 20 to 25 needles.

As your radiation oncologist or urologist proceeds, he will have continuous visualization of your prostate on a monitor via the probe. As he implants each seed into your prostate, at different locations and to different depths, he will see them going in. This is advantageous as it allows him to better guide the placement of the seeds exactly as planned, for maximum effectiveness.

The seeds, each approximately the diameter of a pencil lead and about four millimetres long, are placed in rows and columns in a pre-planned three-dimensional matrix format, throughout the prostate gland. They are kept away from the area directly adjacent to the prostatic urethra, the rectum and the bladder, to avoid radiation damage to those areas.

The seeds are positioned as close as possible to the predetermined target areas, as once they are in, that's where they will remain forever, even after all the radiation has dispersed. Some centres use a special program that allows identification of the actual radiation fields. Thus, if a *cold spot* is detected, a new seed could be implanted to fill the gap. Using this methodology, superior implantation is achieved.

After the implantation phase is completed the **post-implantation phase** begins. By this time, all the seeds are firmly implanted. An X-ray is taken so that the process of counting and recounting the implanted seeds can take place. You are then taken to a recovery room, where an ice bag will be placed between your legs at the perineum, where the needles entered your body, to help reduce any swelling. You will remain in the recovery room until the anaesthetic wears off.

The urinary catheter will then be removed, and you will be sent home.

A follow-up CT Scan is generally done about four to six weeks later to document the distribution of the seeds and the radiation dose in the various parts of the gland.

The implanted seeds will remain in your prostate where they will dispense the prescribed radioactivity over the next 12 months.

High Dose Rate (HDR)

High dose rate (HDR) radiation treatment or rapid interstitial therapy, sometimes referred to as "smart bombed therapy," as popularized by Andy Grove, provides for the safe transfer of a high dose of radiation to the prostate at a fast rate for a fixed period of time. This is accomplished by the delivery of "fractions" of the overall dose for a 5 to 15 minute period, at intervals of six hours over the treatment period, or daily for about three days, depending on the treatment centre.

As with SI, preparing for HDR radiation treatment requires a series of tests, including blood tests and an ultrasound volume, to determine the shape, size, and location of the prostate gland and tumour.

Likewise, if the procedure is being done outside of your community, town or country, you may have to travel to get the tests done or have them done locally and the results forwarded.

Using information from the ultrasound volume, your radiation oncologist will calculate how many needles, or catheters, are required and where they should be placed, as well as what source material should be selected. He will then prepare a template for their insertion.

Part V   Treatment Options

The beginning of the HDR implantation phase is similar to that of the SI, but some specifics and tools may vary.

The procedure is conducted in a hospital or treatment centre. On the night before the treatment you will take a bowel-cleansing drink and subsequently refrain from consuming anything.

To begin the treatment, you will be placed under a local or general anaesthetic. You will lie on your back in the dorsal lithotomy position. Your perineum will be shaved and cleansed with an antiseptic solution and your legs will be draped in sterile gowns. An ultrasound probe, wired to a computer and supported by a cradle to keep it still, will be inserted into your rectum. The probe is adjusted until a good image of the prostate gland is visible on the monitor. A small square template, with 32 two millimetres diameter holes about five millimetres apart is attached to the probe and placed at your perineum. Guided by the ultrasound probe and the template, one non-radioactive seed may be injected into the lowest part of the prostate gland to serve as a reference marker when a CT scan is done later.

Next, using a removable metal insert, five to 32 hollow plastic needles, or catheters, will be inserted through the template and the skin of your perineum, into the prostate gland. The catheters may be about 24 centimetres long by two millimetres in diameter. The number of catheters inserted averages between 14 and 25, but they may be as few as five and as many as 32, depending on the size of the prostate and the practice of the treatment centre.

As the catheters are being placed, your radiation oncologist will see where they are going via the monitor. The goal is to get them placed along the sides and bottom of the prostate gland. They will stay clear of the urethra.

When all the catheters are in place, your oncologist will remove the ultrasound probe and then insert a cystoscope through your penis to your bladder. Your legs will be lowered to a horizontal position. Your radiation oncologist will then push each of the plastic catheters, one by one, until they are in connection with the wall of the bladder, which will be indicated by a bulge in the bladder, seen through the cystoscope. Thus he will know that the needles are pushed all the way through the prostate gland. The cystoscope is then removed and replaced with a urinary catheter.

The catheters will be connected to a computer-controlled remote afterloading machine. The location of each catheter is numbered and recorded in the computerized planning system, which determines the optimal dose of radiation to be delivered to each. Pre-determined dosages of high-energy radioactive source (material) will then be loaded into each catheter. The dosages that are near delicate areas, such as the rectum, bladder and urethra, will be limited to what those areas can tolerate in order to protect them from damage. A catheter that's too close to the urethra or rectum may deliver little or no radiation and one that passes directly through the centre of the tumour will deliver more. The delivery of the radiation to the cancerous cells is optimized by the computer software program, to ensure that it can be "heated up" in some areas, and "cooled off" in the delicate ones. It also ensures that radiation "clouds" from each source cumulatively cover the entire prostate.

During treatment, you will be alone in a shielded room, to protect others from radiation exposure. Your therapist will control the remote afterloading machine and computer from an adjacent room, where he will also monitor you via an audio/video system.

The delivery lasts for about 5 to 15 minutes, then the radioactive source is withdrawn. Thus the delivery of the first fraction of the dose is completed.

You'll then be transferred to the recovery room where you'll remain for about an hour, after which a CT scan of the prostate will be taken, in order to identify the prostate, as well as the rectum, urethra, and location and position of the catheters or needles.

This CT scan is critical for planning the dosages in each catheter, and achieving optimum dose distribution. It allows the radiation oncologist to see where adjustments are needed to each of the implanted catheters and to make final adjustments to each.

You may then be transferred to the hospital ward with the template and needles still in place. You may be told to lie still and not to sit up, in order to not disturb the needles.

Some centres will give a second dose, or fraction, of radiation in six hours, others do so a day later. Then the treatment might be repeated for a third time in six hours, or a day hence, and possibly in another six hours or a day. This is dependent on the schedule and the dosage, or fraction, chosen. With each procedure, a fraction of the total dosage is delivered. The same procedure that was used to transfer the radioactive source into each catheter, and emit the first fractional dose, will be followed each time.

Depending on your particular schedule and dosage – which is largely based on the analysis of your condition and your chosen treatment centre – you may or may not be brought back for the third and possibly a fourth dose. After your final session, the template and the catheters are removed. You will then be discharged within a few hours, and may resume normal activities soon thereafter.

Treatment Variations

Unfortunately, within the field of cancer treatment, there is ongoing debate on which IRT treatment can produce better results. This is so, despite the fact that different modalities may be best suited to specific cancer characteristics. Trying to make a selection can be confusing and frustrating for patients.

There are also variations in technique, technology and material (seeds and sources) from treatment centre to treatment centre. In fact both SI and HDR treatments aren't always offered at the same centre.

Often the choice between HDR and SI is easy to make, as HDR is generally better suited for higher risk cancers. The choice is usually recommended by the radiation oncologist, based on your cancer characteristics.

Monotherapy treatment is done in a few days and recovery and rehabilitation occur swiftly thereafter; however, if hormone therapy is added, it can add months, and sometimes years, to the treatment process. If EBRT is added to the equation, although its dose is only about half of what it would be on its own, it still is delivered over about five weeks. Bear in mind that all the side-effects and after-effects that come with each of these treatments individually, come with them cumulatively as well.

Seed and Material Source Variation

There are several types of radioactive material used for IRT. We'll not discuss them in detail in this book, since the patient hardly has a choice of which one to choose. But some of them are:

- Palladium 103
- Iridium 192 and Iridium 194
- Iodine 125 and Iodine 129
- Gold 198

Each emits a known amount of radioactivity. Some have a long radioactive life, but are weaker and cause less damage to tissues. Others have more energy and emit their radioactivity over a short period of time.

The dose of radiation is not a decision for the patient either. The radiation oncologist must be sure he is providing sufficient radiation to kill all the cancer cells. Generally, he will try to achieve a total dose of about 100 grays (Gy) or 10,000 centigrays (cGy) between the IRT and the EBRT (Grays is a measure of absorption of radiation energy – the absorption of one joule of radiation energy by one kilogram of matter).

What is important to know is that the delicate rectal wall situated just behind the prostate gland can only safely tolerate a limited amount of radioactivity. When that amount is reached, no more radioactivity should be delivered in that area, otherwise severe and permanent damage to the rectal wall will occur.

Armed with this information, the radiation oncologist, in conjunction with a physicist, can calculate exactly how much and what type of radioactive material is needed, and what dose to apply, to effectively treat a specific prostate cancer. The number of seeds implanted are dependent on their type as well as the size and shape of the prostate gland.

Success Rate

Variations of treatment, as well as variations in the radioactive material, are further complicated by the fact that the results aren't all based on the same standard of cure. In fact, very few published cure rates are based on the same conditions prior to treatment, such as age of patient, PSA levels, grade and stage of the cancer. This makes it difficult to get credible statistics on the cure rate and side-effects of each type of treatment.

Data on cure rates published up to the early 1990s vary, and may even be inflated in some instances, mostly because of a lack of standards. And to top it off, the available data only go back to 1992. Today, IRT in other formats, such as combined SI and EBRT, or HDR and EBRT, and even triple modalities are being used to treat high risk patients relatively successfully.

The question is not "Does IRT cure?" but rather, "How good is it in comparison to other treatment modalities in getting all of the cancer?" Some sources say that radioactive SI achieves a survival rate comparable to that of surgery, but others disagree. Some profess that HDR is even better. That begs the questions: "Based on what facts?" and "According to who?"

In a presentation made to the American Cancer Society's 42nd Science Writers Seminar in March 2000, it was reported that an observed 79 percent cure rate at 12 years was achieved for high-risk prostate cancer patients who received a combination of EBRT and brachytherapy.

In a study of 215 brachytherapy patients observed at one institution for up to 12 years, an overall cure rate of 70 percent was achieved. Eighty two of those patients were characterized as high-risk.

A leading radiotherapy clinic in Georgia presents the following statistics on five and 10-year cure rates achieved using a process called prostRcision, which is a combination of brachytherapy followed by EBRT, using a PSA level of 0.2 ng/ml as a *nadir* benchmark:

Part V   Treatment Options

PSA level Before Treatment	percent Cure after 5 years	percent Cure after 10 years
0 – 4 ng/ml	96	85
4+ – 10 ng/ml	94	85
10+ – 20 ng/ml	79	67
20+ ng/ml	71	34
Overall	89	72

According to Andy Grove, in his 1996 Fortune Magazine article:

- Surgery has a recurrence rate of about 31 percent
- EBRT has a recurrence rate of 27 percent
- SI Brachytherapy has a recurrence rate of 19 percent
- HDR rapid interstitial therapy has a recurrence rate of 14 percent

One must be very cautious in utilizing these data as we do not know who developed them or under what conditions. It may be like comparing apples to oranges.

Technology and techniques have also been improved and refined since Andy Grove's investigation, as has the expertise of the doctors, and the methods of collecting, reviewing and analyzing data. Also, we do not know the age of the patients, the PSA levels, and the grade and stage of the cancers prior to treatment. Nor do we know the elapsed time used to establish the data. There is still not sufficient years of track record available to come to a good comparative conclusion on these treatments.

So when you are quoted a cure or success rate for a recommended treatment, it's important to understand the benchmark used. You should also find out:

- If your radiation oncologist is experienced in administering the treatment.
- How long has your treatment centre been performing the procedure you are contemplating.
- If your radiation oncologist is quoting benchmark PSA nadir of 0.2 ng/ml.
- If the performance data you are being quoted is their own performance data or that of the industry.

And you should understand exactly what therapy is being recommended. Is it monotherapy, combined therapy or triple modality treatment? There are different consequences and time involvement attached to each.

Take the statistics for what they are worth. Practitioners of SI and HDR and other related treatments may be biased in choosing their patients, particularly in a free enterprise environment. Moreover, the numbers are reportedly based on the results of experts who may, because of popularity and expertise, have the opportunity to cherry-pick their patients. Furthermore, they aren't necessarily all using the same standards or benchmark for cure or success, nor exactly the same treatment.

Recently a steady PSA level of less than 0.5 ng/ml, and in some cases even as low as 0.2 ng/ml, for at least 10 years after treatment has become the standard benchmark for cure (PSA Nadir). In Canada many urologists work toward an undetectable level, meaning nearing zero. It would be even more beneficial for patients if consideration was also given to standards for continued erectile function, continued capability of successful sexual intercourse, and ability to maintain urinary control.

Post-Implementation Guidelines

Your radiation oncologist will provide you with post-implantation guidelines specific to your case and particularly for SI recipients, some of which may include:

- Do not let children sit on your lap.
- Avoid prolonged contact directly with, or within about six feet of, pregnant women.
- Expect to experience some level of sexual dysfunction toward the end of the radiation period.
- Do not be surprised if a few seeds spew out in the early days after implantation, particularly in your urine or occasionally in your semen during intercourse (It has been known to happen).
- Expect some urination difficulties, such as slow stream or difficulty starting. Your physician may prescribe medication, such as an alpha-blocker for a few weeks, to help with this.

> An acquaintance of mine who opted for SI Brachytherapy had 76 seeds implanted. Within four weeks, he spewed out three of those seeds in his semen during ejaculation. Yes! He was able to function normally and adequately for months after. However, as he anticipated, his level of erectile functioning began to wane by the end of six months. The question to ask is: "Could the removal of these three seeds create a pocket for cancer cells to hide themselves safely from the radiation?"

Advantages

IRT procedures have several advantages over some of the other treatments, which include:

1. The radiation material used can deliver much more concentrated radiation than EBRT.
2. SI is a one-time procedure.

3. SI procedure is done in short order and with only a brief hospitalization to recover from anaesthesia. In fact, it can be conducted in an out-patient setting and within two to three days you can be back to your normal routine.
4. SI kills cells as they are dividing. This is because the implanted seeds give off radioactivity continuously for several months, instead of giving off a one-time radioactive blast. So the radioactivity gets the cancer cells as they multiply.
5. Lesser chance of erectile dysfunction, incontinence and urinary side-effects, initially.
6. As monotherapy, IRT procedures result in virtually no incontinence, except occasionally due to weakening of the urethral sphincter muscle; however, when SI is combined with EBRT, incontinence may be more severe.
7. IRT procedures do not destroy the seminal vesicles or other reproductive organs. This means that ejaculation can be achieved during intercourse subsequent to treatment, even though your capability of having an erection might be diminished in later years.
8. No surgical incision is required, so bleeding is minimal, and therefore there is practically no requirement for blood transfusion (note: even with surgery, requirement for blood transfusion is uncommon, usually only about one in 50 to 100 cases) – I was one of those. However, since needles are inserted up to 30 times in the perineum, there is a chance of some bleeding.
9. The doses of applied radiation are concentrated in very small areas, therefore the volume of tissue treated is limited, and the surrounding normal tissues and organs receive a lower dose of radiation than they would with EBRT; thus no damage is expected to these areas.
10. The HDR radioactive source are also capable of reaching extra-capsular cancer that has broken through the prostate gland and into the neighbouring tissue, or extended up in the seminal vesicles.
11. With HDR the radioactive source as well as the catheters or needles are removed at the completion of the application, thus nothing is left in the body after the procedure.
12. Side-effects, such as nausea, hair loss, or diarrhea, which commonly result with other treatments, are non-existence with IS or HDR.
13. No special dietary considerations or major pre-treatment preparation is required.
14. Recovery time is minimal.

Disadvantages

Some identified disadvantages of IRT procedures include:

1. SI seeds cannot be removed after they are implanted.
2. Some SI seeds may migrate to other areas of the body via the blood stream, or out of the body via the urine or semen.
3. SI seeds that aren't injected into the planned position cannot be compensated for, which can result in "cold spots" and reduce chances of a cure.

4. With SI, there is not much control over where the dose goes, which may result in an inability to give more radiation to the tumour itself, as well as to treat outside the prostate gland.
5. The possibility of erectile dysfunction exists 25 to 61 percent of the time, and may increase with time, although this generally surfaces after treatment is completed.
6. There is a strong possibility of irritation of the bladder and rectum, especially during the first few weeks for the bladder, resulting in voiding difficulties.
7. The lymph nodes aren't evaluated for presence of cancer, which could prove serious, if they are later found to be cancerous.
8. The back wall of the rectum can take only a limited amount of radiation, dictating the quantity of radiation given in that area.
9. After the procedure the treatment may still have to be supplemented with EBRT and/or hormone treatment.
10. Long-term results are still unknown, especially for HDR, since the track record is still too short for adequate analysis. About 12 to 15 years is required to establish a track record.

Possible Side-Effects

Possible side-effects resulting from IRT, include:

- Early incontinence
- Daily fatigue
- Some bloating
- Erectile dysfunction (Even though this may not begin to show for months after treatment This might be because of the time it takes for the radiation to reach, and do harm to, the neurovascular nerve bundles outside the prostate.)
- Local discomfort from swelling and bruising of the perineum

Concerns

The major concern reported regarding IRT is that, because of the spacing of the seeds and radiation sources, and the variability of human delivery and movement of the prostate, it sometimes produces "cold spots," small areas that may get missed by the radiation cloud and where cancer cells may survive.

Testimonials

When I investigated IRT brachytherapy as an possible treatment for myself, I was informed that my PSA level, which had jumped above 10 ng/ml, to 11.5 ng/ml, disqualified me. Thus, I was discouraged from further investigating it as a possible treatment. Later, I discovered that I would have been accepted at other clinics, particularly in the U.S. In fact, at some treatment centres I would have been given HDR and in others, a combined treatment. That's not to say that I would have been cured, because they would probably have used a different type of energy source, which could have made the results less certain.

One man reported that he had *radioactive seeds implanted* in October 1998. By June 1999, his PSA had dropped to its lowest reading of 2.5 ng/ml. In October 1999, it had risen to 3.1 ng/ml and a reading in January 2000 showed 5.1 ng/ml. In April 2000, it was 7.1 ng/ml. Obviously, he was not cured and was experiencing a recurrence. In an ideal world, one would be able to feel that when the treatment is complete, he is cured. Unfortunately, none of the therapies can offer such a guarantee.

Several other men, particularly those who experienced HDR treatments, and others who had a combination of HDR and EBRT, have maintained an undetectable or low PSA level for years after treatment.

Many experts feel that HDR radioactive treatment is a good option for younger men with more aggressive or high-risk localized cancer.

A colleague, who maintains a very busy schedule, had the HDR treatment or "smart bombing" at a clinic in Seattle, Washington in 1996. Today, more than 10 years later, he's doing well and is very satisfied, with no sign of recurrence. However, it should be stressed, that his experience alone is not sufficient for generalization.

Some other experts feel that, overall, HDR followed by EBRT is even more effective. HDR followed by EBRT is designed to treat intermediate or high-risk cancers. Monotherapy is used only for low risk cancer. Remember that the side-effects of the combined SI or HDR and EBRT, may be cumulative. Also remember that the EBRT procedure is the same as previously described, except that in this case the dose is substantially less. So you will experience all those side-effects.

Where Is IRT Performed?

IRT is performed at several major health centres in the United States and Canada. However, if you feel that you would like to have IRT as your treatment and you are turned down by one centre, because of the stage of your cancer or the level of your PSA, you may want to investigate further at another centre, since each might have different criteria or may offer combinations of therapies.

Be reminded that the health care systems of Canada and the United States differ vastly, and their approaches to treatment and marketing their services differ accordingly. The health care system in the U.S. encourages free enterprise, resulting in private for-profit institutions which aggressively market their services. The Canadian system is not based on free enterprise and does not encourage aggressive marketing of services. The approach in other countries may also differ. If nothing else, the U.S system lends itself to innovative approaches and establishes a challenge for its Canadian counterpart, which sometimes loses prospective patients to alternative treatments across the border.

Cost

The cost of IRT in 2008 was approximately $20,000 U.S. for monotherapy to $45,000 U.S. for HDR triple modality. Your health care plan may cover this expense; however, it might be wise to check this first, particularly if you will be having the triple modality done in another country.

Chapter 33

HORMONE THERAPY

"Champions aren't made in gyms. Champions are made from something they have deep inside them – a desire, a dream, and a vision. They have to have the skill, and the will. But the will must be stronger than the skill."

Muhammad Ali

The Magic of Testosterone

Hormone therapy, also known as "androgen-deprivation therapy (ADT)," or "androgen suppression therapy," is one of the older forms of treatment for prostate cancer at various stages. It's accomplished by the surgical removal of the testicles (orchiectomy, more commonly known as "surgical castration" or simply "castration"), or the use of drugs.

Hormone therapy is based on the premise that prostate cancer cells survive by feeding on the testosterone – eliminate the testosterone and most of the cancer cells will die. Almost 95 percent of a man's testosterone is produced by his testicles. The other approximately five percent is produced by his *adrenal glands*, which are two small glands located on top of the kidneys.

The two methods of administering hormone therapy are:

- Surgical removal of the testicles (orchiectomy or castration).
- Using drugs (non-surgical methodology), taken orally or by injection, to:

  i) Stop the production of the male hormone testosterone, produced by the testicles
  ii) Reduce the production of testosterone produced by the testicles
  iii) Block the action of the testosterone

Each contributes to extending life and relieving symptoms although with different side-effects.

Testosterone's major functions are to:

1. Develop male sex characteristics, such as growth of body hair, deep voice, develop the penis, provide libido (sex drive) and the maturation of sperm.
2. Accelerate muscle build-up, regeneration, help with recovery after injuries and burning of body fat.
3. Stimulate bone growth.
4. Regulate prostate gland.

Unfortunately testosterone also feeds cancer cells.

The level of testosterone production peaks during puberty and begins to decline at about age 23, although its decline is slower than its rise.

Since testosterone also provides the libido that creates sexual desire, when you eliminate the testosterone, you also eliminate the man's sexual desire or sex drive.

History

Hormone therapy dates back many decades, when orchiectomy, or surgical castration, was the primary method of treating patients whose prostate cancer had metastasized. Since most testosterone is produced in the testicles, doctors sometimes simply cut out the testicles as a cure. Its goal was to stop the production of testosterone and thus stop feeding the cancer with testosterone produced in the testicles. The premise was that by removing the testicles, you are removing the source of 95 about percent of the cancer's "food," which effectively resulted in reduction of testicular androgens. Unfortunately, surgical castration resulted in some side-effects, including adverse psychological factors.

Some patients misunderstand when it's suggested that their testicles be removed as hormone therapy for their prostate cancer. They quickly think it's suggested because the cancer may have spread, or is spreading, to the testicles.

Orchiectomy or surgical castration, is still done today; however, approaches to hormonal therapy have evolved significantly over the last several decades and we now have several drugs that can achieve the same results – counteracting the testosterone produced in the testes. These drugs essentially cause an equivalent to castration, thus chemical castration. The major advantage is that unlike surgical castration, chemical castration can be reversed by simply discontinuing the drug treatment.

Part V   Treatment Options

To get to the stage where we could invent and develop those drugs, researchers had to first learn how to isolate the testosterone. That was achieved in 1935 by German biochemist, Dr. Adolf Butenandt (1903 – 1995). Then, in the 1940s new discoveries provided enhancements in the use of hormone drug therapy which offered a ray of hope for survival or prolonged life to patients with advanced prostate cancer.

Starting with Canadian-born Dr. Charles Brenton Huggins (1901 – 1997), born in Halifax, Nova Scotia and a professor of surgery at the University of Chicago, who made medical history by successfully interrupting the body's hormonal interactions to slow or stop the growth of cancer cells. He showed that surgically removing the testicles or suppressing their testosterone action with medication, such as the female hormone estrogen, could turn off the hormonal fuel that feeds the malignant cells.

Dr. Huggins and a colleague, Dr. Clarence V. Hodges, applied their hypothesis to the benign enlarged prostates of dogs, the only other animal known to develop cancerous tumours in the prostate. They removed the dogs' testicles to have their prostate glands shrunk, then injected them with hormones, before measuring their re-growth. Their findings not only confirmed testosterone's role in the growth of the dogs' glands, but also suggested that men's prostates could be similarly manipulated.

In clinical research that followed, Huggins, Hodges and others confirmed that malignant prostate cells had a similar dependence on hormones. Castration and/or doses of female hormones, such as estrogen, suppress the testosterone action and slow or check the growth of the tumour. Estrogen fools the brain, by telling it, there is enough sex hormones in the system, which drives the body to stop producing male hormones.

Although Huggins introduced the use of female hormones or estrogens, which also suppress androgen production, it's not often used today, despite its effectiveness and economic advantage over other anti-androgens. It works just as well as the other hormones and is much cheaper, but the side-effects are more significant, including: higher risk of heart problems, blood clots in the legs, high blood pressure, and fluid retention (usually ankle swelling).

In a paper entitled, "The Effect of Castration, Estrogen, and Androgen Injection on Serum Phosphatases in Metastatic *Carcinoma*s of the Prostate," Drs. Huggins and Hodges introduced androgen deprivation as therapy for advanced prostate cancer, confirming the hormonal influence on the cancer and the dependence of the male hormone especially testosterone, by the human malignant cell. This opened a whole new world of treatment, knowledge and further research which resulted in hormone therapy becoming, more or less, the definitive approach to prostate cancer therapy.

This historic discovery benefited many terminally ill patients who, previously without recourse, were given some temporary, even prolonged, symptomatic relief. It also earned Drs. Huggins and Hodges the 1966 Nobel Prize in Medicine.

Hormone therapy remained the gold standard of prostate cancer treatment for almost 25 years, but even with this enhancement, the death rate did not appear to decline. Then it was discovered that prostate cancer is composed of both "hormone-dependent" and "hormone-resistant" cells. Deaths were continuing as a result of the hormone-resistant cells.

The Veterans Administration Cooperative Urological Research Group (VACURG) in the U.S. provided data and guidelines for the use of orchiectomy (surgical) and estrogen (non-surgical) treatment, based on observation of a large number of men between the years 1960 and 1975.

One of the first non-surgical treatment option was a semi-synthetic estrogen compound called diethylstilbestrol (DES); however, due to the potential for significant cardiovascular toxicity in higher doses, its use has been limited.

Then in the 1980s, *luteinizing hormone-releasing hormone* (LHRH) agonists and

anti-androgens were developed and introduced. These compounds have been evaluated for use in advanced disease therapy as well as in *adjuvant therapy* (following major therapy) and neoadjuvant therapy (prior to major therapy).

Hormone therapy drugs, such as LH-RH agonists, are administered to reduce or prevent the production of testosterone and are injected, into the patient's buttocks or abdomen, monthly or quarterly, or implanted yearly. They act on the *pituitary gland* in the brain, which controls hormone production, to prevent it from releasing hormones that stimulate the production of testosterone in the testicles. The injections can be done in the doctor's office or at a cancer treatment centre and may be supplemented by anti-androgen drugs (pills), taken daily to block the body's ability to use other testosterone produced by the adrenal glands.

The introduction of the LH-RH agonists, the two most common being "leuprolide" and "goserelin," revolutionized the treatment of advanced prostate cancer and provided an enhancement to chemical castration; however, it also resulted in a side-effect – testosterone "flare" or "surge" which, most times, resulted in a worsening of bone pain, urinary obstruction, or other symptoms attributable to rapid cancer growth.

The testosterone flare or surge is, a short period of apparent cancer growth, caused from the "agonist" compounds stimulating the body to release more male hormones, for that period of time. Soon thereafter they disrupt the brain's control of androgen release, which results in stoppage of testosterone production.

Part V Treatment Options

In Canada, a steroidal progestational anti-androgen, called "cyproterone acetate" (CPA) is used as monotherapy or as an agent to prevent the flare during initiation of LHRH agonist therapy. CPA blocks the androgen-receptor interaction and reduces serum testosterone through a weak anti-gonadotropic action. Unfortunately, it's also associated with cardiovascular complications, although it's generally well tolerated.

Recently, *gonadotropin-releasing hormone* (GnRH) antagonists, have been investigated for use. Abarelix, one of the new, modified GnRH antagonists, is a pure GnRH antagonist that blocks the anterior pituitary receptor, resulting in prompt and significant reduction of luteinizing hormone. This results in castration levels of testosterone while avoiding the testosterone flare.

Based on observations, it's been suggested that androgen deprivation may induce a remission in about 80 to 90 percent of men with advanced prostate cancer and may result in a median progression-free survival of one to almost three years, at which time, an apparent androgen-independent condition may emerge, which then leads to a slightly extended overall survival of a little over three years from the start of androgen deprivation treatment.

As it did in the days of Dr. Huggins, 65 years later prostate cancer still progresses to a *hormone-refractory* stage and among the current debates are the value of the use of:

- Monotherapy (one drug or form of treatment – drug or surgical-castration) versus Combined Hormone Therapy
- Early versus late hormonal deprivation
- Continuous versus *intermittent androgen deprivation.*

However, as indicated earlier, the cancer will eventually become resistant to the drugs. This is because a small number of prostate cancer cells aren't responsive to hormones.

The theory is that the majority of the cancer cells do respond and die, leaving behind some "insensitive" cells which then grow unchecked. Those are the cancer cells that become resistant to hormones. Therefore, hormone therapy is not actually a cure, but rather a temporary measure to stop the cancer growth, effective for an average of three to five years before the cells becomes hormone-resistant.

One would most likely see a fast drop in the PSA level with hormone treatment, but that would not signify a cure. When the PSA starts to rise again, in spite of the hormones, it usually means the cancer is now hormone-resistant.

Hormone therapy works anywhere in the body and therefore is most commonly used on cancer that has spread outside, or well beyond, the prostate gland (Stages N+ and M+ or T3 and T4). It's the first line of treatment, for metastasized prostate cancer.

In some cases, hormone therapy is used in combination with other treatments. For example, in advanced stages, when the cancer has spread beyond the prostate (Stages N+ and M+ or T3 and T4), it can be used in combination with palliative radiation therapy. At these stages, surgical removal of the prostate is not advisable.

Hormone therapy is also applied to reduce the size of the tumour and the prostate itself, in preparation for brachytherapy, EBRT, radical prostatectomy or cryotherapy (see next chapter).

It's also used sometimes in combination with radiation on patients with high risk (high Gleason score) cancers that are still considered confined to the prostate. It may be given for two to three years and then discontinued for observation.

Research has shown that aggressive treatment of the prostate cancer with combined hormone therapy and EBRT, plus long-term hormonal suppression, will significantly increase life expectancy and cancer-free survival.

Intermittent Approach

Because prostate cancers treated with drugs become resistant to the drugs over a few years and occasionally in as little as a few months, some doctors stop the treatment temporarily after the PSA drops to a very low level and remains stable for awhile. This therapy "interruption" allows the testosterone levels to recover, although its main aim is to relieve the patient of the side-effects for a period of time. It's referred to as a "drug holiday," as it provides some relief from side-effects such as erectile dysfunction, hot flashes, and loss of sex drive. The interruption may also provide the benefit of prolonging the usefulness of therapy.

If the PSA level begins to rise again, the drug delivery is resumed. This off again – on again, or "intermittent" therapy is considered experimental. It's a relatively new approach and it's still too early to say if it's more advantageous than the "continuous" approach. It may still be applicable to patients with prostate cancer who have to undergo long-term therapy.

Early studies of the intermittent approach show that patients with advanced prostate cancer found this method acceptable. It did not appear to have an adverse impact on survival and the majority of patients who had experienced erectile dysfunction as a result of the standard treatment resumed sexual activity during the "drug holiday."

Side-Effects and After-Effects

The down side of hormone therapy is that, whether you retain your testicles or not, it deprives you of the effects of testosterone, and produces undesirable physical and psychological after-effects. For example, as a result of decreased testosterone, men may:

- Lose libido (sex drive)
- Lose their ability to achieve and /or keep an erection.
- Lose muscle mass.
- Gain breast tissues (breast swelling), a symptom referred to as "gynecomastia."
- Suffer from fatigue.
- Experience hot flashes.
- Experience blood clot in the legs
- Suffer from mood changes.
- Experience long-term problems resulting from loss of bone mass, leading to osteoporosis or brittle bones
- Experience anemia (low blood counts).
- Change in the blood lipid picture (less favourable with more bad cholesterol and triglycerides).

Patients, who receive anti-androgen drugs, may also experience nausea, vomiting, tenderness and swelling of the breasts. You must follow the direction of your specialist, because some of these drugs may increase risk of heart problems, particularly if you have a history of heart disease.

Advantages

Some advantages of hormone therapy are its:

- Capability to reduce the size of the prostate
- Potential to help extend life
- Potential to help enhance the success of other treatment
- Ability to quickly halt the cancer growth
- Ability to provide symptomatic relief from pain and obstruction of the urinary tract.

Disadvantages

In addition to the side-effects mentioned, some adverse effects of hormone therapy, include:

- Diarrhea
- Insomnia

- Liver function change
- Psychological effects
- Perceived low quality of life

Precaution

A major concern of prostate cancer treatment is the potential under-estimation of the condition. Based on results of pathology tests done on surgically removed prostates, up to 40 percent of all cancers, which were thought to be confined within the gland, had actually penetrated the capsule. Therefore, the successes of radical prostatectomy, EBRT, IRT, and cryotherapy may be compromised by the inaccuracy of the cancer staging. As a precautionary measure, some doctors who use these treatments complement them with hormone therapy, depending on the risk factor, especially for high grade aggressive cancers with Gleason score of 8, 9 or 10..

Hormone Therapy is offered at almost every major hospital throughout the world.

Cost

The cost of hormone therapy in 2008 is approximately $20,000 U.S. per year for LHRH agonist injections and about $7,000 per year for anti-androgen pills. In Canada and the United States, it's usually covered by health care plans, private drug plans or seniors' drug plans. Some provinces in Canada may restrict the use of certain "brands" of LHRH agonists.

Hormone therapy is one of the biggest single expenses to the health care systems, as many patients are on medication for long periods. In contrast, surgery or radiation are one-time expenses.

Chapter 34

CRYOTHERAPY

*"When we learn to say a deep, passionate 'yes' to the things that really matter...
then peace begins to settle onto our lives like golden sunlight sifting to a forest floor."*

THOMAS KINKADE

Freeze It

Cryotherapy, or *cryosurgery*, or *cryoablation*, also known as "freeze therapy," is a procedure that destroys cancerous and non-cancerous tissues by exposing them to extreme cold temperatures.

Cryotherapy has been performed on tissues, such as the skin (most common), liver, kidney, prostate, and breast. In some cases, such as the liver, an incision is made and the cold temperature is applied directly to the tissue.

For prostate cancer, cryotherapy is a minimally invasive treatment. It's the freezing of prostatic cells, normal and abnormal, by subjecting them directly and swiftly to subzero temperatures.

Brief History

Cryotherapy had its early beginning in Brighton, England in the 1840s, when Dr. James Arnott applied ice-salt mixtures to breast and cervical cancer through hollow tubes, to reduce complications, particularly pain.

It was applied transurethrally a hundred years later, in the 1960s, to treat BPH. Soon after, it was offered as a treatment for prostate cancer as what has been referred to as "first generation of cryotherapy." That was subsequently followed by the open transperineal (through the skin at the perineum) approach in 1972. Because of serious technical and physical complications, the open transperineal approach was abandoned, but re-introduced in 1988, taking advantage of technological advances making up the "second generation of cryotherapy," including:

- transrectal ultrasonography, to visualize the placement of cryo probes (hollow needles) or cryo-needles and monitoring the freezing, and
- a more reliable liquid nitrogen circulation system.

Since then, the technique has been further refined to "third generation of cryotherapy," using:

- advanced transrectal ultrasound visualization guidance techniques,
- advanced cryo technologies,
- liquid argon (for freezing) and helium gas (for thawing),
- thinner cryoprobes or needles (17 gauge or 1.5 mm), and
- sophiscated prostate ultrasound scanning techniques.

Qualifications

Although it's a minimally invasive procedure, it requires expertise in prostatic ultrasound scanning, cryo-needle placement and ice-ball formation monitoring.

Prostate cryotherapy, or cryosurgery, is sometimes referred to as "percutaneous (through the skin) cryosurgery of the prostate."

It's considered appropriate for:

i) Men with prostate cancer that's confined to the gland. (It's not recognized as first-line treatment in Canada, as long-term results aren't available. However, it's fairly widely accessible as first-line treatment in the U.S.)
ii) Men who haven't had prostate surgery previously, including TURP.
iii) Men with certain serious medical conditions that make them unable to tolerate surgery or radiation.
iv) Men whose prostates are 40 grams or less, as measured by ultrasound.
v) Older men for whom radical prostatectomy might prove too risky.
vi) Men whose prostate cancer indicates high risk factors, such as a stage T1 – T3, PSA>10, and Gleason score >6.
vii) Treatment of recurrent prostate cancer, after initial treatment with EBRT, SI or SDR has failed. It's then considered as an alternative to: surgical removal of the gland, hormonal treatment, and watchful waiting and is referred to as "*salvage therapy*." (See the last chapter in this book on "Recurrent Prostate Cancer.")

It should be noted that patients with distant metastasis or lymph node involvement do not qualify.

The Procedure

Cryotherapy involves freezing the prostate gland to a solid mass, which is expected to kill all the tissue in the frozen gland. Various experiments have shown that minus 40 degrees centigrade is the level of temperature that kills cells. As the cells freeze, ice crystals begin to form inside them, drawing out water, which ultimately leads to cellular dehydration and their ultimate destruction. As thaw takes place, the ice melts and the water's position shifts, causing cell damage, destruction or death.

As simple as that procedure may sound, it's essential that proper pre-planning and preparation take place.

Prior to the procedure, x-rays and ultrasounds are taken to determine the exact size of the prostate gland, the extent and location of the tumour, and the status of structures such as the seminal vesicles. Routine preoperative blood work and a chest X-ray are also required. Similarly, a bone scan and a CT scan of the pelvis are necessary – to confirm that the cancer has not spread. In some cases, sampling of the lymph nodes is also recommended.

If the prostate gland is larger than the preferred working volume of 40 grams, you may be placed on three to six months of hormonal agents to shrink it before cryotherapy is performed.

You will be asked to refrain from consuming anything after a certain time the previous day. You will also be asked to take a bowel-cleanser the previous night and to empty your bowels before you are admitted.

Your surgical team, made up of an anaesthetist, a urologist, and sometimes a radiologist and ultrasound technician, will conduct the same type of ultrasound volume study as is done for radiation treatment. They will then develop a plan, mapping out the exact placement, including the depth, for each cryo-needle.

The anaesthetist will put you under either a "spinal" or "general" anaesthetic. Many doctors prefer the spinal for this procedure as a general anaesthetic results in a longer-lasting sedative effect and longer recovery.

You will lie on your back in the dorsal lithotomy position with your legs raised and your ankles supported in stirrups. Your skin, at the perineum, will be shaved and cleansed. A warming catheter will be inserted through the urethra, via the penis, and a heating substance, consisting of warm salt water, or equivalent, will be circulated through it. This is to prevent damage from the freezing to the urethra and its neighbouring muscles, including the external sphincter muscle.

The bladder will be kept drained via a tube called a *suprapubic* catheter, inserted through a skin incision on the abdomen and into the bladder. This is done so that if the prostate swells and squeezes the urethra after the procedure, urine can be drained through this tube.

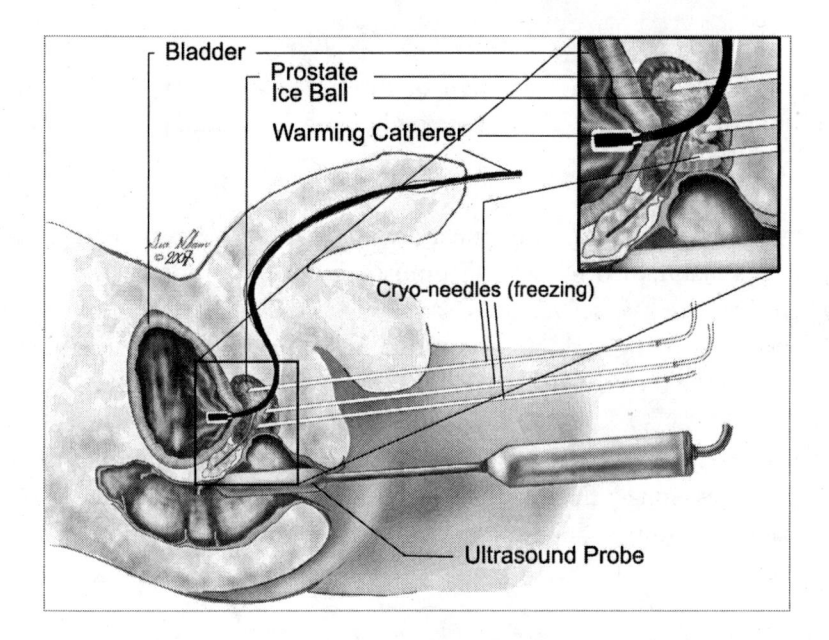

Your physician will insert an ultrasound probe, connected to a computer, into your rectum. Guided by the transrectal ultrasound (TRUS), he will insert five to eight (sometimes even more) cryo-needles transperineally into your prostate, using a template guide similar to the one used for brachytherapy. The locations of the needles are pre-selected, according to the contour and size of the prostate, and the location and extent of the cancer. With the older type of equipment used in first and second generations, a special guide wire was placed through each of the cryo-needles and then each needle was removed and replaced by a slim plastic straw. However, with the newer, third generation equipment, that step is obsolete.

About five thermocouples (thermal sensors) are placed at various pre-selected locations, internally and around the periphery of the gland, to monitor the process, as follows:

- Around the external sphincter muscle below the prostate,
- Near the urethra and the walls of the rectum to ensure that temperature does not exceed what they can tolerate and to avoid damage to them, and
- Into the left and right nerve bundles to monitor that temperature, in an effort to preserve them and maintain erectile function.

Part V Treatment Options

Cryotherapy freezing is accomplished by inserting thin cryo-needles with sharp tips, through the skin at the perineum and into the prostate gland. High-pressured gas, such as argon or liquid nitrogen with freezing properties, used according to Joule-Thompson theory, is applied through the needles, to the normal and abnormal tissues of the prostate. As the gas comes in contact with the prostate tissue at each needle, the area become extremely cold and freezes. Soon, the surrounding areas of the prostate freeze also, forming several small balls of ice and then one big ball of ice.

The placement of the needles and the extent of the freeze are controlled by visualizing the gland and the tumour through the TRUS thereby helping to avoid damage to the rectum and sphincter.

This freezing process continues until a temperature of minus 40 degrees centigrade is reached. This required level is maintained for several minutes, followed by about 10 minutes of thawing, primarily using helium gas, delivered the same way as the argon, through the same needles. To defrost or thaw the frozen gland, high-pressured helium gas will be delivered at high speed through the needles to the prostate gland similarly as was done for the freezing.

A second similar freeze-thaw cycle is applied, then all instruments, including the needles, are removed. If the prostate is longer than 27 millimetres, which is the effective length of the ice-ball isotherm, a pullback procedure is done and two more freeze-thaw applications are conducted to cover the length to the apex.

The goal is to freeze the entire prostate, or as much of it as possible, killing all the cancer cells, at the expense of destroying the entire gland, including the normal cells. This freeze-thaw cycle shatters the outer walls of the cancer cells and destroys them. With time, the dead tissues are eventually absorbed into the body, leaving a shrunken prostate gland behind.

The entire procedure, including preparation, takes approximately two hours.

You will be discharged within about 24 hours with either an inserted Foley catheter or the suprapubic catheter, depending on the choice of the therapist. Whichever is chosen, will remain inserted for two to three weeks, until the prostate heals sufficiently to allow voiding. Most normal activities can usually be resumed within a few days. You will also be prescribed antibiotics to take for at least the next seven days.

When cryotherapy is chosen to correct recurrence due to radiation failure, as recognized by a rising PSA level, the radiologist or urologist needs to first confirm that cancer is in the prostate and not somewhere else. Thus a biopsy is needed. See last chapter in this book on recurrent prostate cancer.

Protection

Protection of the rectal wall, the urethra and the external sphincter muscle is of paramount importance in the freezing process and whenever possible the same goes for the nerve bundles.

The nerve bundles, which provide erection capability, are located on the outside surface of the prostate, adjacent to the rectum and are difficult to protect from freezing. Thus, they are permanently damaged in the process. Notwithstanding this awareness, some physicians do advocate partial "nerve-sparing" for some patients by selectively freezing part of the nerve bundles and monitoring this using the placement of thermocouples as explained above, in an attempt to preserve erectile function. Unfortunately, according to some specialists, that technique presents a risk of incomplete destruction of the cancer cells, making the approach highly controversial. It's therefore not universally recommended.

Some centres in the U.S. have also introduced "focal" cryosurgery, identifying and treating only the tumour within the gland. This is still under review, although early results appear promising in lowering the rate of erectile dysfunction.

Enhancements

Several recent enhancements in delivery techniques and technology have brought about improved application of cryotherapy to prostate cancer.

One of these involves increasing the number of cryo-needles. The standard number inserted for total ablation is five, creating more than five overlapping ice balls and resulting in a gland that's virtually one solid ice ball. However, some specialists have increased the number of needles to as many as eight, in an effort to improve the destruction of the entire gland. The idea is that more needles may give a better shape and more precise freeze with less chance of "pocket" formation. Therapists who have utilized this approach believe that the increased number of needles results in more total destruction and thus improved outcomes.

With the advent of the third generation of cryotherapy, including the much thinner 17 gauge needles, there have been a few experiments in the U.S. to insert up to 15 needles into the prostate, one centimetre apart, depending on the size of the prostate. The goal is to achieve 100 percent destruction. As the freezing occurs, ice seeds, instead of ice balls, are formed around the tip of the needles. Results are as yet unknown with this approach, but concerns have been expressed that spaces may be left between the ice seeds, which could result in cracks or crevices that aren't ideally frozen and leave behind live cancer cells.

Sometimes, the surgeon may perform a cystoscopy, after the cryo-needles are placed, but before the warming catheter is inserted, to ensure none of the needles have penetrated the urethra.

Cure

Once again, it's important to be cognizant of the criteria used for survival or cure. In general, a PSA nadir of 0.4 ng/ml is considered cured. Most published data about cryotherapy results are relatively recent, based on just a few years of practice – particularly for third generation. Although it appears promising, the procedure is still controversial. It's approved as standard therapy in the United States, but not in Canada.

Since its approval in the U.S. there has been increased demand for its use, which has led to more experience, research and delivery enhancements.

Cryotherapy is offered at several centres in the U.S. with, apparently, reasonably good results, although some have abandoned the procedure due to unsatisfactory results and unacceptable complications. Notwithstanding those circumstances, there is still a certain amount of popularity for it in the U.S. as "primary therapy."

Some centres, including a few in Canada, may offer it as salvage cryotherapy after EBRT, IS or HDR have failed.

Based on records of some of the thousands of men who have undergone cryosurgery for prostate cancer in the U.S. 97 percent were cancer free at the end of the first year following surgery, and 82% at the end of five years. Among high risk patients who were treated for recurrence, as a result of failed radiation therapy, 65 percent remained cancer free after three years following cryosurgery.

Caution

Although the description appears simple enough, cryotherapy should be considered a difficult and complex procedure and you should ensure the experts with whom you talk, or who will perform this treatment on you, have sufficient hands-on experience and knowledge of the third generation cryotherapy and any additional enhancements – otherwise, seek another specialist. It requires knowledge of ultrasound imaging, of the prostate and rectal anatomy and pathology, and skills with the cryoprobe equipment. Obtaining the necessary expertise, takes time.

If cryotherapy is an option you wish to pursue, you should review the option with your urologist, because its development continues to be dynamic; every day brings new developments.

Ensure that you understand:

- How it will affect your quality of life, including erection capability and incontinence.
- Who are the experts in this field.
- Who can best perform this treatment for you.

It's very likely your urologist may lack the necessary knowledge and skill to perform this procedure, or he might discourage you from pursuing it. It would be wise to visit a reputable urologist who will discuss it with knowledge and empathy.

Risks

Major risks associated with cryosurgery are:

- Erectile dysfunction, as a result of freezing the nerve bundles. This may cause permanent damage, but occasionally it may be transient with recovery taking place in a year or two as the nerves regenerate.
- The possibility of not completely destroying the cancer cells.
- Potential formation of a fistula – an abnormal connection between the urethra and rectum (or between two hollow organs). It occurs as a result of tissue damage from the freezing.
- Bladder outlet obstruction (BOO) – a narrowing of the urethra at the bladder neck, obstructing the flow of urine.

Side-Effects

Side effects as a result of cryotherapy include:

- Erectile dysfunction
- Incontinence
- Urethral scarring
- Some pelvic pain
- Blood in the urine
- Urinary urgency
- Scrotal swelling
- Damage to rectal wall
- Damage to the urethra
- Bruising around the site where the needles entered the skin.

Advantages

As a treatment for prostate cancer, cryotherapy's advantages may include:

- No open surgery or surgical incision
- Minimal blood loss (therefore no requirement for transfusion)
- Little discomfort / Less pain than other treatments (little post-operative pain)
- Short hospital stay (two days maximum)
- Fast recovery (up and about quickly following the procedure)
- Can be repeated if not totally successful
- Can be performed on patients for whom radiation therapy was not previously successful (recurrent cancer – salvage cryotherapy).
- No serious problem with incontinence
- Relatively inexpensive
- Can be used for focal cryosurgery

Disadvantages

Disadvantages may include all the side-effects mentioned previously, plus those below. It should be mentioned, however, that third generation cryotherapy provides several enhancements that seem to minimize many of these:

- Unavailability of long-term (10 to 15 years) studies of its effectiveness.
- A risk of causing a fistula between the prostate and the rectum (although rare).
- A small risk of incontinence (approximately one to two percent).
- May leave a urinary obstruction due to scar tissue or sloughed "dead" tissue.
- High possibility of erectile dysfunction (about 80 to 85 percent).
- Inability to ejaculate during orgasm.
- Irritation of the bowels.
- A burning sensation during urination.
- May not get all the cancer cells, particularly around the urethra.
- Concern that some cancer cells may escape the freezing and then proliferate.
- Concerns that some cells may have unknowingly escape from the gland and not treated.
- No insurance coverage in Canada.

Some swelling of the penis and scrotum may also be experienced for about two weeks.

Where is Cryotherapy Offered

As stated, cryotherapy had lost its excitement, but recently there has been some resurgence of interest, since it appears to show new promise. There are a fair number of doctors at hospitals throughout the U.S. who perform the procedure. However, it's still considered at the investigational stage in Canada. This means that it may not be covered by health insurance. Although it may be justified in patients who have failed primary radiation therapy, as a salvage treatment, it will be considered a non-standard form of therapy for awhile by Canadian insurance companies, particularly given the lack of information on long-term results.

Because of the uncertainties surrounding long-term effectiveness, distrust for its utilization as a standard treatment for prostate cancer lingers on in the minds of many experts. No doubt, if it were to be accepted across the continent, we could see some very interesting further enhancements

Cost

The cost of cryotherapy treatment in 2008 was approximately $18,000 U.S.

Medicare in the U.S. has had a national policy in place since July, 1999, approving cryoablation therapy (cryotherapy) as a primary treatment for localized prostate cancer. Thus it's covered by Medicare and some private insurance companies. It's not approved in Canada.

Chapter 35

HIGH INTENSITY FOCUSED ULTRASOUND (HIFU)

"Risk! Risk anything! Care no more for the opinions of others, for those voices. Do the hardest thing on earth for you. Act for yourself. Face the truth."

Katherine Mansfield

Deliver the Sound Waves

High Intensity Focused Ultrasound (HIFU) is used to treat localized prostate cancer by directing high-frequency sound waves to a target, rapidly inducing heat at the target and destroying it.

It is considered a *non-invasive* (no incision) surgical treatment. Energy generated from the waves is absorbed at the target, where it's converted to heat. When the target becomes hot enough, the tissue is destroyed. With the waves being *focused*, a very small targeted area can be accessed deep within the tissue.

This procedure is characterized by its ability to penetrate tissue inside the body and reach a distant target with minimal impact on the penetrated tissue.

HIFU has reportedly been used successfully in China, Japan, Europe and Latin America. However, the technique is not approved for use to treat prostate cancer in Canada and the U.S. except on a trial basis. Its easy access, apparent safety and newly available tools, have increased its popularity and raised curiosity worldwide.

There are two prominent HIFU devices competing for the world market:

- Ablatherm, manufactured by EDAP – Technomed (based in France)
- Sonablate 500 (SB500), developed by Focus Surgery, Inc. of Indianapolis, IN and manufactured by Misonix, Inc., of Farmingdale, N.Y.

Both devices have the same purposes:

- to use ultrasound to guide the surgeon during the procedure;
- to destroy the cancer cells using intense heat generated by the high intensity focused ultrasound waves.

However, differences in their component parts bring different advantages and disadvantages.

One must be careful in reading and interpreting available material on HIFU, in that:

- Many of the articles originate from the same initial or original source.
- Many of the articles are based on the early days of using the procedure – the first five years.
- Many of the articles are written by, or based on articles about, the manufacturers of the devices.
- Many of the articles may be forward-looking, based on manufacturers' hopes and expectations and could include risks and uncertainties which may or may not materialize.
- The devices and techniques used have gone through considerable enhancements since their early usage, particularly in the area of nerve sparing.

History

For many years scientists have recognized that cancer cells are more sensitive to heat than are normal cells. At high temperatures cancer cells break down. In the 1960s heat began to receive attention as a potentially effective therapy for cancer when it was recognized that it could work synergistically with other therapies.

In 1984, after medical scientists like Haim (James) I. Bicher, M.D., of Valley Cancer Institute, Los Angeles, California, and others had worked for decades to provide a cohesive body of clinical research and testing, heat treatment was given legal status as an approved medical procedure. Although the principles of tumour heating were recognized for years, the technology to direct the heat in a focused way was absent. As a result, its use for prostate cancer treatment was abandoned in the Western world.

However, the advent of ultrasound waves at high frequency to generate heat and the ability to focus those waves at a distant point generated much interest and accelerated progress in these areas.

Part V   Treatment Options

The development of ultrasound *transducers* started with the work of French physicist Paul Langevin (1872 – 1946). During World War I, Langevin led a team of engineers and other specialists, using the piezo-electric (discovered by Pierre and Jacques Curie in 1880) properties of quartz crystal (excellent ultrasound emitter and detector) to build the first submarine sonar (used to detect submarines by the reflection of their ultrasound waves).

The first investigation of high intensity focused ultrasound for non-invasive ablation was reported by John G. Lynn et al, in the early 1940s – "A New Method for the Generation and Use of Focused Ultrasound in Experimental Biology, Lynn et al., Journal of General Physiology, 1943, pp. 179-193." In the 1950s physicist William Fry, at the University of Illinois, theorize application of ultrasonic waves as a non-invasive surgical technique. Then together with his brother Francis Fry and Regional C. Eggleton, they developed a transducer system that culminated in clinical treatment of neurological disorders, particularly Parkinson's disease. A paper was published as part of the Scientific Program of the Third Annual Conference of the American Institute of Ultrasonics in Medicine, Washington D.C., September 4, 1954, pp. 413-423.

The initial work in utilization of high intensity focused ultrasound and devising a machine (Sonablate 500) to focus the ultrasound waves at a cancer inside the prostate gland began in the 1980s at Indiana University Medical Centre, following the development of transrectal ultrasound probe. This was quickly followed by research centres in the U.S., Europe and Japan.

In 1987, feasibility studies demonstrated that focused ultrasound was capable of ablating prostate tissue, including in treatment for BPH.

In 1989, three European research groups – French National Institute for Health and Medical Research (INSERM unit U281), the Urology service of the Edouard Herriot Hospital in Lyon, France and EDAP Technomed – combined their efforts and initiated a project to develop a special device (Ablatherm) to treat localized prostate cancer using high intensity focused ultrasound. Within 10 years their efforts materialized into a product that was given approval in Europe. Much of the early work was carried out in France and the device received a CE (European approval) mark in 2002. It has been used in China and Japan since the late 1990s and in Europe since the early 2000s.

HIFU is being studied in several countries around the world to treat all types of cancer and other soft tissue diseases. Its technology is currently approved to treat localized prostate cancer and BPH in Europe, Russia, parts of Asia (China and Japan), the Dominican Republic and Mexico. It's utilized for experimental purposes in Canada and the U.S. It's approved in the U.S. for investigational purposes in ongoing clinical trials as further studies are needed, for FDA approval for general use.

How Does HIFU Work?

The real interest in the technique comes from the fact that the urologist can plan the treatment under ultrasound image guidance, target the prostate and monitor the therapy, all using a single combined probe and transducer.

In HIFU therapy, a shower of ultrasound waves, originating at the transducer – which is embedded in the rectum – and directed toward a selected small targeted area of tissue, converge on and intersect at, the target. As the waves meet and intersect they create significant energy, causing *acoustic ablation*, which then rapidly creates a rising temperature within the tissue to about 90 degrees Centigrade or 195 degrees Fahrenheit, instantly destroying the tissue by *coagulation necrosis*. Each shower of waves treats a precisely defined portion of the tissue referred to as "target" or "target lesion."

Because this therapy accomplishes its task of destroying the tissue non-invasively, it's also referred to as "non-invasive HIFU surgery," and the method as "non-invasive acoustic ablation technique." It offers certain prostate cancer patients a surgical solution to remove the cancer, without incision.

The body eliminates the dead cancer and tissue, progressively, in the same way as it does for other dead tissue. It may eventually be replaced with scar tissue.

HIFU application has been likened to the transmission of a ray of the sun's energy through a magnifying glass onto a specific point on a dry leaf or wood chip to start a fire. The ray of energy is safe and harmless throughout the entire area until it reaches the leaf or wood chip and burns it.

HIFU devices consist of the following key components, which may vary by manufacturer:

- A table, like an operating table or, similar to the examining table in a doctor's office, for the patent to lie on during treatment.
- An ultrasound (transducer) imaging probe and an ultrasound treatment transducer, which emits the focused beam transrectally. These two units may be built separately or combined within each other then placed in a condom-like latex balloon filled with cooled liquid.
- An ultrasound imaging system which provides the urologist with the image of the prostate.
- A real-time integrated computer, which aims, emits and controls the high intensity beam, from the surface of the transducer to the lesion, according to the treatment plan, systematically moving the target from lesion to lesion, zone by zone, as established by the plan.
- A detector to ensure the patient lies still and the prostate stays in target. This provides automatic pause of the procedure if the patient moves – which may also shift the gland.

The current machines have computerized programs to shift the focus from one target lesion to the next, in a precisely timed orderly fashion. The sequential focusing and ablation of the successive adjacent target lesions eventually result in complete ablation of the prostate gland. The urologist's role is to image the prostate with transrectal ultrasound, define the target lesions and set the treatment parameters – durations, voltage, and others.

How Is HIFU Administered

Patients qualify for HIFU based on their age (best suited for those older than 70, although some urologists treat younger patients), health condition, PSA blood level (under 15 ng/ml), Gleason score (7 or less), the clinical stage (low risk T1c/T2b), the extent of their cancer based on the Partin tables (or other nomograms), a prostate volume of 40 cubic centimetres or less and confirmation that the cancer is localized.

Prior preparation includes consultation with the urologist and an anaesthesiologist to review information and to answer any questions. This may be done the day prior to the procedure or just before. An enema for internal cleansing is done before treatment begins.

The treatment is performed transrectally (through the rectum) under general or spinal (epidural) anaesthesia to ensure complete immobility, which is necessary to keep the prostate target still. Depending on the device used, the patient either lies on his back in the dorsal lithotomy position (SB500) or on his right side in a lateral fetal position (Ablatherm).

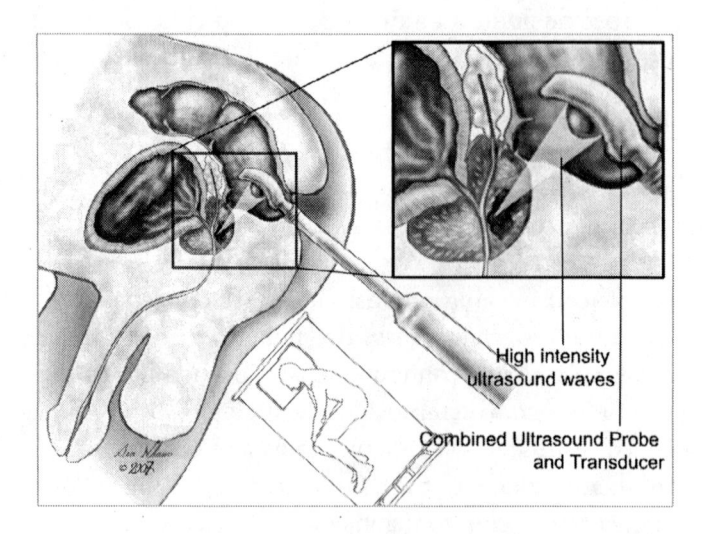

The ultrasound probe, which incorporates a standard transrectal ultrasound transducer and the treatment transducer, coated with gel and placed in a condom or balloon filled with the cooling liquid, is inserted into the rectum. Multiple ultrasound images are then taken and reviewed to determine the shape, size, and location of the prostate gland. This may have been done when the biopsy was taken, but may be repeated at this time for on-site planning and treatment purposes.

The shape and size of the entire prostate is determined because it's not possible to accurately see and treat just the tumour within the gland; the entire prostate gland has to be divided into treatment zones. The treatment zones and target lesions are then defined and logged into the computer. The probe is adjusted so that the waves emitted from the transducer are directed precisely at the target lesion. Multiple beams of high intensity ultrasound waves are emitted at different angles from the surface of the transducer (slightly larger than the size of a marble), to converge precisely at the target lesion.

As the treatment begins, the surgeon selects a small portion of tissue (target lesion) – within a zone (block) – about the size and shape of a grain of rice, and directs a shower of high intensity ultrasound waves to converge precisely at that target lesion. Controlled and guided by the computer, showers of convergent waves systematically converge on, and attack, rice sized and shaped target lesion after target lesion, in all the zones. The waves are delivered to all the lesions that make up the entire gland, including cancerous and non-cancerous tissues, until the gland is completely destroyed. The zones and target lesions are defined so as to spare the prostate capsule and possibly the nerve bundles from damage. The procedure requires only one treatment and can be done in an out-patient setting.

Each rice size and shaped target lesion takes about three seconds to heat and destroy and it takes about six seconds to move on to the next lesion. A 40 cubic centimetre prostate gland accommodates about 600 of these lesions and it takes about three hours to completely destroy them all on an individual basis. Larger glands may be impeded by bone structure which ultrasound cannot penetrate.

Little damage is done to anything in the path of the beam, including the rectal wall and the nerve bundles, as the beam is not focused on those. To ensure that the desired temperature is reached and maintained, without being exceeded, the temperature being delivered may be monitored constantly. Also, the surrounding tissue and the rectum are protected from heat damage by special mechanism; however, extreme caution has to be taken as the heat and tissue destruction can damage the tissue situated between the prostate and the rectum. Damage to this area can result in sloughing of the tissue, which then leads to an abnormal communication between the rectum (fecal stream) and the prostatic urethra (urine stream). This is called a fistula and is a serious problem with poor healing.

During treatment, certain controls and monitoring are established to ensure the patient's safety and the treatment effectiveness. Special devices are connected to the equipment to achieve the following:

- Continuous control of the position of the probe in relation to the rectal wall, to avoid damage to the rectum..
- Constant control of the power delivered to the patient, to prevent surges which would cause damage to surrounding structures.
- Constant monitoring of the rectal temperature to avoid heating and damaging the rectum.
- Continuous monitoring of the target stillness to ensure it does not move and to automatically stop the procedures in the event of such movement.

The prostate itself may become temporarily swollen, as a result of the heating process. This swelling or *oedema* (the medical word for any swelling in the body) may compress the urethra and cause some temporary restriction in passing urine. To help this situation during this brief healing period, approximately seven to 21 days, until the edema recedes, a suprapubic catheter is often inserted via the lower abdomen into the bladder or a Foley catheter via the penis/urethra, to allow urine to drain.

Antibiotics are usually prescribed for a few days immediately following the procedure, to prevent urinary infection. It's essential that the full complement of the antibiotics be taken as prescribed.

Research and Development

The Journal of Urology published an article entitled "High-Intensity Focused Ultrasound for the Treatment of Localized Prostate Cancer: 5-year Experience," in 2004 (Urology 63 (2), p.297-300, 2004), written by A. Blana, B. Walter, S. Rogenhofer, W.F. Wieland of the Departmant of Urology, University of Regensburg, Germany. In the article, the physicians showed clinical results at five to 10 years using Ablatherm HIFU technology for the treatment of localized prostate cancer.

The study included 137 patients who were treated, with five-year follow-up, and showed 93.4 percent constant negative control biopsies. About 87 percent of the patients had constant PSA levels of less than 1.0 ng/ml. and 1.5 percent (two patients) had a PSA level that rose to greater than 4.0 ng/ml.

Research results published by Dr. Toyoaki Uchida (urologist), from Takai (Kitasato) University in Tokyo, Japan and John C. Rewcastle Ph.D from the Department of Radiology, University of Calgary in Canada, of a Japanese survey of 132 men treated with HIFU found that almost 70 percent had very low or undetected PSA level, after five years (similar to conventional surgery and radiotherapy).

Also, the results of a large European multi-centre study, involving 402 patients, reported after five years 80 percent of subjects with a normal PSA level and no evidence of recurrence. An estimated 10 percent needed additional treatment such as repeat HIFU or salvage radiation.

Armed with these promising results, other countries such as Britain, Canada and the United States have started trials.

The use of HIFU for prostate cancer treatment, although potentially promising and despite the apparent successful use in several countries outside North America, leaves many questions unanswered to satisfy authorities in Canada and the U.S. That's not unusual, since all new therapies on being introduced for use have to be tested in a controlled manner within the context of clinical trials and by an appropriate review process by Health Canada and/or the FDA (Food and drug administration) in the U.S.

Clinical trials are research studies conducted to test the safety and *efficacy* of the product or treatment. If the product or treatment is found to be safe, based on the clinical trials, then they are approved for public use. These trials answer important scientific questions and lead to future research and enhancements. Even the most promising scientific findings must first withstand the safety and effectiveness tests of clinical trials.

Most trials start with basic cancer research in a laboratory. If a new approach appears promising, it may be tested on animals, then have people participate. Four main kinds of clinical trials in cancer research, are:

- Cancer prevention trials
- Cancer screening trials
- Quality-of-life trials
- Cancer treatment trials

Cancer treatment trials incorporate four progressive phases, I, II, III and IV, each designed to answer specific questions.

Phase I trials look mainly at how safe a treatment is and what the best approach might be. They generally involve about 15 to 30 people and seek to answer some basic questions.

Phase II trials focus on the effectiveness against the disease. Less than 100 people are usually involved and side-effect information is collected.

Phase III trials provide a detailed evaluation of a promising new treatment that was identified during a phase II trial. They involve a large number of people and comparison is made against the best current standard treatment available. These utilize a process called randomization, by which patients are randomly assigned to one of two groups, the experimental group and the control group.

Part V   Treatment Options

Some in-depth questions are considered, such as:

- Are patients who get the new treatment less likely to have their cancer spread?
- Are patients who get the new treatment likely to live longer?
- Do patients have fewer side-effects from the new treatment?
- What is their quality of life like after the new treatment?

Phase IV trials are conducted to follow patients who have been through phase III trials, to gain information about possible long-term risks and benefits.

A phase I clinical trial for the SB500 was approved by the FDA in 2004. It was completed at Indiana University School of Medicine in Indianapolis. The results were submitted in May 2005.

The FDA has subsequently granted an Investigational Device Exemption (IDE) to allow the SB500 to be used for HIFU as primary prostate cancer treatment in a multi-centre combined phase II/III clinical trial for low risk (T1c/T2b) localized prostate cancer. This study will look at 266 patients in about 24 locations.

A Phase III clinical trial using the Ablatherm device (equipment and technology) for HIFU therapy as primary prostate cancer treatment is also underway in Canada and the U.S.. The purpose of this study is to obtain FDA approval for the use of the device in treatment of low-risk localized prostate cancer. The FDA is requiring the trial to compare HIFU versus cryosurgery, thus there are two arms of the study – HIFU and cryosurgery. The treatment phase of the trial cannot be completed until both arms have treated the required number of patients.

There are several other Phase III multi-centre clinical trials being conducted, on HIFU therapy as primary prostate cancer treatment, around the world, including a combined trial in the United Kingdom, Italy, Germany and Austria, to collect long-term safety and efficacy data.

There is also an FDA Phase I clinical trial in process to apply HIFU therapy to patients who have failed radiation therapy for prostate cancer. Criteria for inclusion in this trial include:

- Positive biopsy after radiation treatment.
- PSA still in the low range.
- No evidence of cancer elsewhere.
- Prostate must be under 40 grams.
- No significant rectal problems such as radiation damage.
- No inflammatory bowel disease.
- No rectal wall invasion by tumour.
- No previous brachytherapy or cryosurgery treatment.

A recent trial at the University College London Hospitals in the U.K., approved by the UK National Cancer Research Network and funded by Cancer Research U.K., was conducted on the first known *hemi-ablation* procedure (ablation of cancer limited to one side of the prostate).

Similar "focal HIFU" experimental studies are underway elsewhere of which results are pending.

Unknowns

HIFU, being a relatively new procedure for prostate cancer, particularly in Canada and the U.S., represents what could become the next generation of minimally invasive or non-invasive treatment for this condition. According to some specialists, it appears to be a promising, non-invasive treatment for prostate cancer, capable of destroying cancerous tissue with good precision and selective sparing of surrounding tissue. For some specialists, although clinical data and information is still limited, the technology has been extensively studied and developed to the point where it serves the purpose and meets the objective. However, there are still many clinically relevant unanswered questions regarding the long-term effects, such as:

- What represents a detectable PSA or PSA nadir, after HIFU?
- Will the PSA remain at nadir level?
- Will residual tissues not destroyed by HIFU eventually start to grow and metastasize?
- Can the effectiveness be improved with further improvement in the technology?
- Should HIFU be offered as primary therapy for previously untreated prostate cancer or should it be limited to the radiation failure group?

There will undoubtedly be further improvements in the device and the technique.

It's also important to be cautious and recognize that much of the published data profess that HIFU is as successful, or better than, other methods of treating small, slow-growing prostate cancer. As much as it may be tempting to accept those, the long-term evidence is still not in.

Who Qualifies for HIFU

With insufficient long-term efficacy data, determination of who might benefit from HIFU is based on extrapolation from other treatment outcome data.

In France, initial treatment is reserved for patients over 70 with localized prostate cancer. This is because HIFU being a recent treatment, has less than 10 years follow-up, which means that it's intended for patients who have an average life expectancy of 10 years.

It may also be used on some younger men who aren't candidates for surgery. Their tumour must be at a clinical stage lower than or equal to T2b, with a PSA value lower than 15 ng/ml and a Gleason score lower than or equal to 7 (3+4). The prostate volume must be lower than 40 ml.

The National Institute of Clinical Excellence (NICE), which advises health professionals in England and Wales on providing patients with the highest attainable standards of care, has reviewed all the early data on prostate HIFU and has recommended that HIFU should be made available as a prostate cancer treatment, so long as the normal procedures of consent, audit and clinical governance are in place.

After-Effects

Some of the after-effects which might be experienced are:

- Swelling of the prostate gland, resulting in difficulty passing urine during the first few days after the procedure.
- Potential for infection – antibiotics are provided for this purpose.
- Potential for urinary incontinence – perhaps from temporary damage to the internal sphincter muscle.
- Damage to the rectum. – probably from heat generated during ablation of neighbouring tissue.
- Potential for failure to destroy all the prostate tissue, thus possible leaving behind some untreated tissue.
- Potential for erectile dysfunction, if sparing of nerve bundles is unsuccessful.
- Lack of ejaculation and fertility, since the entire prostate gland will be destroyed and it will no longer be functional.

Advantages

Advantages of HIFU treatment on localized prostate cancer are:

- It's a relatively simple procedure.
- Treatment performed in one session.
- No radiation required.
- Non-invasive – no incision required.
- May be performed in an out-patient setting.
- Patient can return to a normal lifestyle within a couple of days.
- Capacity to generate in-depth, precise tissue ablation using external applicator, with no short-term adverse effect on surrounding structures.
- Can be repeated, if necessary (other conventional treatment can still be applied later).

- Available short-term studies show low rate of incontinence (approximately eight percent).
- Available short-term studies show relatively low rate of erectile dysfunction.

Disadvantages

Some disadvantages of HIFU are:

- The lack of long-term results, thus uncertainty of complete cancer elimination.
- If the prostate is larger than 40 cubic centimetres, it may first require hormone treatment to reduce its size and in some instances even TRUS, before HIFU.
- Inability to ejaculate during climax, thus infertility.
- Not suitable for treating cancer that has spread outside the gland.
- Requires a catheter for up to two weeks following treatment.
- Possibility of erectile dysfunction.
- A relatively long procedure of close to three hours.

Where is HIFU Offered?

Despite the short-comings, there are several clinics and hospitals in Europe, Asia and Mexico that offer this treatment on a regular basis. In Canada and the U.S., it would be offered for investigational purposes only, except for a few private facilities which offer it separate from the clinical investigation protocol.

Cost

The cost of HIFU treatment in 2008, in places where it is offered, mostly private facilities or outside of Canada and the U.S., would be in the order of $16,000 to $20,000 U.S. Like other treatments that are still considered investigational, HIFU treatment would not be covered by most health care plans. When it is offered as part of a clinical trial or investigation protocol, the research grant would likely cover the costs.

Chapter 36

CHEMOTHERAPY

"You have powers you never dreamed of. You can do things you never thought you could do. There are no limitations in what you can do except the limitations of your own mind."

DARWIN P. KINGSLEY

It's a Regimen – Stick to It

Chemotherapy is the use of chemical substances (cytotoxic or anti-cancer drugs) to stop cancer cells from growing. It's designed to destroy and kill cancer cells and is considered a systemic treatment as it can eliminate cells even at distant sites from the cancer origination.

There are many types of chemotherapy drugs available for use to affect cancer cells, each works differently to meet specific criteria in terms of timing and life cycle of the targeted cells. They may be administered intravenously through a vein, by injection or orally in the form of a pill.

A chemotherapy *regimen* (a treatment plan of drugs, cycle and schedule) generally includes drugs to fight cancer, plus drugs to help support completion of the cancer treatment, at the full dose, on schedule and at specific intervals. To get the most from chemotherapy, it's important to stick to that regimen

History

The birth of chemotherapy may be traced to pharmacists Louis Goodman and Alfred Gilman, who in 1943, during World War II, discovered that nitrogen mustard was an effective treatment

Chapter 36 | Chemotherapy

for cancer, specifically non-Hodgkin's lymphoma.

A few years later, in 1947, based on a theory that antifolates could suppress proliferation of malignant cells, work was carried out by pathologist Sidney Farber at Harvard Medical School, Harriett Kilto and chemists at Lederle Laboratories (then a Division of American Cyanamid of Pearl River, New York – now owned by Wyeth Pharmaceuticals of New Jersey), on the effects of various synthesized folate (folic acid) analogues – such as methotrexate – to perform as antagonists to folic acid. This was reported in New England Journal of Medicine, June 3, 1948. Although this theory was not widespread accepted at the time, these analogues became the first drugs to induce remission in children with acute lymphoblastic leukemia.

A decade later, in 1958, Roy Hertz and Min Chiu Li at the National Cancer Institute (NCI), discovered that methotrexate treatment alone could cure choriocarcinoma, a germ-cell malignancy that originates in cells of the placenta. Thus, the christening of chemotherapy came about.

In 1955, the U.S. congress created a National Cancer Chemotherapy Services Centre (NCCSC) at the NCI to promote drug discovery for cancer. The NCCSC developed methodologies and tools for chemotherapeutic process.

A giant leap was made in 1965, when a hypothesis was put forward, that cancer chemotherapy should parallel the tuberculosis antibiotics theory of drugs combinations, with different sites of action. It was believed that cancer cells mutate to become resistant to a single agent but by using several drugs simultaneously, the cells would not develop resistance to all of them at the same time. As a result, today most successful chemotherapy regimens use the paradigm of simultaneous multiple drugs delivery.

Later, it was discovered that drugs were more effective on smaller tumours. Out of this was born the adjuvant theory – that if the tumour burden could be reduced by surgery, chemotherapy might be able to clear away any remaining malignant cells.

Similarly, since some cells grow or divide rapidly and some do so slowly, different drugs are offered to target the different growth pattern of these cells as well.

However, there are also rapid growing healthy cells, and most forms of chemotherapy target rapid growing cells in general, without distinguishing the difference between a cancer cell and some healthy cells – as a result, the drugs destroy not only the rapid growing cancer cells but also the rapid growing healthy cells, such as hair and blood cells.

Several effective chemotherapeutic drugs or agents have been subsequently developed, as researchers came to understand the genetic nature of cancer and cell biology. They uncovered signaling networks in cancer cells that were radically altered and that regulate cellular activities such as proliferation and survival. Thus, chemotherapy took the form of targeted therapy using drugs that inhibit a signaling molecule.

Even with the initial successes of cancer chemotherapy, they still fell short of the high expectations of curing the most common cancers: lung, breast, prostate, bowel and melanoma. This is an ongoing challenge for doctors and researchers.

Whereas chemotherapy may cure some forms of cancer, such as *testicular* cancer, currently available chemotherapy agents do not cure prostate cancer. Nevertheless, they may help to improve quality of life by reducing pain. They can also temporarily control tumour growth.

With the success of combination chemotherapy and the discovery of several new drugs, it's now believed that all cancers can be treated, if the correct combination of drugs, in the correct doses and intervals could be decided upon.

Knowledge about molecular biology of cancer and tools to specifically target abnormal (structurally altered) proteins are opening up new possibilities.

Research and Development

The use of chemotherapy in prostate cancer is continuously being studied. It's believed by some doctors and researchers that two competing strategies of cancer therapy will emerge on the road to cure cancer: small molecular inhibitors and adaptive immunotherapy with re-programmed effector cells.

Doctors continue to study different combinations of chemotherapy drugs, as well as different doses and different sequences in which they are delivered, in an effort to find more effective ways of treating prostate cancer with chemotherapy.

Men who are on chemotherapy are encouraged to talk to their doctors about experimental trials. There are advantages and disadvantages to each of the regimens your oncologist will discuss with you. Based on your own health, personal values, wishes, and side-effects you may wish to avoid, you can work with your doctor to come up with the best regimen for your lifestyle.

Results of recent trials have shown that prostate cancer responds to the well-known drugs, mitoxantrone and taxotere, although the latter is considered better for prostate cancer that has continued to grow despite hormone therapy. Taxotere is also believed to provide a small increase in survival time, as well as reduced bone pain.

Chapter 36 | Chemotherapy

Taxotere, pronounced tax-o-teer, has shown to be effective in 30 to 50 percent of patients. Its introduction, has altered the treatment approach for advanced prostate cancer.

In May 2004 the U.S. Food and Drug Administration (FDA) approved the use of taxotere, injected in combination with prednisone (a steroid), for the treatment of patients with advanced metastatic prostate cancer. It was the first drug approved for hormone-refractory prostate cancer that has shown a survival benefit. It was approved because it had proven to help some patients live longer. The FDA felt that it offers hope to certain patients who have not responded to other treatments.

Taxotere, belongs to a class of chemotherapy drugs called taxanes, from the taxoid family. The chemical used to make taxotere is a semi-synthetic derivative of the needles of the European yew tree (taxus baccata). Taxol, the first commercial taxoid, was discovered in the early 1970s as part of the National Cancer Institute's screening of higher plant species for anticancer activity. Taxotere was brought to market by the French pharmaceutical firm Rhone-Poulene, which was later acquired by Aventis Pharmaceuticals. Subsequently, Aventis was acquired by Sanofi to form Sanofi-Aventis, the world's third largest pharmaceutical company.

According to the FDA, the safety and effectiveness of taxotere was established in a randomized, multi-centre clinical trial with more than 1,000 patients, which compared the use of "taxotere and prednisone" combination to "mitoxantrone and prednisone" combination in men with androgen-independent (hormone-refractory) metastatic prostate cancer. The former, given every three weeks, showed a survival advantage of approximately 2.5 months over the control group. Details of that study were presented to the American Society for Clinical Oncology on June 7, 2004 in New Orleans, Louisana.

In a presentation on October 1, 2005 to the 12th Annual Prostate Cancer Foundation Scientific Retreat in Phoenix, Arizona, the Cytogen Corporation of Princeton, New Jersey, reported the positive results of their Phase II (comparative study using randomly selected patients) clinical trial on treatment of advanced refractory prostate cancer using taxotere and their flagship product quadramet, which resulted in reduced PSA levels.

Quadramet, which is approved by the FDA to treat pain associated with bone cancer, is a radioactive small molecule that's injected to suppress bone marrow function. Its prime objective is to relieve pain.

There are also trials being conducted on bisphosphonate agents (a class of drugs used to strengthen bone), such as clodronate (Benefos or Loron), ibandronate and zoledronic acid (zoledronate or zometa) which help control bone thinning (osteoporosis) and pain, and also slow down, prevent or delay damage to the bone or completely stop the spread of cancer to the bones.

How does Chemotherapy Work?

According to the experts, chemotherapy works best when cells are dividing rapidly. The chemicals and anti-cancer drugs, when introduced into the bloodstream, destroy or kill the rapidly growing cancer cells.

Although chemotherapy may not destroy all cancer cells, it will likely slow their growth or multiplier effect. Unfortunately, the drugs also damage some healthy rapid growing cells in the process.

All cells in the body contain microtubules, which form a supporting structure, like a skeleton, for the cell. Damage to this skeleton can stop cell growth and/or reproduction. The introduction of taxotere makes the microtubules, in some susceptible cancer cells, very stiff. This prevents the cells from growing, dividing and reproducing.

Who Qualifies for Chemotherapy?

At one time, it was believed that prostate cancer did not respond well to chemotherapy; however, clinical trials, such as those mentioned above, and others, using some of the well known drugs, such as mitoxantrone (mitozantrone) and docetaxel (Taxotere), have proved this wrong. Those studies should put to rest the notion that advanced prostate cancer would not respond to chemotherapy.

According to Mario Eisenberger, M.D., a principal investigator from John Hopkins University, in another study, " … a treatment must be very effective to achieve a two to three months increase in median survival."

Chemotherapy treatment may be recommended for prostate cancer patients:

- whose cancer has spread to other areas of the body;
- whose cancer has failed to respond to hormone therapy (usually after an initial response to hormones); or
- who are experiencing recurrence,

Chemotherapy reduces the growth of the tumour and can ease symptoms such as pain. Because it does not cure the cancer and has a potentially small effect, it's not recommended as a treatment for localized prostate cancer.

Thus, chemotherapy is usually the last line of defense when other treatments have failed and it's generally reserved for advanced cancers that are no longer responsive to hormonal therapy.

However, some newer forms, which are less toxic, are now being tried in earlier stages of the disease and showing promise.

How is Chemotherapy Administered?

There are many different chemotherapy drugs and, as mentioned above, they often work in combination. Some of these may work for you while others may not. Just because certain drugs work on one person's cancer is no guarantee that they will work on another's. Each cancer is different. A few particular drugs, however, have shown more potential against prostate cancer than others.

Most chemotherapy drugs are administered daily, weekly, or monthly and in one of the following ways:

- By mouth (orally – pills, capsular liquid).
- *Intravenous*ly, with a thin needle (to travel through the bloodstream).
- By injection into tissues such as muscles (under the skin, or directly into the cancerous area).
- Topically (on the surface of the skin).

Generally, two or more drugs are administered simultaneously to reduce the likelihood of the cancer cells becoming resistant to the chemotherapy.

It's very important to maintain a proper balance between the drugs, in order to reduce damage to healthy cells. For this reason, doctors generally plan and administer a well-balanced dose that's strong enough to kill the cancer cells, but not so strong to destroy or damage too many healthy cells.

The effectiveness of the chemotherapy may be measured by the lowering of the PSA level and/or a decrease in pain, or other symptoms. It's generally effective in about 30 to 40 percent of cases.

Chemotherapy is given in cycles, meaning that it's administered for a few weeks, followed by a break of a few weeks, then the cycle is repeated again. Your health care team will decide on your cycle. The entire treatment generally lasts for a period of four to six months.

Side-Effects

Chemotherapy drugs work by destroying very active cells that divide rapidly. Unfortunately, that includes healthy cells as well as the intended cancer cells that actively divide, including those healthy cells in:

- The blood forming in your bone marrow,

- Your hair follicles,
- The inside of your mouth, and
- Your intestines.

When any of those occur, side-effects, such as those below, follow.

Depending on the type of drugs used, chemotherapy recipients may experience:

- pain,
- fatigue,
- hair loss,
- nausea and vomiting (termed chemotherapy-induced nausea and vomiting),
- anemia,
- sore mouth,
- diarrhea,
- loss of appetite,
- loss of sex drive,
- temporary bloating, or
- a low white blood count.

These side-effects generally disappear after chemotherapy is stopped, although some may take awhile to recover.

Supportive medication is generally given to help offset the side-effects. There are even some new medications that may prevent the nausea and vomiting.

Bone pain and fracture may also be a problem in advanced cases where the cancer has spread to the bone.

Advantages

Some advantages of chemotherapy as a treatment for prostate cancer include:

- may relieve bone pain;
- slows the growth of the tumour;
- non-invasive;
- may improve quality of life;
- may be of value for men with advanced high stage prostate cancer who have failed hormone therapy

Disadvantages

Some disadvantages of chemotherapy as a treatment for prostate cancer are:
- serious side-effects, some which may be irreversible (dependent on the drug used);
- it's usually not curative;
- it's still experimental and of little or no proven value for survival.

Cautions

Cancer chemotherapy drugs are essentially poisons. Patients receiving them may experience severe side-effects. As a result, the doses are limited, as are the beneficial effects.

It's important to know that chemotherapy does not cure prostate cancer and is considered palliative only. It can cure some cancers, such as testicular, as it did for cyclist Lance Armstrong. Prostate cancer is simply not as chemo-sensitive as some other forms of cancer.

Where is Chemotherapy Treatment Offered?

Chemotherapy is offered at major hospitals and treatment centres, and by some physicians in their offices. At times a hospital stay may be required if there is a need for close monitoring.

Cost

Cost of chemotherapy treatment in 2008 varied, depending on the type of treatment, drugs and the centre. It's almost always covered by health insurance plans.

PART VI

The Surgery Experience

Chapter 37

MAKING MY DECISION – OPTING FOR SURGERY

"If you wait for inspiration, you'll be standing on the corner after the parade is a mile down the street."

Ben Nicholas

Traditional and Alternative Treatment Options

After using up valuable time denying to myself that I had prostate cancer, I finally followed my wife's advice and started investigating what this condition meant. Did it mean the end of my manhood, my enthusiasm, the quality of life I had become accustomed to? I found out that it was none of those, unless I chose to allow it to affect me in those ways.

I researched and amassed some valuable information, much of which I am sharing in this book. I experimented and spent a lot of money unwisely, on various types of non-traditional consultation and treatments before I spontaneously – cold turkey, as the saying goes – one day stopped and analyzed my situation, based on the information I had gathered. I soon realized I could not completely commit to any of those non-traditional practices. From my perspective, they involved too many different activities to be concerned about simultaneously and at tremendous cost. I knew that I would not be able to keep up with all their requirements forever, especially considering my busy schedule and financial resources. This had nothing to do with being positive or negative. It was simply smart analysis and calculations, and prudent decision. The time involved was more than what a full-time job would demand, the cost was more than the salary of a full-time job and neither the treatments nor the prescriptions were covered by insurance.

Chapter 37 | Making My Decision – Opting for Surgery

I also felt that if such treatments worked at all, there was no guarantee the cancer would be cured. I felt that it might only go into remission temporarily. I wondered what would happen if later, I found myself reducing my activities, which would surely happen, given my busy schedule. Would the cancer then recur? There were no answers to these questions. The information was simply not available, hence, for me, the risks seemed much too great.

Most treatment directives will tell you it takes time for the treatment to take effect, and based on my conversations with many patients, I agree. But what if the cancer continues to grow and spread during that time? I realize that the saying, "Rome was not built in a day," may apply in using these non-traditional practices or healing methods, but gambling with my life was not a risk I was prepared to take.

I will not dispute the probable effectiveness of some non-traditional alternative treatments, because I know some of them have worked for some people. But they do not necessarily work for all people. There are many stories and hypotheses written about them, but only a few trials that prove the hypotheses. It's also my impression that you must be totally committed to the treatment for the rest of your life. To me, that's like being a prisoner in my own body.

More and more the traditional alternatives – surgery, radiation, seed implant (brachytherapy), and cryotherapy – were more attractive to me. And when I considered, that no two prostate cancers are the same, I became even more convinced that what was good for others may not necessarily be good for me.

My preferred treatment option, initially was seed implant, alone or in combination with EBRT. I believe that, together, they would have cured my cancer while leaving my continence and erectile function intact. Unfortunately, neither seed implant alone, nor the combination, were commonly offered in my area and I did not have the money to travel outside of the country for treatment. Also, according to the necessary qualification that was presented to me to have seed implant, my PSA level was in excess of the eligibility criteria.

Once I had satisfied myself that the preferred radiation alternatives were virtually out of the question, because of distance and cost, I began to think more seriously about surgery as the most responsible and viable alternative. I began to seek more information in order to understand the risks and after-effects, what was involved in administering the treatment and the potential for success. I seriously considered the after-effects, including the quality of life that would result due to the possible incontinence and erectile dysfunction, and the fact that I would never be able to ejaculate again. What I was not aware of, and therefore did not factor into the equation, was the resultant reduced penis size, in length and girth that several men have miserably experienced after surgery.

Although surgery was not my first choice, I did find the idea of the removal of the entire cancer, once and for all, very attractive. And its availability in my home city made it more economical and convenient. Being in familiar surroundings, close to home, family and friends, and within easy access to excellent health care made it even more attractive.

Several people offered me their opinions, for which I am grateful. However, they were not unanimously in favour of any particular alternative, so I had to weigh the various opinions and balance them with my personal knowledge, disposition and concerns.

Surgery Was My Answer

So, finally, I opted for surgery! Not with a lot of enthusiasm or exuberance. In fact, I submitted to it out of the fears expressed above, as well as the fear of continuously delaying my decision. I did not think that delay was doing me any good.

Once I had decided on surgery and set the date, it was a relief for many, myself included. I simply stayed the course, putting all my faith in my urologist/surgeon who convinced me that he was very experienced in performing bilateral nerve-sparing radical prostatectomy.

One of the favourable reasons I opted for surgery was because my urologist/surgeon recommended it as the most promising of the conventional treatments for my condition. His recommendation was based on several factors, namely:

- my relatively young age (under 72 – I was 58 at the time);
- my good health;
- my good physical condition;
- the grade of my cancer – Gleason score 4;
- the stage of my cancer – T2a (B1)
- my PSA levels and movement – <10;
- the probability that the cancer was still contained within my prostate, based on the Partin Tables.

I was assured that I had a reasonably good chance of cure, as well as of continued erection capability (after all he had done hundreds of the nerve-sparing procedures before) and only a short period of incontinence. I did not want to continue searching for alternatives, particularly unproven alternatives. I wanted a proven way. At the same time, I wanted the treatment that would give me the best possible chance for urinary control and erection capability. It was put to me that with my young age, my cancer's stage and grade, and my urologist's vast experience, I stood a good chance of a successful outcome in every aspect.

Furthermore, I was concerned, not so much about the cancer within my prostate itself, but rather about the risk of it spreading through the bloodstream with each passing minute. I was prepared to take the risk of waiting for a while, but not forever. In fact, even waiting for a while might be too long.

I was also very concerned about my family, some of whom were becoming increasingly worried. "What good would you be to us dead?" they asked.

So I went into acceptance phase with a certain amount of trepidation, knowing that it was time to make a final decision. At the same time, I wished that there was something available that I could just swallow and it would make the cancer go away.

If you were to ask me about my level of comfort in choosing surgery as my treatment option, I would have to say that it was a 7 on a scale of 1 to 10. I was not fully convinced that I knew exactly what was involved. For example, I had no idea what my surgeon would cut out and what he would leave intact. I was also not fully convinced that I would be able to continue with my sexual activities, which were very important to me. I never really felt that I was given complete assurance that I would continue to be fully functioning in that aspect of my life. I felt however, that it was implied that I would continue to function normally, otherwise.

Setting the Date

On December 13, 1999, immediately following separate discussions with my urologist and his research associate, I decided to go with surgery. The discussions took place at a follow-up visit to one I had in October when my urologist had expressed grave concern about my delay in making a decision and had sent me for a bone scan. In both discussions he and his research associate got me thinking more about the almost two years that had elapsed since I was diagnosed. So on that very day, I made my decision and set the date for surgery.

I should point out that my discussion with the research associate was strictly unofficial and initiated on my part simple as a friendly discussion. It was not arranged by my urologist, but rather because she was an acquaintance of mine. However, it does support my notion that consultation of this type might be a good thing for newly diagnosed patients and should be incorporated into the program and made available officially to all patients. It would allow the urologists more flexibility to spend time on diagnosis and examination.

The earliest date available for my surgery, based on my urologist's busy schedule, was March 3, 2000. My urologist performs this surgery two to three times two days per week. He probably performs more radical prostatectomies than anyone else in Canada. That further delay of three months was a relief for me. It meant that I had some time to put some things in order, fulfill certain commitments for January and February, cancel appointments for March and April, and then plan on fulfilling other commitments later in the year.

Part VI   The Surgery Experience

I marked the date in my calendar, and decided to forget about it temporarily by getting on with my life. After all, the world was not going to stop just because I was going to have surgery. I made arrangements for my "pre-admission" clinic visit to the hospital.

Most men I spoke with, both those who had experienced prostate cancer and others who had not, were of the opinion that surgery, external beam radiation, hormone therapy and chemotherapy were the only treatments available for this cancer. They had never heard of internal radiation treatment, cryosurgery, HIFU, or others. In fact, many of those people thought that any problem with the prostate eventually leads to cancer. Likewise they thought that removing the prostate was a simple procedure. Some compared it with removing the appendix. I have undergone both procedures and they aren't remotely similar. The appendix is an organ that serves absolutely no purpose. Without it, you are still the same, whereas the prostate is a major functioning organ, which participate in ejaculation, siring children and even having an erection. Those are major differences.

My choice of surgery was not because I considered that it would provide the best overall cure and quality of life, but rather because it was the best alternative that was available, based on cost and location of health care facilities. The hospital where I had my surgery done was just five minutes drive or 15 minutes walk from my home. My government's insurance covered most of the cost and my private insurance covered everything else, except a required pair of tight-fitted stockings, necessary to help prevent blood clots from developing in my legs.

Now, looking back to the time of my surgery, I am satisfied with my decision. I am also happy that I was forced into searching for more information. The level of understanding I needed to come to that decision was more than what anyone could have afforded the time to provide, so I sought it on my own. And I have only just scratched the surface. But what I found was enough for me to make an informed decision.

One final note: Remember that your cancer combined with your situation might be different than mine, so your ultimate decision could be different.

Chapter 38

PRE-ADMISSION CLINIC

*I expect to pass this way but once.
Any good therefore that I can do, or any kindness that I can show to any fellow creature,
let me do it now. Let me not defer or neglect it for I shall not pass this way again.*

STEPHEN GRELLET

Admittance to a hospital for surgery involves some very necessary advance preparation. Most hospitals conduct *pre-admission* consultations with patients a few weeks prior to admittance. These consultations are sometimes called pre-admit clinics. Based on personal experience, this is a valuable exercise for both the hospital and the patient. It enables the patient to arrive at the hospitals, be admitted, undergo surgery, be transferred to the recovery room and later to a ward and to start rehabilitation, all in the same day.

The purposes of the pre-admission clinic are to:

- Sort out administrative details prior to admission; and
- Inform the patient of the procedures and hospital care policies.

If the pre-admission clinic is part of your hospital procedure – and I hope that it is – it will probably be held about two weeks prior to admittance. If you do not attend this clinic, you will not be admitted and your time slot will be given to someone else.

If your hospital does not conduct a pre-admission clinic, you will probably learn all of this just as you are about to undergo treatment. Sometimes, you are admitted the day before the treatment, for the equivalent of the pre-admittance clinic. I prefer to be prepared in advance.

Part VI   The Surgery Experience

The clinic itself takes about three hours. The first 15 minutes are used by the hospital staff to gather administrative information from the patient. That's followed by a waiting period of up to 45 minutes, then a one-on-one consultation with a nurse. Sometimes, this includes tests and a physical examination.

The administrative information gathering includes:

- registering your insurance coverage;
- being advised of the type of room you are entitled to, such as, ward, semi-private or private;
- identifying your method of payment;
- establishing the date and time of surgery;
- registering your family doctor and surgeon's names; and
- identifying your significant other, or next of kin, in case of emergency.

My suggestion is to approach the clinic or process with an open mind, a positive attitude and a willingness to listen and respond to questions. I was fortunate to have a very polite, calm, compassionate and empathic nurse. I arrived feeling a little apprehensive and left feeling very confident.

During my consultation, my nurse explained what would happen on admission into the hospital and thereafter, as well as everything I had to do in order to prepare. By the end of the consultation I felt mentally prepared. I felt that I knew what to expect and was ready to face it.

A helpful part of the consultation, for me, was the portion on managing pain. I am a coward and do not like pain, including a needle puncturing my skin. My nurse explained why pain management was an important part of the recovery process, and various approaches to help its success, such as pills, liquid, suppositories, injections, and patient controlled analgesia (P.C.A.). That put me at ease.

Another useful piece of information concerned the anaesthetic. My nurse told me what to expect, and gave me a brochure which explained it further.

Some other information she reviewed with me were:

- I would be admitted to hospital two hours prior to surgery.
- Instructions on adjusting my diet, and emptying and cleansing my bowel prior to admittance, starting two days before, then one day before, then midday before, then the night before. It's important that you do not eat or drink anything after midnight before surgery.
- To call my surgeon if I developed a cold or any other illness, as those could be cause for rescheduling the surgery.
- I should start exercising my legs immediately after regaining consciousness from surgery. She instructed me to point my toes toward my head, then towards the foot of the bed, then twirl

my feet around in circles five or six times, approximately every hour. I should also bend and straighten my legs one after the other.
- I should start deep-breathing exercises immediately, by taking three deep breaths, inhaling through my nose and exhaling through my mouth.
- I should cough two or three times hourly, during my recovery and rehabilitation.
- I should expect and know how to handle the many discomforts which come with rehabilitation.
- Be aware of and understand the "after surgery" procedures, including recovery room monitoring, intravenous, pain killers, medication and transfer to surgical unit.
- My discharge from the hospital would incorporate a transition to home care, and follow-up appointments.

You can make an appointment for the pre-admission clinic by telephone. Likely, your urologist/surgeon's staff will advise you where to call.

When attending the clinic, you will need to have the following (or equivalent) with you:
- all pills or medicine you are currently taking;
- your government issued health insurance card;
- any supplementary insurance information, such as Blue Cross or Green Shield, or others;
- completed admission form;
- any forms given to you by your doctor/surgeon for admission purposes;

Other things that you may want to consider:
- ensure that you have a will and/or power of attorney
- there is no necessity for fasting prior to this visit.
- bring a family member, if you wish.
- bring an interpreter with you, if necessary.

When I left the pre-admission clinic I was ready to take on the challenges of surgery.

Chapter 39

ADMISSION

You are the only person alive who has sole custody of your life.
Your particular life. Your entire life.
Not just your life at a desk, or your life on the bus,
or in the car, or at the computer.
Not just the life of your mind, but the life of your heart.
Not just your bank account, but your soul.

ANNA QUINDLEN

On the day of my admission I had grown anxious and scared. This was major surgery and because I was still not completely sure that I had made the right choice, something kept gnawing at me, telling me my life could easily take a drastic turn for the worse as a result of this choice. However, I kept that feeling to myself and tried to look on the positive side. I was going to be cured. I definitely did not want to make my wife overly concerned. I knew that if I could be brave, she would be, also. I also knew that if I showed or express fear, she would become three times more so. Thus I pretended to be fearless. As a result, she showed bravery and confidence and was able to share her strong positive support. She was the wind beneath my wings.

My admission time was 1:00 p.m. on Friday March 3, 2000. I drove to the hospital, accompanied by my wife, parked my car in the hospital's parking lot and in good spirits, making humourous small talk, we walked boldly for three minutes to the admissions office. I had pretty well convinced myself that there was no turning back. I was physically, mentally and spiritually prepared. As we approached the office, I said to my wife, "I feel like a lamb walking to the alter to give itself up to be slaughtered."

Chapter 39 | Admission

We arrived at the administration office on the ground floor of the hospital at precisely 1:00 p.m. and were met by a staff member. After preliminary identification, my file was retrieved and I was directed to an area on the fifth floor. There we were met by a nurse who instructed me to disrobe, put on a hospital gown, and lie on a nearby gurney (rolling-bed). Then the realization of my purpose there hit me. As I lay there the nurse pulled a pair of tight fitting TED stockings on to my legs, from ankle to crotch. These were to help prevent blood clots. I wore them for the entire time I was in the hospital. Actually, apart from the parking fee, a few parting "thank you" to the nurses when I was discharged, the cost of those $30 stockings was the only out-of-pocket expense I incurred for this surgery. That's the Canadian way of health care.

Soon, after a kiss and a hug from my wife, I was wheeled away to another area which appeared to be a corridor near the operating room. My wife went off to the waiting room where she spent the next six and a half hours. As I laid there in the quiet corridor, several people in white robes passed by and chatted briefly with me, as if trying to cheer me up. I remember one person in particular – I believe he was the anesthesiologist – said to me, "Don't worry, it will feel as if it only takes two minutes." I found that encouraging, because I realized immediately that I would not know or feel anything until it was over. I recalled immediately when I had two of my wisdom teeth taken out: one minute I was awake, and the next thing I knew a half hour later, the dental surgeon was telling me that it was all done. I realized then I would be wheeled into the operating room, put to sleep and awake five or six hours later. And it would be done.

Everyone who came by tried to encourage me, although by that time I had resigned myself to the fact that it was going to happen. I was very upbeat and think I was one step ahead of passers-by. As they asked me how I was feeling, my reply would be my standard, "sensational!" In almost all instances, that one word took them by surprise and made them chuckle. Was I worried? Definitely not! I was assured that my surgeon was the best and he had performed this nerve-sparing procedure many times in the past – an average of five per week for the past eight years at least. I had complete confidence in him.

Soon I was wheeled into the operating room, where they lifted me from the gurney onto an operating table. I was positioned directly below some very bright overhead lights. I knew that we were coming closer to the moment when I would be unconscious. The thought did occur to me that it was possible I might never regain consciousness.

Health care professionals surrounded me. One of them tried, unsuccessfully, to find a vein on the back of my left hand, through which she would feed the intravenous liquid. She finally switched to the right hand and found one. I remember that my urologist/surgeon came in to see me and asked how I was feeling, and if my wife was in the waiting room. He informed me he was going out to talk to her, and then they put the mask over my nose and advised me that I was going to start feeling dazed. Almost momentarily I fell into a sound sleep.

Part VI   The Surgery Experience

I regained consciousness about 8:30 that evening. I was in my bed in the hospital ward. My wife was beside me, as well as a nurse who would take care of me throughout the night. I felt relieved to know I had made it through the surgery was still alive.

Chapter 40

SURGERY MADE EASY

*Write the bad things that are done to you in the sand,
but write the good things that happen to you on a piece of marble.*

ARABIAN PARABLE

Cut to Cure

The surgery itself was easy, or so I perceived it to be. One minute I was awake in an operating room, staring up at those bright lights, surrounded by all those people in white robes, caps and masks preparing me for the operation – and the next minute, or more accurately 5 1/2 hours later, I was in a bed in the ward, being care for by a nurse. My prostate gland was gone and with it, hopefully all the cancer. Now I was on my way to recovery and cure.

Radical prostatectomy is undeniably a major operation. Mine was a bilateral nerve-sparing retropubic radical prostatectomy. There is also the less used alternative known as perineal radical prostatectomy. The retropubic approach is basically conducted via an incision. There is also the Laparoscopic radical prostatectomy using five small puncture holes in the abdomen around the navel for the instruments to pass through. The perineal approach is conducted via an incision between the legs, scrotum and anus. Chapter 30 offer more details on these.

As I lay on the operating table staring up at the ceiling and bright lights, the anaesthesiologist placed a plastic mask over my nose, causing me to inhale the anaesthetic. Within seconds I was sound asleep. Then they shaved me, in the area surrounding the incision site – then they sliced my abdomen open. The surgery had begun.

Although it may vary with the individual, my incision started below my navel and continued downward to above my pelvic bone. It was about 15 centimetres or six inches, long and required 25 staples to close. An acquaintance who had similar surgery two years later had only a 10-centimetres or four-inch incision. Current practice utilizes closer to eight-centimetres or three-inches incision.

Some surgeons, including mine, are also utilizing the Laparoscopic method. We'll hear a great deal more about this as it becomes more commonplace.

Imagination Runs Wild

Many people, when facing surgery, find their imaginations working overtime, coming up with strange, even frightening scenarios. I was no exception. I had a vision that when my abdomen was cut open, all my organs – intestines, bladder and others – would instantly jump out of the confinement of the skin and flutter like a roll of tubular gas filled balloons. I was thinking of a time, a few years back, when I witnessed the slaughter of a goat for a family feast in my native country of Belize. My nephew, who slaughtered the goat, sliced open its abdomen with one stroke of a knife, and everything, including its intestines, literally flew out, uncontrollably fast and furious, just like inflated balloons. That was what I envisioned would happen to me, but apparently, nothing like that happened.

As you lie on your back, the prostate gland is hidden beneath tissues and the pelvic bone, just above and adjacent to the rectal wall. Once the incision is made, the surgeon reaches in and clears a path to the prostate by pushing the various organs and tissues to both sides to make way for his hand and instruments.

Fortunately, I am a small person with a relatively small stomach. My surgeon/urologist maintains that he's experienced enough to handle large and small men; however, it seems to me that the smaller you are, the easier it may be for the surgical team to reach through the various organs and tissues to get to the prostate. In my case, I had prepared myself by exercising and smart eating over a period of 20 months prior to surgery. My suggestion is that as soon as you find out you have prostate cancer, start on a special diet, nutrition and exercise program that will help you burn some excess fat. We all have excess fat to burn. That might make it easier for the surgeon, if you choose surgery.

When the path is clear and the gland is found, the surgeon examines and severs the lymph nodes from either sides of the bladder and sends them to the lab for immediate microscopic analysis, to see if they are inflamed or cancerous. This is not always necessary however, since an experienced surgeon could assess the likelihood of lymph node involvement himself, using the Partin Tables. After the lymph nodes are removed, the prostate gland is examined to see if it's inflamed or if the cancer appears to have spread. If there is any indication that the cancer has penetrated the wall of the prostate capsule and escaped to other parts of the body, or metastasized, the surgery would be stopped immediately. A decision would then be made about alternative treatment, such as radiation, hormone therapy or both. Unlike the past, this situation is rarely encountered since doctors are now much better at determining lymph nodes involvement and cancer metastasis before surgery takes place. This helps the experienced surgeon in qualifying patients for surgery before the fact.

I was fortunate in that my cancer had not metastasized, so I was pre-qualified for surgery.

Bear in mind that a non-metastasized malignant tumour is curable, whereas a metastasized malignant tumour is not curable, but treatable.

Saving the Neurovascular Nerve Bundles

If there is no indication of capsular penetration or spread of the cancer, your doctor may set out to preserve the delicate and precious neurovascular nerve bundles around the prostate gland and with them, the cavernous nerves that is responsible for the erection. If your Gleason score is 8, 9, or 10 they would not endeavour to save them, since the likelihood of cancer spread would be great.

The nerves bundles are those nerves that clasp themselves on both sides of the prostate gland like two hands tenderly cupping a baby's face. They are cobweb-thin and delicate. They are part of the nerve system that leads from the brain via the spinal cord to the prostate and the penis. Within them are two tiny important nerves, called the cavernous nerves. They are situated alongside the prostate gland and carry signals to the penis and are responsible for the erection capability. If the cavernous nerves break or become damaged in the treatment process, you can simply kiss good-bye to ever being able to have an erection again. That's a harsh reality. So every effort is made to protect those nerves from damage. Every man wants to have his erection capability intact after surgery. He may or may not be fortunate to have that wish granted.

Saving the nerves bundles on one side only is considered a unilateral nerve-sparing procedure. Saving the nerves on both sides is considered a bilateral nerve-sparing procedure.

Before treatment, you might think that it does not matter if you cannot have an erection, as long as life goes on. But after you are well and back to normal, and the only thing missing from your quality of life, is the ability to have an erection, you will see the effect it can have on you. Quality of life includes erection capability and you may find yourself wishing, time and again that you could have your penis rise and enlarge as your mind commands. You may even wish you had chosen an alternative method of treatment. I have spoken to many men, who have experienced this nerve-sparing procedure, about this, and invariable they express these sentiments.

Your surgeon may successfully save those nerves as long as the cancer is not too advanced and he is experienced enough to do so. Some parts of the nerves may unavoidably go along with the prostate and some may be unavoidably damaged. But those depend largely upon the condition of the gland and how much it has been attacked by the cancer. However, an experienced surgeon will save whatever has not already been damaged. In some cases he may revert to the nerve graft procedure mentioned in "Chapter 29."

Severing the Prostate

Once the surgeon has preserved the nerve, he has the task of severing the prostate gland. He accomplishes this by slicing the urethra tube at its bottom end then lifting it and disengaging it from the surrounding tissues, including the delicate cobweb-thin nerve bundles at both sides, as well as from the rectum wall. Now the gland is left attached only to the base of the bladder, the vas deferens and the seminal vesicles. The seminal vesicles are attached to the prostate like two rabbit ears. These points of attachment are carefully separated.

The surgeon then cuts into the bottom of the bladder and slices the prostate away from it. With that goes the internal sphincter, the mechanism that helps the bladder control the flow of the urine, leaving the bladder with an opening about the size of a small coin at its base.

When the separation is done, the prostate is lifted out of the body.

After the surgery, the specimen is forwarded to the pathologist for microscopic examination. The pathologist dissects the prostate gland into several slices and cuts them into smaller pieces, examining each thoroughly to determine the stage and grade of the cancer.

The condition of my prostate, was described as follows:

On February 9, 1998, based on biopsy:

"right base Gleason score 2+2=4 with neural invasion."

On March 3, 2000, based on the whole prostate, after it was removed:

"prostate carcinoma, Gleason 3 + 3 = 6, very focal capsular invasion, no vascular invasion."

Now the urethra has to be reconnected to the bladder. In order to do this, the surgeon inserts a Foley catheter via the opening at the head of the penis, through the penis and the urethra, to the bladder. The end of the catheter, which fits inside the bladder, is fitted with a balloon which, when it's in place, is inflated by pumping 10 to 15 cubic centimetres of water into it. This water does not interfere with the tubular passageway. By inflating that end, the catheter becomes secured inside the bladder and cannot be pulled out. At the outside end, it's connected to a plastic bag for the deposit of urine drained from the bladder.

The surgeon then sews up the base of the bladder, leaving a small opening that fits the urethra tube; then he pulls the remaining urethra toward the bladder entrance and sews them together. It's very important that the surgeon achieves a complete reunion of the urethra and the base of the bladder. After that, nature takes it course and seals them permanently. Remember, about an inch and a half of the urethra is taken away with the prostate.

The clean-up process is done with the Foley catheter still in place. Another tube is placed through another part of your stomach to drain any excess fluid such as lymph, serum or small amounts of blood from the surgery site.

You are then sealed up. Your incision is closed and stapled together and you are taken to the recovery room, where you are closely observed by a nurse for about an hour and a half. Later, you are taken to the ward where you will start your rehabilitation process with the help of some very efficient and caring nurses and doctors, over the next two to three days. That's a marked improvement over my time of five to six days.

Chapter 41

HOSPITAL STAY

*Nothing is more precious than good health;
and when health problems arise, nothing is more important than excellent care.*

2000 – 2001 Annual Report
Community Care Access Centre
London – Middlesex, Ontario CANADA

In Appreciation

This chapter is written in appreciation of those wonderful hospital staff members who cared for me and made me feel secure and comfortable during the period that I was confined in the hospital, recovering. Individually and collectively, they are special.

Caring Staff

The nursing staff and other medical and service personnel at the London Health Sciences Centre, where I was admitted and operated on, were knowledgeable, friendly, caring, empathic and compassionate. I put my trust completely in their hands and they never let me down. Being a patient in the hospital under such circumstances did not allow me to be bashful or cowardly. I was there to be cared for and to recover and I wanted to make it easy for those administering the care. Being co-operative, to the best of my ability, was my intention. I started by being positive and upbeat. I think the staff appreciated that. I followed their instructions completely and avoided being a pest.

I had a private room, which was over and above the semi-private that my health insurance covers. I enjoyed the privacy and individuality.

Chapter 41 | Hospital Stay

Tubes! Tubes! Everywhere

It all started when I was wheeled into my hospital room about 8:30 p.m. on the evening of the day of my surgery. After about a half hour, I began to realize there were people around me. As I awoke from the sedative state I had been in since 2:30 that afternoon, I saw my wife at the foot of my bed along with one of the several nurses who would subsequently care for me.

One of the things that I feared before the surgery was to awaken and find myself wrapped in a multitude of tubes. I had a vision of finding a tube leading through my mouth and down my throat. It was a relief to find that was not the case.

I did, however, have a number of rubber tubes connected from a few transparent plastic bags to various parts of my body. The bags, hung by several different hooks on a portable steel intravenous (IV) rack, contained liquids that provided me with life support, comfort and energy. This IV rack was supported by five legs on wheels which made it difficult to move about and steer in a straight line.

A Y shaped "nasal cannula" tube was in my nose, connected to an oxygen tank hung on the IV rack. Oxygen was delivered to me from the oxygen tank through tubing attached to the nasal cannula – a tubing that was placed a short distance into my nose.

There was a tube (suprapubic catheter) from one of the bags, inserted through a skin incision on the right side of my abdomen leading into my bladder.

A Foley catheter entered my bladder from my penis through my urethra. Together, this Foley catheter and the suprapubic catheter formed an irrigation system that helped to wash the blood out of my bladder and discharge urine. My urologist/surgeon told me that, in most cases today, only one drainage tube (catheter) is used, and no irrigation is done. In my case, these two catheter were to be transformed into a very necessary irrigation system, as you will read later.

There was a tube leading from a skin incision on the left side of my abdomen to a plastic, hamburger-shaped, compact that lay beside me. This tube was draining excess serum from my abdominal cavity into the compact.

Another tube, connected to the IV bag hanging from the rack, was attached to the IV needle that was inserted in the back of my right hand.

Two of the tubes led from a glass jar containing pain-killing substance. One flowed into the IV line and the other was attached to a tube that led to a cylindrical, patient-controlled analgesia (PCA) hand-size pump that laid beside me on the bed. This allowed me to supply myself with the pain-killer whenever I needed some relief from pain. It worked like magic!

The PCA pump is a computerized pump that safely permits you to push a button and deliver small amounts of pain medicine into your IV line. There is no injection of needles into your muscle. PCA provides stable pain relief in most situations. This gives the patients a sense of control over their pain management.

It's hard to believe that I put up with those for six days. Today, they have shortened that hospital stay in most treatment centres, to approximately three days. Following is my experience.

Friday's Care – 1st Night

The atmosphere in the hospital at nights was creepy but tranquil. My room was situated beside the nurses station. When the lights in my room were turned off and the door closed, I sensed a lot of activity outside of the room, in the hallway leading to the nurses station, as noise and lights crept under the door and moving shadows consistently interrupting them. I felt as if angels were guarding my room from the outside.

After my wife left for home at about 9:30 on the first night, I went off to sleep quickly. I remember being awakened several times throughout the night by the nurse. She came in and took my temperature and blood pressure, checked my tubes and internal drainage system, and gave me antibiotics. Each time she came in, I awoke and chatted with her. I was glad to know that I was alive, conscious and could recognize and appreciate things happening around me, even if I was still dazed. I felt really excited about successfully making it through such major surgery and still feeling so well. I had imagined myself being so weak that I would not even recognize members of my family.

The nurse that first night instructed me, as the nurse had at the pre-admit clinic, to twirl my feet around, and raise and stretch my legs one at a time. She reminded me to take a few deep breaths and cough a few times every hour. That was difficult to do, but I was told it would help to prevent my lungs from collapsing and contracting pneumonia. I did my breathing regularly, and with the help of a small instrument which I breathed into, was able to set goals for the amount of power I put into my breathing.

Saturday's Care – 2nd Day

I thought that as morning rolled around, I would have been weak from the loss of blood. However, it started out as a very exciting day. Much to my surprise I was painless, exhilarated and happy about feeling so good. It even occurred to me that I felt so good that they might want to send me home early. Unfortunately, this changed later.

Chapter 41 | Hospital Stay

At 7:00 a.m. I met the second nurse who cared for me. She was the day nurse on duty that Saturday and the first of only two who dressed in white. Her immaculate uniform and businesslike approach gave me the impression that she was a seasoned professional in her field, who was there to do her job. It was not long before she demonstrated that she knew exactly what she was doing and what I needed. She gave me a bed bath and got me a bed-pan and water so that I could clean my teeth. I had already started the foot exercise and the breathing and coughing routine.

Later in the morning, with that nurse's help, I took my first walk. Can you believe that, less than 24 hours after major surgery? Well, believe it because today that first walk takes place even sooner.

The walk was short, and I had to push my portable IV rack that was supporting the oxygen tank, the jar and all those bags of liquids connected to me via the tubes. It was probably the most difficult walk I have ever taken. At that moment I was not very strong, but the nurse accompanied me. We walked out of my room down the hall for about six metres, or 20 feet, and turned back. It was exciting to me that I was capable of walking so soon after the surgery. On my return, I sat down in a chair and watched my nurse change the bed linen. Soon after the walk my nasal cannula tube was removed from my nose along with the tube to the oxygen tank. That was one down, with still a few remaining.

On an hourly basis throughout Saturday the nurse took my temperature, checked my blood pressure, and checked the instruments and bags. She particularly checked the bag leading from my bladder to ensure the cleansing was working. I was still bleeding internally, as could be seen by all the red liquid waste draining from my insides, but I did not worry as it was obvious to me I was in good hands.

My wife and eldest daughter, Natalie, along with her one-year-old daughter, Sierra, visited me later that day. The most touching gift that I received while hospitalized was the one I received from Sierra that day. It was a picture of my grandchildren with a statement saying: **"We can't wait to play again grandpa – we love you!"** There were two pictures on the single sheet – one of Sierra and the other of the children of my second daughter, Stephanie, her three-year-old daughter, Isabelle, and her five-month-old twins, Mathieu and Michelle. The pictures were scanned into a computer, printed and framed. If you think things like these aren't real consolation at times like these, think again!

That afternoon, I had my first visit from a resident doctor. He asked me a few questions, and examined all the contraptions attached to my body. After he had assured himself – and me – that all was well, he left.

Part VI   The Surgery Experience

An anesthetist also visited me that afternoon. He asked me a few questions and when he was convinced that I was recovering safely from the anaesthetic, he left. Later, a physiotherapist visited. In fact, she visited me twice during my stay to ensure that I was doing the appropriate exercises with my feet and lungs.

That day, the communications salespeople came and offered to rent me telephone and television services. Renting the telephone and rejecting the television was perhaps the best decision I made that day. If I had rented the television I would have missed the opportunity to get to know all of the wonderful nurses and others who cared for me. I would have read less and never received and recognized the inspiration to write this book. Let me explain.

My Inspiration – Conversations With God

A week before my surgery a friend lent me a book entitled "Conversations with God – an uncommon dialogue, Book 1," written by Neale Donald Walsch. I took the book with me to the hospital and it became a conversation piece with my many visitors and subsequently my inspiration for writing this. As I was reading the story of dialogue between God and a man, the thought crossed my mind that what was written was simply the author's imagination and that he must have been inspired to put down on paper the thoughts or dreams that he had. It occurred to me that even factual information can be passed on if one is inspired to write it down. There and then I decided to record factual information about my stay and treatment in the hospital, to make it easier for others who would be admitted. That paper turned into this chapter and, later, the inspiration to share more researched information. I have henceforth expanded the project to what you are holding, by including the many things I learned.

The book, "Conversations with God," as it sat there on my bedside table, also gave the people in the hospital a certain perception of, and admiration for, me. I personally think that God gave me the inspiration to put all this on paper for the benefit of others. I have always remembered one of Benjamin Disraeli's (1804 – 1881, twice prime minister of Great Britain) quotations: "The secret of success in life is for a person to be ready when his opportunity comes." By the way, he also said that "the best way to become acquainted about a subject is to write a book about it." I believe you and I are fortunate that I recognized that call and received the inspiration, and the opportunity to write this book.

Changing Nurses

My day nurse, on that Saturday, cared for me until near four o'clock, when she was called away to the bedside of her nephew, who had been in a serious automobile accident. Her replacement was a nurse who was very excited about her upcoming trip to Cozumel. She was going there on a diving and snorkeling vacation. Being born and raised in Belize, I knew a little about snorkeling and diving and certainly about Cozumel, which is in neighbouring Mexico. In fact it shares the same barrier reef with Belize. She talked about her excitement about upcoming trip and I shared that excitement with her and mentioned some of the wonderful experiences she would encounter. Then my energy began to wane. I began to feel weak and suspected that something was affecting me. Perhaps my pain-killer was wearing off.

On Saturday evening a new night nurse arrived. Interestingly, I had never met this nurse before but immediately felt an affinity with her, as if I had known her all my life. She came into my room early to introduce herself and as soon as she saw the pictures of my grandchildren, exclaimed, in an excited high pitched voice: "Oh, look at the babies!" and walked over to admire the pictures. I liked her immediately and felt that I was in good hands.

She cared for me until 7:00 a.m. Sunday. The procedure was the same as before, taking my temperature and pressure, checking my pulse and drains, ensuring that sufficient liquids were in the various bags, and giving me my antibiotics. As usual, in my high-spirited friendly way, I was always talking to her, asking her about herself, her family, work and recreational activities. I learned that she was a full time nurse who shared her job half and half with another nurse – and was very happy with the arrangement. She had two young children and it gave her time to spend with them and her husband. Her job-share colleague was in the same situation and felt the same way.

Sunday's Care – 3rd Day

My nurse who looked after me most of Saturday was back on Sunday morning. She treated me in the same professional and respectful manner as she had the previous day. I felt safe and secure with her and followed her instructions completely. She sent me on the walk down the corridor and challenged me to increase the distance. I proudly walked twice the distance. In fact, I walked twice that day, for a distance of about 18 metres, or 60 feet, in the morning, and about 30 metres, or 100 feet, in the afternoon. It was even better in the afternoon, because my wife was there to accompany me.

About mid-morning, four resident doctors, including the one who had visited me on Saturday, and two interns called on me, accompanied by the nurse. They came marching in like a small army, all perfectly in single line behind each other, led by the senior resident, who was specializing in urologic surgery. The chief resident had a demeanour and voice that commanded respect and attention. He asked me a few questions, examined me, checked the tubes and gave some instructions to the nurse. That was a very reassuring visit because he left making me feel that I was recovering nicely.

Part VI The Surgery Experience

My urologist/surgeon, who has more of a serious demeanour and who appears to be always focused on his work, although he also runs marathons, also visited me Sunday afternoon. As he walked into the room he asked in his very low pitch voice how I was. I replied happily: "Sensational!" He laughed (I had never seen him laugh before) and with a smile said, "You must be the only person on this ward who is sensational." His visit was most reassuring, since he was the one who had diagnosed me and encouraged me to have surgery. On that visit, he advised me that the cancer appeared contained within the prostate and he was able to remove it all. He subsequently became the co-author of this book.

Throughout Sunday I continued to feel down, weaker, and in more pain, particularly in the area of my bladder. I used the PCA pump for relief.

I had several visitors, but as the day wore on, I began to feel less and less energetic and enthusiastic, and more and more exhausted. By four o'clock, it was so bad, I was incapable of entertaining my visitors. My daughter Natalie, with Sierra playing around on the floor, stayed with me for the evening. My wife stayed until 9:30.

On Sunday night the friendly nurse, who attended to me the previous evening returned. The first thing she did was to stop by my room to say hello. She had no idea what she was going to experience that night. Having been such an easy and friendly patient up to now, I am sure she expected everything to go smoothly. So did I. Unfortunately, that was not to be.

I awoke at about 11:30 that night, trembling and experiencing severe pain in my bladder. I called my nurse to tell her about the trembling, but the pain was becoming so excruciating that by the time she arrived, the pain took precedence. She examined the Foley catheter and immediately realized that nothing was flowing through it. She attributed that to the fact there might be a blood clot blocking the tubes.

She obtained a plastic bottle with a *syringe* inside and filled it with liquid, then, disconnecting the tubes at my abdomen from the bag, she pushed the mouth of the syringe into the suprapubic catheter tube and manually pumped the liquid through the tube into my bladder. That action forced the assumed blood clot to move and unblock the Foley catheter tube.

The liquid immediately began to flow through the Foley catheter and simultaneously my pain began to subside. What a relief! Along with the liquid came several clots of blood as well as a very red mixture. It was necessary to allow the flow to continue in order to irrigate all the blood and clots, so she pumped liquid in at one end via the suprapubic catheter, which pushed it out at the other end through the Foley catheter. To make this operable on a continuous basis, she needed a pump that would continuously provide pressure to produce the flow, and simultaneously control and measure its quantity and speed. There was no such pump in this ward so she decided to go to another ward to borrow one.

Chapter 41 | Hospital Stay

Within 10 minutes after she, my body began to shiver again. It became worse by the second and soon I was shaking and trembling uncontrollable. It was frightened. I called for a nurse to come and help me again. Since my nurse had not yet returned another nurse came to my rescue. I was shaking so badly that I could hardly talk. The nurse became concerned and ran to fetch my nurse who was in another department negotiating the loan of a pump.

On their return I was in a convulsive state of trembling. They tried to get me to settle down so that they could take my temperature and blood pressure, but that proved impossible. They calmly asked me to try to settle down. I can still remember my nurse's voice, pleading with me gently, sensitively and with empathy, as she held my shoulders, saying: "Harold, try to keep still so that we can get a reading of your pressure and temperature." I tried, I tried hard, but try as I might, I could not. I was getting more and more frightened, because I had never experienced anything like this before. My shaking and trembling went on for about 30 minutes before they finally succeeded in calming me.

My temperature increased dramatically. Within that short period, it rose from a near normal of 36.9 degrees Centigrade to a high of 39.8 degrees Centigrade C. When they finally got me to settle down, my body felt exhausted. Immediately after that incident, the nurse reconnected the oxygen tube and placed them into my nose once again

She set up the pressure pump, which she had brought from the other department, and within minutes a constant stream of liquid was flowing through my bladder, irrigating it. The liquid was pumped from a new bottle hung on the IV rack. The flow of the liquid was initially set at 75 millilitres per hour. Later, in the early morning, she reduced that to 35 millilitres per hour. The liquid from the bottle was crystal clear, but by the time it passed through the bladder and urethra and into the plastic bag, it was red. I was obviously still bleeding.

The nurse continued to observe my condition throughout the rest of the night, taking my temperature, blood pressure and pulse. She even took a blood sample. I am sure she must have been relieved that my severe shaking and trembling did not reoccur. By dawn I had sweated the fever away and felt much better and relieved. The pressure pump that was now irrigating my bladder was kept in place for the duration of my stay in the hospital. The doctors and my other nurses observed it continuously and adjusted its rate of flow from time to time.

I was embarrassed that I had given these nurses such a scare, but what better way to leave a lasting impression. I bet they will never forget me. I know that I will always be grateful to them for caring so well for me that night.

Following that incident, I had a few more blockages caused by blood clots in my bladder, but those were pumped out using the bottle and syringe procedure. They felt much less painful than that first blockage.

Part VI   The Surgery Experience

Monday's Care – 4th Day

On Monday morning, the fourth day of my hospital stay, I met another incredible day nurse. Sometimes I swear these folks are simply magicians. The senior resident and his entourage dropped by again as part of their rounds. They were informed, by the nursing report, of my previous night's trauma and they discussed it with me. I found that reassuring.

Up to this time I had been on a liquid diet. That morning, the senior resident decided that I could eat food that was a little more solid. He advised the dietitians accordingly. I was still bleeding internally, as was evident by the red liquid coming through the Foley catheter. I walked three times that day, increasing the distance each time, and still pushing my IV rack ahead of me.

On this day I also used my private bathroom, for the first time, to wash myself.

I walked to the bathroom situated at the end of my small private room, pushing my rack as an extension of myself. Everything that I needed for my washing, such as soap, wash cloth, towels and hospital robe were inside the bathroom. They were within reach of where I stood. I carried my personal grooming accessories including shampoo, toothpaste, toothbrush and comb, in with me.

Bleeding

Later in the day, something interesting happened. One of the resident interns returned to examine the liquid coming through the Foley catheter. He increased the flow of the liquid flowing through my bladder from 35 to 100 millilitres per hour. Later, I overheard him talking on the telephone – he told them what he had done and then spent a long time justifying his action. Much to his credit, later in the day, my urologist/surgeon came in and increased the flow again, this time to a whooping 300 millilitres per hour. That increase helped tremendously and within a short time the liquid began to change colour from very red to clear and transparent, which seemed to indicate that the bleeding had slowed or stopped. Several times through the day the intern came in to monitor the flow and the colour.

My Hemoglobin Watch

Another interesting occurrence that morning was the senior resident advised me that my *hemoglobin* was low, at 100, and likely the ongoing bleeding was responsible. He advised that he would have it monitored and if it fell to as low as 70, he would arrange for a blood transfusion. In order to monitor it, the nurses took blood samples every few hours throughout that day, Monday and the following Tuesday morning. My left arm became very bruised from the assault of the needles. I did not relish those at all, as I hate pain, and those needles were large.

Monday night I had a new nurse. She was the other half of the Saturday and Sunday night nurse. Great person! She was very lucky, because I was an improved patient.

Tuesday's Care – 5th Day

My Tuesday day nurse was the same one as Monday. This day turned out to be an eventful one. My hemoglobin fell to a low of 73 and as a result, it was decided that a blood transfusion was required. I was given solid food, starting with breakfast, and also began taking my nutritional supplements. I was discharged from physiotherapy because I was improving so well. The physiotherapist instructed me to continue with the exercises, the coughing and the deep breathing. She then wished me well, then left.

My nurse disconnected and removed the IV tube and needle from the back of my hand, as well as the PCA pump.

That afternoon, they pumped two units of somebody else's blood into me to raise my hemoglobin.

In order for the staff to observe the acceptance of the transfused blood and ensure that I experienced no side-effects or decrease in hemoglobin, it became necessary for me to stay in the hospital for an extra day, to be observed – for a total of six days.

According to my urologist, it's rare for a person to need a blood transfusion after radical prostatectomy. It's only about one out of every 50 to 100 patients who needs it. Apparently, it did not appear that I had lost too much blood during the procedure but rather after it had been completed.

My nurse that night was the same one who had cared for me on Monday night.

The rest of my hospital stay was focused on steady rehabilitation with the same observations and activities taking place. My daily walks increased in frequency and distance. Sometimes, my daughter or my wife would accompany me.

Wednesday's Care – 6th Day

I spent most of Wednesday walking and doing other activities. The nurses observed my blood condition to ensure that my body would accept the transfused blood. That required taking several blood samples intermittently throughout the day. I was also allowed to order regular food from the hospital. That morning the nurse – the first male nurse I had – disconnected the drainage tube from the left side of my abdomen and removed it with one swift pull. "Wow! That hurts!" was all I could say. After all it was imbedded four inches into my abdomen. It burned for a few minutes and then the pain subsided. He dismantled the pumping system and removed the suprapubic catheter (tube) through which liquid flowed to and from my bladder. Now, there were two 3/8 inch diameter wounds in my abdomen, which had to be sealed and healed.

He did not bandage these. He said that he wanted them to close and heal quickly. Now, the only thing left in place was the Foley catheter, and I felt so much freer. Now I felt more like I was staying in a hotel than a hospital.

Oh, I did not mentioned, the male nurse was an acquaintance of mine whom I had known for a few years previously and I had previously informed him that I was coming to be his patient.

Thursday's Care – 7th and Final Day

On Thursday morning I was ready to go home. I felt I had recuperated enough and gained enough strength to face the outside world. I expected that I would be discharged that day, so I took a shower for the first time. My biggest challenge was preparing to get into the shower stall and under the low shower head.

I had to disconnect a plastic urine collector bag, which was attached to the Foley catheter. Ah, that dreadful catheter.

Disconnecting that bag, emptying it and rinsing it out was a chore that had to be done carefully and slowly, especially that first time. But I conquered it. It's something that I had to learn to do patiently, because I had to do it every morning and every night for the next two weeks.

With the catheter tube hanging from my penis without the bag, but like a long narrow penis extension, and a long incision down the front of my lower abdomen, held together by 25 staples, I carefully stepped into the shower stall, turned on the shower and washed my entire body, including shampooing my hair, for the first time in seven days. It felt strange. My penis had never felt so heavy, delicate, tender, intolerable and uncomfortable.

After showering, I prepared myself for the outside world. I attached a smaller plastic urine collector bag to the catheter. This replaced the larger plastic bag, which I had disconnected. I strapped this smaller bag around one of my legs. With that in place, conveniently hidden inside my pajamas, I was able to easily walk around. Then I slowly slipped into my pajamas and waited for a final visit from the doctors. Now instead of having this bag attached to the rack, it was strapped to my leg. Of course I had to empty its contents about every hour.

Ear Problems

A irritating side-effect that concerned me was a pressure in my left ear. It was painful and uncomfortable and I complained about it. The ear, nose and throat specialist came to see me. She attributed it to the antibiotics used at the beginning of my treatment. She assured me that it was temporary. I felt that pressure for weeks after my discharge. My ear drums were subsequently checked again about a month later and found to be in good order. The pain lingered for about three months and eventually faded away.

Discharged

On the seventh day, after an unusually long stay in the hospital, it was time for me to go home, and I was ready! Others had to stay only five days but they did not have a blood transfusion. Five days in the hospital is enough! Today, two to three days is the norm.

Before I was discharged the interns examined me one last time. They checked my hemoglobin level and were satisfied that my blood count was stable. I was discharged at 12:30 p.m.

So I had lunch, called my wife, changed into my clothes, and spent some time saying "goodbyes" and showing my gratitude to the nurses. I gave each of them one of my trademark pins that said "ATTITUDE." I followed those later with a "thank you," cards.

When I left that hospital, I knew the names of every doctor, intern, nurse and service support staff, who attended to me, cleaned my room, brought me food and made my bed. Most other patients only knew the names of a few people. Not me! I knew them all by name. They were special to me. Nevertheless, I was really glad to be seeing the outside world again.

What I Needed in the Hospital

Several people have asked me what they should take with them to the hospital. My answer is: "Take very little." I took one book to read, a light robe, a pair of slippers, toothbrush, toothpaste, comb, my watch and some family photographs. In other words, dress appropriately and pack light. Of course, my home was just around the corner.

The experience of my hospital stay and care is one that words cannot adequately express. I will

Part VI   The Surgery Experience

never forget the people, the occasion, nor the care. I will forever be appreciative of their dedication, empathy and friendliness. I say this today, even after all the years that have passed.

I had many wonderful nurses, interns and specialists to whom I owe a great deal of gratitude. I could never forget the wonderful treatment by the service staff who looked after me and my room. They all talked to me on such friendly terms. They made me feel like a human being and made my stay very special.

Without a doubt, they were the best.

Chapter 42

POST-SURGERY CARE

All conditions and all circumstances in our lives are a result of a certain level of thinking. When we want to change the conditions and the circumstances, we have to change the level of thinking that's responsible for them.

ALBERT EINSTEIN

Homecoming

I was discharged from the hospital just after mid-day on the Thursday. My blood transfusion was successful and I was feeling sensational. My wife arrived to take me home, and at 1:30 that afternoon we left the hospital for the four-minute drive to our home.

Upon arrival, I had a feeling of joy and apprehension. The joy resulted from being back within the walls of my home and closer to my family. The apprehension was because I had to give up the safety and security of the wonderful caring nurses at the hospital. They were always available and now suddenly, they were not. On the other hand, I felt that nobody knew me as well as my wife, and I knew that she was reliable and would take good care of me. Of course, it soon became clear to me that I was the one who had to take care of me. Others can only help. This is an important message, because we'll only feel as good as we make ourselves feel. We cannot go around feeling that others will take care of us.

Having said that, I cannot emphasize enough that everyone is different when it comes to speed of recovery. Some people will take what seems like forever, others will bounce back quickly. I have no doubt that my nutritional supplements and positive mental attitude contributed considerably to my speedy recovery and rehabilitation.

Part VI   The Surgery Experience

That Dreadful Catheter

I came home with the catheter still attached. It was a long tube embedded inside my bladder, where it was inflated so that it could not pull out. From there, it extended down through my urethra, and out through the head of my penis. My penis looked pathetic with this tube protruding from it, like a worm trying to free itself. The interchangeable plastic urine collector bag was attached to the tube at the lower end.

I had to move around with this tube and bag hanging from the head of my penis. The daytime bag was small and strapped around my leg, inside my trousers. It was replaced at night by a larger bag, designed to be carried outside of my clothes and to be hung somewhere as I lay in bed.

It was amazingly easy to travel around with my small bag during the day without it being noticed. On one occasion, I had a speaking engagement at a community centre. I rose from my seat, walked to a lectern in the front of the auditorium and delivered my speech. Nobody knew that I had a bag tied to my leg collecting urine. Even the few people there who were aware that I had surgery did not know.

As I prepared to retire to bed at night, I would change the plastic bag attached to the catheter, from the small daytime bag to the larger night time bag. Then in the morning I would do the reverse.

The procedure for extracting the bag and connecting it again was a delicate one, at least for me. That first night at home, as I removed the bag which was strapped to my leg, I felt tender and sore in the most delicate and sensitive parts of my body, especially while washing them. Even while connecting the night bag and putting on my pajamas, I had to be careful and gentle in order to avoid hurting myself. I had to avoid any pull on the catheter hanging from my bladder through my penis, to prevent pain and discomfort. The slightest pull felt like a hundred pound force tugging at my bladder.

Changing the bags before retiring to bed at night was done in two stages: the removal of the small bag and the attachment of the larger bag.

To remove the small bag, I would empty it of its contents first, then unstrap it and disconnect it from the tube. This was accomplished by pulling on a plastic lever attached to the neck of the bag. This lever controlled a clamp that closed off or opened the flow of the liquid. When pulled down, it opened the clamp and allowed the discharge of the contents (urine). I would then unbutton two buttons on the two latex rubber belts, used to strap the bag to my leg and disconnect the bag from the catheter, by pulling off the rubber tube connected to it. I would rinse the inside of the bag with diluted vinegar and hang it out to dry for use the next day.

To attach the larger bag, I would climb into my pajamas, then bring the catheter tube through the front opening and connect the larger bag to the catheter by pushing the rubber tube over the plastic mouth of the bag. It could be hung on the drawer of my bedside table, or on the side of the bed frame. Either way it had to be hung at a lower level than my mattress to allow gravity flow.

The next morning the entire procedure would be reversed. The only difference between the routine at nights and in the mornings is that, when I disconnected the night bag in the morning, I stepped right into the shower.

Once I mastered this procedure and discomfort it became easier. Eventually, as the tenderness and sensitivity wore off in the penis, the urethra and inside the bladder, I was able to conduct the procedure much more quickly.

One of the problems I encountered was that the latex strap burned into my flesh and created blisters, which turned to sores, and left some scars during the later days. I reduced the pain and discomfort from those blisters and sores by using a cloth bandage under the strap. Unfortunately, those scars remained visible for a long time.

As time passed, I found it easier to use the night bag around the house during the day, when I was alone at home. I just tolerated it and carried it around with me, hanging from one of my fingers. Of course, if someone should come to my door, I would not answer it, because there is absolutely no way that I would stand there with a large bag containing my urine with a tube leading through my trousers to my penis. Fortunately no one visited.

Extended Nursing Care

Extended nursing care was offered during my first two days at home. On the first day, the visiting nurse removed the staples from my incision. Her visit lasted only a few minutes. On the second day she advised me and my wife on how to use the bottle with syringe inside, in the event there was any blockage to my catheter. Her second visit was even shorter and in my opinion, somewhat of a waste of time, since it seemed like everything could have been accomplished on the first day. Perhaps that was because I had seen that syringe used so many times in the hospital that it was very familiar to me. Nevertheless, it was nice to have two visits – after all, anything could have happened

My wife stayed home from work for a week, after my return home. Since her workplace was only a 10-minute drive away, we concluded that I could look after myself. If I needed her she could quickly come home.

Part VI   The Surgery Experience

Becoming Active

On the Friday, my second day at home, I went out for a slow walk, accompanied by my wife. We walked for 10 minutes away from home then turned back. We walked that distance again on Saturday – twice. I repeated the walk, alone, on Sunday, Monday, Tuesday, and Wednesday. On Thursday I walked twice the previous distance, and repeated that on the Friday through to the following Thursday. On that day, 20 days after my operation, I went for my scheduled visit with my urologist. He removed the catheter – I'll tell you more about that later. What a relief! Suddenly I felt lighter and more enthusiastic about recuperating.

I tried desperately to do some Kegel type exercises while I had the catheter in me, but I didn't feel it was very successfully done, so I stopped. After the catheter was removed, I resumed the exercises, which are very important. More about that in the next Chapter.

Chapter 43

TIPS FOR CARE AND MAINTENANCE

*How wonderful it is that
nobody need wait a single moment before starting to improve the world.*

ANNE FRANK

On Caring

I could not write this without offering some tips on caring for yourself while recuperating, first in the hospital, then at home. After all, this was my initial objective in putting my feelings into words, which resulted in this book. I appreciate that you may have heard most of these things before, but a little reinforcement will not hurt. In fact it may even make life a little easier for you and your condition more tolerable.

Positive Attitude

It's important to develop a positive mental attitude. Accept the fact that this is not the end of the world, and that you will feel better. You will heal and begin to live a normal life again. You may have to learn to accept certain deficiencies, maybe even a lesser quality of life for a time, but you will become accustomed to them.

Ultimately, what you want is to become healthy, regain your strength and live the best quality life you can achieve. It will not happen overnight nor will it happen if you just sit around the house and sulk. It will happen much faster if you have a positive mental attitude and go about your normal chores, without overdoing it too soon. I think you will find that your Creator has many other plans for you.

Healthy Lifestyle

You should strive to eat healthy, sleep well, exercise, rest and relax. That includes nourishing your body and nurturing yourself. Eat nutritious foods and supplement those with good grade vitamins and minerals. Re-read the first section of this book. Any nutritionist will tell you that the more vegetables and fruits you eat, the healthier you will become. Also less consumption of sugar and fat, particularly saturated fat, trans fat and hydrogenated fat, will help in this regard.

In the Hospital

In order to improve your blood circulation, start doing the following immediately after you regain consciousness (Some or all these may be explained to you at the pre-admission clinic, prior to surgery):

- While lying on your back, twirl your feet around in circles, using your ankles as the pivot.
- While lying on your back, raise your legs and bend them at the knees, one at a time, straighten and bend, straighten and bend, straighten and bend, for about 10 repetitions every hour.
- Walk. Start walking as soon as possible after surgery, and increase the distance each time. This is also good cardiovascular exercise.

In order to exercise the lungs and help prevent pneumonia:

- Breathe. Take deep breaths six to 10 times per hour. Breathe in through your nostrils and breathe out through your mouth. Breathe in, as if you are trying to suck in all the air around you.
- Cough. Cough three to four times every hour.

In order to avoid getting blood clots in the feet:

- Avoid crossing feet, especially at the ankle. I had to keep reminding myself of that constantly.
- Keep bending and straightening your feet at your knee, while laying down.

At Home

Avoid feeling sorry for yourself, and expecting others to feel sorry for you. Instead, become active.

Using comfortable walking shoes with good traction:

- On your first and second day, walk around inside.

- On your second to fourth days, venture outside, first on the deck/balcony, then on the sidewalk.
- On your third through to seventh days, take 10 minute walks at a slow pace three times a day.
- From the eighth day to the 15th, increase the walking time to 20 minutes, two or three times a day.
- From your 15th to 42nd day and thereafter, increase your distance and walk every other day.
- From your ninth week, start some light aerobics, swimming, or light weight-bearing exercises.
- From your ninth week onward, continue to walk and exercise every other day.

Take all prescribed medication regularly, until finished.

- Eat, but eat wisely, and not too much at a time.
- Eating several small meals is better than eating one or two large meals.
- Avoid consuming too much fat, especially saturated, trans fat or hydrogenated fats. They are killers.
- Add some Omega 3 to your diet. Try some salmon, flaxseed, walnuts or helm seeds.
- Eat at least three fruits per day and servings of vegetables two or three times per day.
- Add some extra fibre – both soluble and insoluble
- Always have some fast-acting laxative handy.

Supplements

I cannot say enough to encourage you to supplement what you eat, with additional nutrients in the form of vitamins, minerals and trace elements. It's virtually impossible for you and me to get sufficient nourishment and necessary anti-oxidants, simply from food, particularly while rehabilitating.

- Vitamin and mineral supplements, up to a certain limit, do not hurt and can do much good, particularly during the recuperation period.
- Ensure that whatever nutritional supplements you take include a complete spectrum of vitamins, minerals and trace elements, preferably balanced and bioavailable.
- If you have difficulty making a selection, consult a registered dietitian who recognizes their benefits.

Getting Rest

You will need rest, plenty of it.

- Your body is still very weak, and will be for a long time.
- Try to get at least two short power naps during the day, preferably after exercising, walking and/or meals. Try to get six to eight hours sleep nightly. If you find that you have trouble falling asleep, then at least lie down, rest and relax.

You may experience discomfort when you lie flat on your back in bed. Do not hesitate to adjust your bed to a suitable slanting position. Be creative.

Some people find that during their first few weeks, when laying down, they need to have their upper body slightly elevated and their legs slightly raised, in order to be comfortable.

My wife reconstructed our bed, by placing a thin mattress from a folding bed, horizontally, under the head portion of our mattress, between the bed's mattress and the box spring. This folding bed mattress protruded out on one side, but it was a small penalty to pay for a few weeks of comfort. In addition, I used a number of pillows to prop me up to a comfortable angled position. I also placed a pillow under my legs just above the knees. With these in place I rested and slept comfortably.

Incontinence

Incontinence will affect you regardless of which treatment you choose, because your internal sphincter muscles will be damaged, weakened (by radiation and cryosurgery) and maybe even destroyed (by surgery). Here are a few suggestions for coping:

- Sleep on your back until you feel that you are in control of your *urine retention* muscle (external sphincter muscle).
- Avoid alcoholic beverages, especially beer and wine. They will make you sleep soundly in all positions and you might end up wetting your bed unknowingly. Wine will produce more frictionless urine that flows easily.
- Spread a plastic sheet or garbage bag over your mattress near the lower part of your bed, and spread a towel over the plastic material, before you spread your sheet. These will protect your mattress from becoming soiled in the event you urinate while sleeping.
- Get up and empty your bladder whenever you wake up and feel the urge. Do not be lazy about it, it's far better to get up for a few seconds than to wet the bed.
- If you had surgery, you no longer have an internal sphincter muscle to control urination. You have a little-used external sphincter to depend on. You will have to help it to work effectively by exercising it regularly.
- Similarly, if you had any of the other traditional treatments, your internal sphincter muscle may have been weakened and you need to put the lesser used sphincter to work.
- Like any muscle, if you do not exercise the one you are depending on, it will weaken, and you will experience some embarrassing moments.

Note: Even when you think you have overcome incontinence, there may be occasions, even years later, when you will have a sudden spurt. This might result from a sudden cough, sneeze, strenuous passing of wind, or sitting cross-legged meditation style. Eating too much fruit, especially melons, could produce a more frictionless urine (similarly to drinking wine) that flows easily.

Absorption Pads

In order to avoid embarrassing moments, especially in public places, it's advisable to use absorption pads or briefs, inside your trousers for awhile, during your early days of rehabilitation. In fact, you should even wear them while sleeping. These are adult diapers, but they can make a tremendous difference in your comfort and self-confidence.

Here are some other things to bear in mind about absorption pads or briefs:

- Nobody needs to know that you are wearing them.
- They come in different shapes, sizes and absorbencies.
- You may have to do a search to find those that are most comfortable and suitable for you. (See suggestions below.)
- Until you are fully in control of your external sphincter muscle, you will need to wear them, so get accustomed to the idea.
- Do not be embarrassed about wearing them; this can happen to any man.

After much personal investigation, trials, discomforts and some waste of money, I found I was not comfortable using just any pad or brief during my first few weeks at home. Here are some suggestions, based on my personal experience:

- **At nights to sleep in – up to three to six weeks after coming home:**

    – Use "Tena" ultra briefs (diapers) #67200, or equivalent.
    They have a double protector for heavier night time absorption and are fast drying.
    They are guaranteed to prevent you from wetting the bed.
    They are easy to put on and fit comfortably.
    They have an elastic waist and legs.
    They have fastenable tape for proper fit and quick removal.

- **Around the house during the day – up to three to four weeks after coming home:**

    – Use "Tena" absorbent day-plus pads #62414, or equivalent.
    These are larger pads designed to fit a broad range of sizes and levels of incontinence.
    They can be used with regular briefs or with mesh pants #31401, or equivalent.

- **To go out walking or shopping – up to first six weeks after coming home:**

  – Use "Tena" absorbent day-plus pads #62414 as above, or "Harmonie" duo male pouch #340.
    These are soft, comfortable pads that fit snugly and comfortably.
    They are especially designed to surround and accommodate the genitals.
    They are fully contained and help to prevent leakage to your outer garments.

- **To go out to restaurants and among crowds – up to six weeks after coming home:**

  – Male incontinence pouch #62251, or equivalent.
    These are comfortable pouches that fit around and accommodate the genitals comfortably and neatly.
    These pouches are very comfortable for sitting down.

- **As incontinence improves – up to six weeks and beyond:**

  – Use "Depend" guard protectors for men, or equivalent.
    These are soft and comfortable.
    They are used inside briefs or tight-fitted underwear.

In the early stages of recuperation you may need large-sized diaper pads at nights. The Tena, or similar types will serve well for this purpose. By wearing these larger pads, you will sleep better, knowing that you will not wet the bed.

Having said all this, do not run out and purchase a whole lot of pads or briefs all at once. One pack is enough. You will find that soon you will not need them or that the smaller "Depend" pads, will serve.

You will probably use the smaller pads or pouches in the daytime for awhile. Until you feel that you have completely conquered your incontinence, it would be wise to always have a few smaller pads available for quick and easy retrieval. During my first four months, I never went to a function that would last longer than an hour without wearing a pad. One never knows when a sneeze, cough, or passing of wind will cause a little spurt, or more, of urine leaving embarrassing wet spots on the front of one's trousers.

I stopped wearing any kind of absorption pads about six months after my surgery; however, when I felt the urge to empty my bladder, I did so immediately. When I had to stand in front of an audience for hours to deliver a presentation or facilitate a course, I announced a break whenever I felt the urge to urinate.

Today, I still go and empty my bladder whenever I have the urge. When I eat fruits, particularly juicy fruits such as watermelon, or drink wine, the urge to empty my bladder occurs more frequently. I have become very aware of that.

On Maintenance

Remember that according to experts, your incontinence could last up to a year or more in varying degrees. You might be close to 100 percent, but I doubt that you will ever be completely cured of incontinence. So be aware.

During the early days of recuperation, if you go to public functions, make sure that you know exactly where the washrooms are located. Check it out for location, size and cleanliness. When you have to go, you may have to go quickly. That's the lifestyle you may have to live, in the beginning. Get accustomed to it until you are in control.

During those early months you may also want to consider carrying an extra pad with you, even if it's only in your car. For months, I carried an extra pad in my briefcase. Only once did I use it, and that was because the room I was in was cold and the washroom was far away, and I was afraid that I would not make it in time; however, it gave me confidence that I would not embarrass myself.

Another good idea is to wear darker colour trousers that don't show wet spots. If you feel you are still incontinent, do yourself a favour and wear the pads.

Kegel Exercise

A set of exercises to strengthen the external sphincter muscle are the Kegel exercises. These were developed in 1948 by Dr. Arnold H. Kegel, an obstetrician/gynecologist at the University of California, originally for women with incontinence problems, particularly after giving birth. They work for men also.

I was taught to do Kegel (Pelvic Floor) exercises, as follows:

- Sit in a chair or stand straight or even lie down flat on your back – relax.
- Pretend you are about to pass gas or have a bowel movement then make an effort to hold it back, by tightening your buttocks – you should feel the opening of your rectum contract.
- Tighten the muscle and hold it for about five to 10 seconds while you tilt your pelvis up toward the ceiling and simultaneously sort of pull in as if you are trying to breath in, using your rectum.
- Let go and relax for about five to 10 seconds."
- Repeat the sequence 20 to 25 times at one sitting or laying

Do that about 10 times every hour, six times a day, for the first eight weeks, then fewer times thereafter. The exercise can be done while watching television, or at any time. Other people around you don't have to know you're doing them.

These muscle exercises can give you considerable control over the retention of your urine.

Erectile Dysfunction

Now let us talk a little bit about erectile dysfunction, because you will experience it and you need to understand, accept and live with it.

If you were promised that you will retain the capability of having an erection, understand what that means. That nerve-sparing promise may not be what you expect. You probably will not be told that:

- it might be up to a year or more before you start experiencing erection again, if you ever do;
- your erection will not be as hard as it used to be, ever again, especially at the head of the penis;
- your erection will never last as long as it used to last, ever again;
- your erected penis will never be as large or as long as it used to be, ever again.

The muscles of the penis have experienced some major suffering, resulting in shrinkage. So the thing to do is to begin to understand yourself, your capabilities, your limitations and your short-comings.

Of all the men I spoke to who had nerve-sparing surgery, not one agreed that he has a totally functioning erection, as he did before surgery. The same holds true for men who have had other treatments. This indicates that we should not expect a fully functioning erection and especially not too soon. The nerve bundles have to undergo some healing. That could take upwards of two years, maybe even as long as three years.

Involving your significant other in dealing with these matters would be a wise idea. Between both of you, try to understand and accommodate these capabilities and limitations. Understand each other's needs. Men like to believe, that they must be able to function and perform in order to please their spouses/partners. Well, in many cases, they may be fooling themselves. Many women agree that at this stage in their lives, sex is less an issue than it once was and that the overall relationship is more important.

Libido, Orgasm and Ejaculation

If you were capable of becoming excited as a result of a healthy libido before your treatment, the chances are that you will continue to experience it afterwards. It might come with some frustrations, because you may not be able to satisfy it or achieve release of it, to the same degree as you used to. You might be able to reach an orgasm, but not follow through with ejaculation of semen. It will be a dry ejaculation, sometimes from a soft, rubbery penis. Remember that without the prostate gland and seminal vesicles there could be no ejaculation, but there could be some fluid secreted from the bulbourethral (or Cowper) gland. With some treatments, particularly TURP for BPH, where the prostate gland remains in place but was treated, one may experience "retrograde ejaculation."

After prostatectomy, when you have an orgasm, you might sometimes discharge a liquid, some of which might be urine and some of the fluid from the bulbourethral glands. If the bladder is not drained before embarking on sexual activity, some of the urine might be released, or discharged, during the orgasm. The amount will depend on how long it was since you last urinated and the amount of liquid you had consumed.

It appears that when you have an erection, the external sphincter muscle relaxes and opens up. When you have an orgasm the bladder experiences a spasm and pushes out urine. This urine passes through the urethra and the external sphincter muscle without any resistance and shoots toward the tip of the penis, then spurts out.

If you drink a lot of water, in the order of eight glasses each day, your urine may be relatively diluted. If you do not drink enough water, your urine may be relatively concentrated and have a strong, pungent smell.

You should understand these circumstances and ensure that your partner does also.

Getting it Hard

In the event you are unable to have an erection, you should consult your urologist. There are several ways of achieving erection. Four that are very effective, although not necessarily desirable, are:

1. Medication, such as Viagra, Cialis and Levitra. Others are being developed momentarily. (Note: It's suggested that you never take these if you are on other medication that contains **nitrates,** such as nitroglycerine for angina). For best effect, these should be taken without food.
2. *Penile injection* (Some men say this is not as painful as it sounds).

3. Penile implant (Some men say it provides some extension to the otherwise reduced sized penis).
4. Suction devices.

Each of these is more cumbersome to administer than the preceding one. I suggest that you ask your urologist, or have him send you to a specialist.

If you are affected by erectile dysfunction, see your specialist. Do not be shy. Make the move. No one else will do it for you.

Most people with whom I have spoken, who find themselves in this condition and have sought help, have been surprisingly satisfied with their treatment, particularly medication, and testified it has improved their quality of life.

With respect to the above treatments for erectile dysfunction, you may want to check with your health insurance company to see if they cover the costs and with what conditions. Some insurance programs cover them while others do not. Some will cover them with, a letter from a urologist and prior approval on an annual basis. Some may cover the medication but not the other treatments. So know the facts.

Some Essential Don'ts

Don't

- Travel long distances within eight weeks of treatment.
- Do heavy exercises, or lift heavy weights, within at least 12 weeks of treatment.
- Walk too fast too early.
- Sit upright for too long within six weeks of surgery, such as while sitting at a computer.
- Drive around for too long within six weeks of surgery.
- Go out without wearing a protective pad or brief, until you are almost 100 percent cured of incontinence.
- Let the security of the pads stop you from doing the Kegel exercises or any exercise.
- Use tight fitted pants or underwear within three months of treatment.
- Drink excessive beer, wine or other alcoholic beverages, especially just before retiring to bed, or prior to engaging in sex.
- Drink too much water just before going out during the time you are experiencing incontinence.
- Eat too much watermelon or juicy fruits just before going out in public.
- Smoke.
- Take a tub bath until after you see your doctor at your first appointment after discharge.

Chapter 44

POST-SURGERY MEDICAL CHECK-UP

*To live content with small means,
to seek elegance rather than luxury, and refinement rather than fashion,
to be worthy, not respectable, and wealthy, not rich,
to study hard, think quietly, talk gently, act frankly,
to listen to stars and birds, to babes and sages, with open heart,
to bear all cheerfully, do all bravely, await occasions, hurry never,
in a word to let the spiritual, unbidden and unconscious, grow up through the common,
this is to be my symphony.*

WILLIAM HENRY CHANNING

First Post-Surgery Check-Up

My first post-surgery check-up with my urologist was March 23, 2000, 20 days after my surgery and 14 days after my release from hospital. I was anxious and even somewhat apprehensive.

I was anxious because I knew that I was going to be relieved of the catheter and the bag. Having a penis that was fully functioning made me feel like I was the master of my own fate. However, having something passing through it from inside my bladder to the outside, reduced me to a powerless state of non-confidence and frustration. It was a nuisance and a psychological sentence that made me feel degraded, inept and inadequate.

I was apprehensive because I had no idea what to expect. Would my penis function as it always had? Having the tube hanging there made the once monstrous beast look dwarfed, pathetic and helpless. Looking at it in such a pitiful state, it was difficult to believe that it could ever again perform its functions as adequately as it had throughout my teenage and adult years – functions such as urination and sex, which gave me confidence in my manhood. I was also apprehensive as I anticipated receiving the pathologist's report about the state of my prostate at extraction, fearing that the information may not be so favourable, considering my long delay in deciding on a treatment option.

I decided to brace myself for the worst. Of course, that's easier said than done.

I arrived at the clinic (in the same hospital where my surgery was performed) at 2:00 p.m., registered to see my urologist and checked to see how many people were ahead of me. Realizing there were several, I decided to go upstairs to the ward where I spent my early rehabilitation days to visit the nurses who cared for me so magically during my hospital stay. I was glad that I made that visit, because they greeted me with joy – hugs, laughter and light conversation.

Examination by Urologist

My time of waiting in line at the clinic lasted more than two hours. When my turn finally came to see my urologist, he examined the incision and holes in my abdomen, and asked me to remove my trousers and lie on the examination table so that he could remove the catheter.

Remember, this long rubber tube, slightly more than a quarter inch in diameter, terminated, via my penis and urethra, inside my bladder, leaving about five inches hanging outside to connect to another tube affixed to the plastic bag. The portion inside my bladder was inflatable and deflatable by pumping liquid into or out of it, via a needle-thin entrance. To hold it firmly inside the bladder, it was inflated to form a balloon. Now, to pull it out, it had to be deflated down to its normal size.

Removal of the Catheter

A large diaper was placed under my buttocks and my urologist deflated the balloon by sucking out the water with a syringe. Then, with one swift pull and without warning – swish – he pulled the catheter completely out. It was out of me and into the garbage, before I could feel the resulting sharp pain that followed. Now I was in a whole new world – a world of diapers. I suddenly saw myself as I saw my grandchildren running around in diapers. Yes! I wore a large diaper under my trousers to travel home that day. But I was elated because the catheter was gone. The inconvenience had disappeared. For the first time in 20 days, I thought that my penis might regain its usefulness after all. It felt light and free.

Pathologist's Findings

According to the pathology report, there was no indication the cancer had metastasized. My urologist said there was a spot close to the edge, which he referred to as "very focal capsular invasion," but it had not escaped from the capsule. I felt relieved, although I have a feeling that information could come back to haunt me one day, perhaps in the form of recurrent prostate cancer. I also knew that only time would tell if any cells had escaped into the blood stream.

My urologist also told me that my Gleason score was six (or 3 + 3). I was concerned about that because it was one level higher than the four (2 + 2) from my biopsy sample two years earlier. I was of the opinion that the Gleason score doesn't change and I wondered if someone had made a mistake in interpreting the information. My urologist said the difference of four and six is negligible since they are treated relatively the same; however, if one were to use the Partin Tables, one could make vastly different decision.

There are several possible explanations for the discrepancy. It appears that one person can interpret it as four and somebody else can interpret it as six. They really are that close – and yet so far. Another explanation is that the biopsy result was based on a small sample, whereas the pathology result was based on the entire prostate, or at least a larger sample, which may have areas with Gleason scores of six, four, or even five. It's also possible that, in some cases, the cancer could have gradually become more aggressive.

In my case, I delayed selecting my choice of treatment options, based on a Gleason score of four. If I had been told that it was six, I would had made my decision earlier. After all, a cancer with a Gleason score of six is a more aggressive cancer than one with a score of four.

Nerve-Sparing Success

I was very happy being relieved of the catheter, that I forgot the questions I wanted to ask my urologist. For a short time, I even overlooked the seriousness of the difference in Gleason score. I did ask my urologist if he had succeeded in sparing both sets of nerve bundles. He said "Yes!" To me, at the time, that meant I should be capable of having an erection, without any difficulty, at least no difficulty as a result of the surgery. I learned later that may not necessarily be the case.

Wow! I thought all I had to do was to overcome the incontinence.

That was a mistake! There was still a lot of healing to get through. Those nerves bundles, according to the experts, went through a lot of abuse and perhaps some damage, and nerves do not heal that easily.

So be prepared to be patient, and wait it out. A lot of men are still waiting years after their surgery.

I realize that in the eyes of my urologist, I was just another patient, perhaps another success story. But I was ecstatic. After all, it was my life, my health, my happiness, and my lifestyle. If I could get through this as if it never happened, it would be absolutely sensational.

I left the clinic with a new sense of vigour. I proudly said "Hello" to one of my friends in the clinic. I went upstairs to the ward, one more time, to say hello to the new nurses who had come on duty since I visited a couple of hours earlier. Then I drove home, with much more confidence than when I entered the clinic.

However, there were some new priorities surfacing, such as being able to achieve an erection and conquering my incontinence.

Second Post-Surgery Check-Up

My second post-surgery check-up was June 20, 2000, three and a half months after my surgery.

I arranged to have a blood sample taken two weeks prior to that visit in order to have a PSA reading. In most cases, when you are given an appointment for a subsequent check-up you are also given a requisition form to have the blood test done two to three weeks prior.

On that second visit, I was anxious to know my PSA level. I was also concerned about the two challenges that were troubling me at that time. I was finding it impossible to achieve an erection, and my urine was flowing very slowly and without any force. It seem to take forever to empty. I felt that something was drastically wrong.

The first thing I mentioned to my urologist was the slow urine flow. I was immediately whisked off to another room and prepared for a cystoscopy. I really didn't want this, but it appeared to be inevitable if I were to have the situation corrected. After all, there may have been something blocking the urethra, and indeed, so there was.

As my urologist pushed the cystoscopy tube through my urethra, it felt like a steel pipe was being pushed into my penis, although it was really very flexible. Think about it, this is a body part that has only been used to transport liquid, in the past 60 years. Now suddenly, an object was being forced in the opposite direction to that normal liquid flow. The pain was unbearable.

There was some scar tissue in the urethra, so my urologist said he would have to stretch it. Well, what I thought was painful before, was mild in comparison to what I was about to experience.

I could feel the pressure of an instrument being pushed to stretch the walls of my urethra. It was horribly painful! I thought my penis would pop or burst like a balloon.

To top it off, my urologist decided to place a catheter up my penis, into my bladder again for another couple of days. Well there I was, back to square one. Fortunately, it was only for two days and nights. At the end of those days, I was back at that clinic bright and early, to have it removed. My urine was flowing at an increased speed. That was a relief!

Before I left the clinic during that second visit, I also expressed my concern about my incapability of achieving an erection. Was this a permanent situation? Did he not "spare" the nerve bundles? My urologist explained that it was still too soon and that I needed to give it a little more time. I was a bit disappointed that he could not just give me a pill to swallow that would make it return. But I decided to wait and see what would happen with time.

Looking back now, perhaps my expectation of being able to achieve an erection three to four months after such a major surgery was asking too much. Based on discussion with other men, I have concluded that many are lucky if they can perform satisfactory within a year.

Just before I left that second visit, my urologist announced, in a casual manner, that my PSA was below zero point one (0.1) ng/ml. That, to me, was magnificent. It was good news.

Third Post-Surgery Check-Up

My third check-up was September 26, 2000, six and a half months after surgery. I had a blood sample taken to check my PSA level, two weeks prior to that visit.

My incontinence had vastly improved, perhaps as much as 97 percent cured. There were still a few occasions when I could not hold in my urine and I had to depend on a pad. Those occasions, although few, were still too many for my liking.

I was becoming concerned and growing impatient with my erectile dysfunction. After all, my mind and my libido was saying "stand up boy! stand up!" but the little monster, turned dwarf, remained fiery inside and limp outside. Do not get me wrong, every now and then it showed signs of life by becoming slightly enlarged, but never anywhere close to what used to be its capability of standing erect.

I expressed my frustration about not being able to achieve an erection to my urologist. His reply was: "Well, it's only six months since you were operated on; you have to give it time to heal." I asked how much more time, and he replied: "Anywhere from one to two years." That was news to me, but I think he was just trying to get my mind off the subject. I had never heard or read that anywhere previously. I decided to be patient and occupied myself with other thoughts. In the meantime, the dwarfed penis looked as though it was shrinking from disuse.

Once again, I was told that my PSA reading was less than 0.1 ng/ml.

Fourth Post-Surgery Check-Up

My fourth check-up was April 9, 2001 – one year and five weeks after my surgery. Again, I had a blood test to check my PSA level.

My incontinence was pretty well conquered, except for a very few occasions when I strained to pass wind, sat cross-legged, coughed or sneezed suddenly.

My erectile dysfunction had finally begun to improve with the help of medication. I preferred to achieve the erected state without the use of drugs, simply because the drugs were very expensive and I had not mastered the time management between taking them and arousing myself. It took me a while to master that.

My PSA reading was less than 0.1 ng/ml. That was a good news story. My urologist was very satisfied and set my next visit for six months hence.

Subsequent Post-Surgery Check-Up

Henceforth, my check-ups were set at six months intervals. October 2001, was missed due to hospitalization for a heart attack. March 2002 was favourable, as was October 2002, and all the others since. After my October 2004 check-up, 4 ½ years after my surgery, the six month intervals was changed to yearly intervals. In November 2007, my urologist suggested we can upgrade to a two-year interval for my check-up visits; however, I requested we stay on the yearly interval until 10 years have passed after my surgery.

I am feeling healthy and strong now. I just hope that the deficiencies do not get to me and start to make me feel down or less of a man. I also hope that recurrence will not take place.

After more than eight years, I feel I have overcome the incontinence and the erectile dysfunction, with the aid of medication to a reasonably satisfactory level. But do not kid yourself, there are many men who suffer with these conditions for long periods of time. I encourage you to have patience and fight the good fight with a positive mental attitude, while loving life and living it to its fullest in happiness and health.

Chapter 44 | Post-Surgery Medical Check-Up

My reason for saying these things, is so that you may have the facts, in as plain a language as possible. Remember that in removing the prostate, you also removed a very important piece of the bladder neck and the internal sphincter mechanism. These are very important parts of your urinary control system and, in some respects, a part of your reproductive capability. They both affect quality of life. Be ready to accept your situation! But more importantly, make an effort to understand it. You will probably not be told these by anyone else until after the surgery, when the after-effects slowly creep up on you.

Chapter 45

RECURRENT PROSTATE CANCER

"You aren't built to shrink down to less but to blossom into more."

OPRAH WINFREY

"The goal is to live a full, productive life even with all that ambiguity. No matter what happens, whether the cancer never flares up again or whether you die, the important thing is that the days that you have had you will have lived."

GILDA RADNER (1946-1989)
ACTRESS, COMEDIAN (SNL)
– FROM "IT'S ALWAYS SOMETHING," 1989.

Recognize the Signs

Sometimes, just when you think you are free from cancer and cured because so much time has elapsed since your treatment, signs suddenly begin to surface that indicate "the cancer is showing its ugly head again." Your PSA level begins to rise, and rise, and rise, and you know that spells R-E-C-U-R-R-E-N-C-E.

Recurrence, sometimes referred to as relapse or failure, is when the previously treated cancer returns. It happens to a large number of cancer patients, including many men treated for prostate cancer. Often the recurrent cancer may behave more aggressively than was the case the first time around.

If you think the original realization that you had prostate cancer was devastating, a diagnosis of recurrent prostate cancer is even more so. This is, in part because, at this stage, the cancer is generally considered less likely to be curable. This is when you really need to make your peace with your Creator, be positive, and enjoy your life, family and friends to the best of your ability. Celebrate life.

PSA's Significance in the Identification of Cure

In the pre-PSA era, diagnosis of prostate cancer resulted from symptoms such as pain and urination difficulties. In most cases the cancer had already metastasized to the bones and lymph nodes. Pain in the bones and back was a common complaint.

With the introduction of PSA as part of the medical check-up and subsequently ultrasound biopsy, many prostate cancers are diagnosed early with a high expectation of cure.

After successful surgery (prostatectomy or cryosurgery) to remove or destroy the prostate gland, the PSA drops almost instantly to a very low practically undetected level, well below 0.1 ng/ml.

After successful radiation treatment (EBRT, SI or HDR) to kill the cancer cells, the PSA drops, over a period of time, to a low level, less than 1.00 ng/ml. Sometimes also below 0.1 ng/ml.

Unfortunately, these treatments do not always provide a complete or permanent cure. All it takes is for one cell to have escaped or been left intact and then to multiply for recurrent cancer to occur.

Although it's not easy to tell if cancer has recurred, rising PSA levels are usually the first sign, before any symptoms of pain, urination problems, abnormalities on X-ray, or an abnormality noted in a digital rectal examination.

If your PSA begins to rise persistently, you may be experiencing recurrence. You should undergo some thorough testing, such as further blood tests for additional PSA levels, rectal examinations, a bone scan and CT scan, to see if there is any other evidence of recurrence. If no other evidence is exposed it may be best to observe the PSA movement for a while longer, to verify that there is a definite upward trend.

Once recurrence is confirmed, your oncologist will want to find out exactly where the cancer has recurred. It may recur in any of the following:

- Prostate gland (subsequent to radiation or cryotherapy).
- Prostate region: seminal vesicles, base of bladder, peri-prostatic fat and tissues (usually associated with cancer in the prostate itself).
- Pelvis lymph glands and lymph nodes in other areas of the body.

- Bones, especially the vertebrae, rib-cage, skull, pelvis, long bones of the arms and legs.
- Liver, lungs, brains or other organs.

Types of Recurrences

There are three main types of recurrence: biochemical, local, and distant.

If the PSA is rising and, despite thorough scanning and X-ray, the cancer cannot be seen anywhere, then the recurrence is referred to as *biochemical failure*.

If the cancer is evident in any of the first two bullets above, the recurrence is referred to as *local failure*.

If the cancer is evident in any of the other areas above, the recurrence is referred to as *systemic failure* or *distant disease*.

Evidence of more than one of these types may also be found. In all cases, the PSA level will rise in at least 99 percent of cases.

1. Biochemical recurrence

- Rising PSA level
- PSA level higher than established 0.20 ng/ml for previous surgery treatment, and
- ng/ml for previous radiation treatment
- No evidence of local or systemic failure found, despite a thorough search.

Note: Sometimes, clinicians refer to any rise in PSA levels, after treatment that was intended for cure, as "biochemical failure." It means the evidence of cancer recurrence is found in the blood chemistry test, or PSA.

2. Local recurrence

- Recurrence in the prostate gland or the surrounding tissues – sometimes detected by rectal examination
- No systemic failure found yet
- PSA is most likely rising (This is how any failure is usually detected)

3. Distant (or Systemic) recurrence
   - Recurrence in the lymph nodes, bones or other organs
   - Local failure may or may not be found
   - Almost always have biochemical failure
   - PSA rising

Treatment

It's always advisable to dialogue, assess and manage the situation before considering any specific therapy. This is not something to enter into blindly.

The potential benefits of receiving recurrent prostate cancer treatment must be carefully balanced against the potential risks. You have to ask: "What is the chance that the treatment can cure my recurrent cancer, or at least improve my condition? You may even decide to take no treatment at all.

The purpose of receiving treatment for recurrent or relapsed prostate cancer may be any or all of the following:

- To improve symptoms through local control of the cancer,
- To increase your chances of cure, or
- To prolong your survival

The course of treatment will depend on the previous treatment, the type of failure, the aggressiveness of the cancer, and your overall health. The first things you want to know are:

- Where is the current evidence coming from – PSA, X-ray, scans or other? and
- Where is the recurrent cancer located?

Determining Local and Distant Recurrence

If the information indicates only that it's biochemical recurrence, based on a consistently elevating PSA, you may be assured that there is cancer present somewhere in your body. The question is "Where?" Because of the importance of determining the likelihood of local or distant/systemic recurrence, in the absence of physical evidence, your urologist or oncologist may attempt to ascertain the probability of the recurrence being distant/systemic failure versus local, based on the following considerations:

Table

Factors	Likely Local Recurrence	Likely Distant
Gleason score	6 or less	7 – 10
Time elapsed from initial treatment to the PSA rise	"Late" (more than one year)	"Early" (weeks, months)
Time it takes for PSA level to double	Greater than 6 months	Less than 6 months
Prostatectomy Pathology	Resection margins involved No seminal vesicle involvement No lymph node involvement	Resection margins clear with cancer Seminal vesicle involve Lymph node involved

Local recurrence can be treated again for possible cure by *salvage therapy*, whereas systemic recurrence, which is incurable, can be controlled by hormone therapy.

Hormone therapy, of course, affects the entire body and can cause hot flashes, increased body weight, reduced muscle, reduced bone density, loss of sex drive, erectile dysfuwnction, fatigue, breast growth and tenderness, anemia, possibly memory loss or mood change.

Following are some options for treatment or management of the various types of failures:

Chapter 45 | Recurrent Prostate Cancer

Table

Failures	Management Options
Biochemical	Efforts to distinguish whether it's local or systemic have already been taken Hormone Therapy (This offers no hope for cure, but will keep the cancer in remission) Watchful Waiting (If patient is free of symptoms and if there is no strong reason to start treatment yet) Experimental Therapy (This may include new compounds which have shown promise in the lab. One benefits to defer hormone therapy)
Localized	Local salvage therapy (may be a good option) • after radical prostatectomy – external beam radiation • after external beam radiation – cryotherapy or brachytherapy • after brachytherapy – cryotherapy Watchful Waiting Hormone Therapy Chemotherapy Experimental
Systemic	Hormone therapy Chemotherapy Experimental

Sometimes, physicians faced with an elevated PSA blood count but no evidence of cancer, make the assumption that the elevated PSA is coming from the region of the prostate gland and they proceed with local salvage treatment, such as radiation. This is especially so if the evidence weighs more in favour of local than distant recurrence, and if the patient's general health and age suggest early treatment would be beneficial. If it's felt that treatment would not affect the overall life expectancy or quality of life, or that side-effects outweigh the potential benefits, the physician may recommend surveillance only.

Part VI The Surgery Experience

Salvage Therapy

So what is salvage therapy? One may think of it as picking up the pieces and trying to fix it. Actually, it means trying another treatment option after the initial or primary treatment had not completely worked out. In other words, the cancer has returned or has never been completely eliminated.

Since salvage therapy is intended for another chance at cure, it's only an option when there is local recurrence. It involves a different treatment from the original for the following reasons:

- The recurred cancer may be more aggressive than the original;
- The tissues may be scarred from the previous treatment; and
- The first treatment was not effective.

As a result, salvage therapy also brings with it a higher likelihood of side-effects or after-effects and less possibility of cure. Therefore careful consideration is given to potential benefits versus risks.

You can appreciate that this is now a more risky business. You should not go through salvage therapy with limited information. Your oncologist will have the results of a bone scan and a CT Scan. A transrectal ultrasound and biopsy of the remaining prostate gland or tissues proving that cancer is present may be required.

Occasionally, a *prostascint scan* or other investigative modalities may be used to rule out disease outside of the prostate region. If cancer is detected elsewhere, then local "salvage" treatment would not be an option to pursue.

The "prostascint scan" is a nuclear scan involving injection of a radioactive material into the vein. The radioactive material is chemically linked to an "antibody," which is a compound designed to recognize and seek out the "prostate specific membrane antigen." The idea is to identify cells which are of prostate origin, namely minute groups of cells which may have metastasized but are too small to be picked up by the standard bone and CT scans. The prostascint scan may show minute deposits of cancer cells after radical prostatectomy in the space where the prostate used to be, or it may show them in a distant lymph node.

The procedure involves inserting an IV in your hand or lower arm to inject the radioactive material. You will receive the first scan 30 minutes after the injection. The procedure takes about one to one and a half hours on Day one. Before leaving on Day one, you will be given a bowel prep kit with instructions, to be taken at home prior to returning to the hospital four days later for a final scan.

The prostascint scan sounds very effective in theory, but it has not yet been perfected and, thus is not as reliable as one would like it to be. It's also not widely available due to cost and lack of proven usefulness.

Salvage Therapy after Failure of Radical Prostatectomy

If the PSA rises progressively for a while, say more than a year, after radical prostatectomy, EBRT would be a preferred option as salvage treatment for probable local recurrence.

Such local recurrence may result from a few cancer cells left behind after the gland is removed, which later multiplied and formed recurrence in the prostatic bed. That may happen with locally extensive disease when the surgeon cannot remove any more tissue without damage to the bladder, urethra, rectum or external urinary sphincter muscles. Sometimes in the process of sparing the nerve bundles to preserve erectile function the surgeon may also leave some prostate tissue behind, possibly containing some cancer cells.

Factors which may increase the possibility of local recurrence, include:

- Grade of the cancer
  (a higher grade means it's more likely to spread faster, thus more likely to be extensive)
- Pre-surgery PSA level
  (a higher PSA level means the cancer is more likely to be extensive)
- Size of tumour
- Number of biopsy cores found positive (indicates more extensive cancer)
- Cancer in the seminal vesicles
- Cancer infiltrating the prostatic nerve
- Cancer invading the capsule

Salvage Therapy after Failure of EBRT

Many patients who have recurrence after the cancer has been initially treated by EBRT, undergo some form of "salvage prostatectomy" which is an attempt at complete removal of the prostate gland, notwithstanding the significant side-effects. It's appropriate for highly selected patients, and involves either of the following:

- Those who had their prostate gland removed (salvage prostatectomy), or
- Those who had their prostate gland plus bladder removed (salvage cystoprostatectomy)

The treatment involves extensive surgery, and since the tissue has already been radiated previously, it's not very healthy and thus will heal much more slowly. Complications such as rectal injury, excessive bleeding and incontinence are much more likely to occur in this situation, compared with regular radical prostatectomy without radiation prior. Thus the procedure is offered only to young robust individuals who have been carefully worked up.

Other salvage options include:
- Cryosurgery (cold)
- Brachytherapy
- HIFU

Amongst these, cryosurgery is the most commonly used, although it's only available in a few centres. It, too, has potentially serious side-effects, such as incontinence and rectal damage. However, it does offer another chance for potential cure. In Europe, HIFU is more commonly used.

Salvage Therapy after Failure of SI or HDR

Patients who have recurrence after the prostate cancer has been initially treated by SI or HDR have limited local salvage options. Cryosurgery is one possibility, as is HIFU. Salvage prostatectomy is fraught with significant complications. Hormone therapy remains a viable option.

Salvage Therapy after Failure of Cryotherapy

Patients who have recurrence after treatment with cryotherapy may be treated with repeat cryotherapy, although the chance of problems such as incontinence and rectal damage is higher. Another option is EBRT. HDR and SI would not be possible. Hormone therapy remains a viable option if we are comfortable with the idea of cancer control but not cure.

Summary

Prostate cancer recurrence may occur subsequent to any type of previous treatment. It may happen in the prostate gland, the surrounding tissues, the lymph glands, the bones or other organs. It's important to know the type (local or distant/systemic) of failure and to take into account the patient's age, general health condition, treatment side-effects and effectiveness.

Choosing a treatment is a complicated and difficult task and the decision must be made carefully, in consultation with your urologist and oncologist. I encourage you to utilize the information that is provided in this book and act quickly, in consultation with your urologist, to make a well informed and appropriate decision, unique to you and your condition.

I wish you good health, now go and take good care of yourself and trust in your Creator.

PART VII

Glossary And Resources

Glossary of Terms

5-Alpha Reductase (Enzyme): A catalyst that converts testosterone into an active compound called dihydrotestosterone, which causes the prostate to enlarge – a condition known as benign prostatic hyperplasia or BPH.

A

Ablation: The removal or destruction of a body part or tissue, or its function which may be achieved with surgery, hormones, drugs, radio frequency, heat or other methods. See also "Acoustic Ablation."

Acoustic Ablation: Treatment using high energy sound waves to destroy or kill tissue. See also "Ablation."

Acute Bacterial Prostatitis: Prostate infection characterized by the sudden onset of severe symptoms, such as high fever along with urinary urgency, frequency and a burning sensation. It usually runs its course in a relatively short time, if treated with antibiotics.

Adenocarcinoma: A form of malignant cancer which develops in the cells in the body's glands such as the colon, lung, breast and prostate, usually in the gland's lining or wall. Most prostate cancers are adenocarcinomas.

Adjuvant Therapy: A treatment added after the main therapy. The main treatment may be surgery or radiation and the adjuvant treatment hormone therapy or chemotherapy. See also "neoadjuvant therapy."

Adrenal Glands: A pair of small glands on top of the kidneys, which produce hormones that help control many vital body functions, including heart rate, blood pressure and the way the body uses food.

Alpha Blockers: Medication which relaxes the muscles of the prostate and bladder, thereby allowing easier flow of urine.

Glossary of Terms

Androgens: Hormones that are essential for development and functioning of the male sexual organs and for male characteristics, such as deep voice, facial hair, and muscular build. Testosterone is the most important androgen.

Angina: Chest pain or discomfort that occurs when the heart muscle does not get enough oxygen and blood flow is reduced.

Anti-androgen Drug: Hormone antagonists that work by attaching to "hormone receptors," the proteins on the surface of the cancer cell, thereby preventing male sex hormones such as testosterone from having an effect on the cancer cells.

Antibodies: Proteins produced by white blood cells to neutralize foreign invaders, such as bacteria viruses and toxins.

Antigen: A protein or enzyme produced in the cells of a tissue or gland that's specific to that tissue or gland. It's a biological marker of that cell. See also *"Prostate Specific Antigen."*

Antioxidant: A chemical compound, synthetic or natural, that inhibits oxidation and reacts with and neutralizes free radicals or chemicals that release free radicals, highly reactive molecules that can cause oxidation and subsequent tissue damage. Common antioxidant vitamins include C and E, beta carotene and other phytochemicals in food. See also *"free radicals," " oxidation,"* and *"oxidative stress."*

Arteriosclerosis: A thickening and hardening of the artery walls, sometimes referred to as "hardening of the arteries," which results in a loss of elasticity and restricted blood flow.

Atherosclerosis: A form of arteriosclerosis characterized by the deposition of plaques, containing cholesterol and lipids, on the innermost layer of the walls of large and medium-sized arteries. This is known to occur to some degree with aging, but other factors such as: high cholesterol, high blood pressure, smoking, diabetes and family history for atherosclerotic disease, have been known to accelerate this process. The terms atherosclerosis and arteriosclerosis are often used interchangeably in laymen term.

B

Benign: Term describing a tumour that's non-cancerous or non-malignant. See also *"Malignant."*

Benign Prostatic Hyperplasia (BPH): Condition characterized by enlargement of the prostate gland. Typically, the enlargement encroaches on the urinary passageway, running through the prostate, thus causing a slowing in the urine flow.

Beta Carotene: A form of vitamin A found in many fruits and vegetables.

Bilateral: Term describing a condition or process that pertains to both sides of the body or an organ. See also *"unilateral."*

Bilateral Nerve-Sparing Radical Prostatectomy: Invasive surgery to remove the prostate gland while leaving the nerve bundles on both sides of the prostate behind, intact.

Bioavailable: The ability of a drug or other substance to be absorbed by the tissues of the body and available for use physiologically. This means that the substance is highly absorbable to the cells and therefore bypasses the digestive system until the tissues are fully saturated. The substance is then available for use by the body until it is all used up – it doesn't go to waste.

Biochemical Failure: A situation after cancer treatment and assumed cure, when the PSA is rising and despite scanning and biopsies, the cancer cannot be seen anywhere. See also *"Local Failure,"* and *"Systemic Failure."*

Bioflavonoids: A family of antioxidant compounds that give plants their colours, particularly the red and blue, found in flowers, fruits, vegetables and certain tree barks. They are very helpful in the absorption of Vitamin C, and are sometimes referred to as flavonoids.

Biological Markers: Measurable biological parameters, such as specific enzyme or hormone concentration, which serve as indices for health and physiology related assessments, such as disease risk. Example is prostate specific antigen, which may be detected in the bloodstream during the process of diagnosing prostate problems.

Biopsy: Diagnostic procedure in which a tissue sample is removed from the body, by surgery or needle extraction, and subjected to microscopic analysis, usually to determine whether a growth, such as a tumour, is malignant or benign.

Bladder Outlet Obstruction (BOO): Obstruction caused by blockage or closure at the bladder neck where it joins with the prostate at the internal sphincter muscle. See also *"lower urinary track symptoms" (LUTS).*

Bone Scan: Diagnostic imaging of the skeletal system to determine whether malignancy has spread.

Brachytherapy: A type of radiation therapy, in this case for prostate cancer, that involves the placement of tiny radioactive pellets into the prostate. See also *"interstitial."*

Bulbourethral (or Cowper) Glands: Two small glands (structures) about the size of peas, located below the prostate gland and attached to the urethra, which secrete a few drops of clear, sticky fluid in response to sexual stimulation. See *"Cowper Glands."*

C

Cancer: A family of diseases characterized by uncontrolled cell growth and the ability of these cells to migrate to other parts of the body. Cancer presents a threat to life when growth interferes with, or destroys normal functions of, critical body organs and life-support systems.

Capillary Fragility: Easy bruising and rupture of small blood vessels

Glossary of Terms

Capsule: Term used to refer to a layer of cells surrounding an organ, such as the prostate.

Carbohydrates: A class of food which provides energy to the body. There are two types:
1) Simple carbohydrates, which are easily digested sugars found in fruits and processed foods; and
2) Complex carbohydrates, which are starches found in most plant-based food and usually take longer to digest.

Carcinoma: A malignant cancer that develops in the tissue lining of organs. Prostate cancer is a form of carcinoma.

Cardiovascular: Having to do with the heart and blood vessels.

Castration: Surgical removal of the testicles, medically known as orchiectomy or orchidectomy. The word "bilateral" is added when both testicles are removed. See also *"Orchiectomy."*

Catheter: A flexible tube or needle inserted into the body to provide for the passage of fluid. A catheter may remove waste fluids from the body, such as after bladder or prostate treatment, or it may inject fluids such as intravenous administration or treatment of organs. See also *"Foley Catheter."*

Cell: Smallest self-contained unit of life in our bodies. There are millions of different types of cells. There are brain cells, skin cells, liver cells, stomach cells, prostate cells and the list goes on. Cells make up tissues. They all have recognizable similarities. Cells have a skin called plasma membrane, which protects them from outside environment. The membrane regulates the movement of water, nutrients and wastes into and out of the cell. At the centre of the cell is the nucleus, which contains its DNA. See also *"DNA."*

Cell Membrane: The barrier surrounding the cell that determines what gets in and out of the cell. See also *"Membrane."*

Chelated: Firmly attached – usually an amino acid or other organic compound attached to an atom of metal or mineral, so that the two do not disassociate in the digestive system. See also *"Chelation"* and *"Chelator."*

Chelation: Chemical joining of metallic ions with certain organic compounds or amino acid for easy passage of the metal into the digestive system. See also *"Chelated"* and *"Chelator."*

Chelator: A compound that binds tightly to a metal or mineral atom, thus forcing the atom to go wherever the chelator goes. The bound pair – chelator plus metal atom – is called a "chelate" or chelated mineral. Chelators of nutritional interest include amino acids, organic acids, proteins and occasionally phytochemicals. Chelators carry mineral atoms into the body or into cells in larger amount than the body would normally allow. It is as if the chelators are treated as desirable molecules by the recognition system in all walls and are therefore given entry into the cells, along with their baggage of mineral atoms. When this process occurs in the cells that are lining the digestive tract, the mineral gains entry to the blood stream; when it occurs in the cells that are lining the blood vessels, the mineral gains entry to other body tissues. See also *"Chelated"* and *"Chelation.."*

Chemotherapy: Treatment for cancer using potent drugs that attack and destroy cancer cells. The drugs are injected or taken orally. Often, there are side-effects associated with the treatment.

Cholesterol: A fat-like substance found in certain foods – such as meat, fish, poultry, eggs, and dairy products – and also produced in the body to aid in functions such as the manufacture of hormones. Cholesterol travels through the bloodstream in different packages called lipoproteins. Low-density lipoproteins (LDL or "bad" cholesterol) deliver cholesterol to the body, while high-density lipoproteins (HDL or "good" cholesterol) take cholesterol out of the bloodstream. There is a correlation between high blood cholesterol levels and health problems, including cardiovascular disease.

Chronic: A medical or health condition that is continuously or persistently severe over an extended period of time.

Chronic Bacterial Prostatitis: Persistent form of prostatitis which involves inflammation of the prostate gland lasting for an extended period. Chronic prostatitis usually has fairly mild symptoms that may, become acute.

Climacteric: A period or year of life when physiological changes supposedly take place in the body (like menopause in women).

Clinical Trial: A research study to determine the safety and/or efficacy of new medications and/or treatments, conducted under strict scientifically-controlled conditions.

Coagulation Necrosis: Necrosis in which the affected cells or tissue are converted into a dry, dull, fairly homogeneous mass as a result of the coagulation of protein. Necrosis means death of tissue in the body. This happens when not enough blood is supplied to the tissue, whether from injury, radiation, or chemicals. Necrosis is not reversible.

Cold Spots: Small areas that are missed by the radiation emitted from the radioactive seeds and where cancer cells may survive.

Colon: Large bowel or intestine. The parts leading into the rectum are called "descending colon" and "sigmoid colon." Coliform bacteria are so named owing to their presence in high numbers in the colon.

Cowper Glands: See *Bulbourethral (or Cowper) Glands*.

Cryoablation: A procedure that destroys tissue by freezing.

Cryosurgery: Minimal invasive therapy that employs extreme cold to destroy cancer cells.

CT Scan: Acronym for computerized tomography scan – x-ray technique using computer technology to assimilate multiple images into two-dimensional cross-section image. This can make real many soft tissue structures not shown by conventional x-ray.

Cystoscope: A small telescopic device containing a light and viewing lens, a flexible fibre optic tube, used to view the inside of the bladder and urethra.

Cystoscopy: An examination of the urethra, prostate and bladder, using a cystoscope, inserted through the urethra into the bladder.

D

Degenerative Disc Disease: A gradual deterioration of the discs between the vertebrae of the spine. The discs lose flexibility, elasticity and shock-absorbing characteristics. Although relatively common, this condition is usually not severe enough to warrant medical attention.

Degenerative Disease: Disease or condition that attacks an organ or body and its immune system and life support system, and gradually and slowly worsens or deteriorates over time, until the organ or body is withered to an unrecognizable state.

Detoxifying: The process of reducing the build-up of poisonous substances in the body.

Diabetes: A chronic disease of pancreatic origin that's characterized by insulin deficiency. Sometimes referred to as *diabetes mellitus*. Another type of diabetes is "diabetes insipidus (DI)," an endocrine disorder involving deficient production, or lack of effective action of, an antidiuretic hormone (ADH) in the brain, causing constant thirst, large volume of urine output, dehydration, and low blood pressure.

Diabetic: A person afflicted with diabetes mellitus.

Diabetic Retinopathy: A disease of the retina resulting from adverse effects on the blood vessels supplying the retina – major cause of blindness in diabetics.

Differentiation: Refers to how organized, arranged and well-shaped the cancer cells in a tumour are. Well-differentiated tumour cells resemble normal cells and tend to grow and spread at a slower rate than poorly differentiated tumour cells, which lack the structure, shape, organization and function of normal cells and grow uncontrollably.

Digital Rectal Examination (DRE): An examination performed by a physician inserting a gloved index finger into the rectum to feel its walls and adjacent structures such as the prostate.

Dihydrotestosterone (DHT): A very potent form of the male hormone testosterone. Testosterone converts to DHT with the aid of the enzyme 5-Alpha reductase. DHT causes the prostate to enlarge resulting in Benign Prostatic Hyperplasia (BPH).

Distant Disease: Cancer that recurs away from the primary disease site.

DNA: Deoxyribonucleic acid, the substance in the nucleus of the cell that contains its genetic blueprint and determines the type of cell that will develop. See also *"Cell."*

Part VII   Glossary And Resources

Dorsal Lithotomy Position: A position with the legs elevated and feet supported in stirrups above the head. The position provides a clear view of the perineum.

Dysfunction: A state of inability to function normally.

E

Efficacy: The impact of an intervention, such as medicine, therapy or something else – in a clinical trial. In medical context, it is the acceptability of the therapeutic effect of a given intervention, or that a consensus has been reached that the intervention is as good or better than other available intervention to which it has been compared to in a clinical trial.

Ejaculatory Ducts: The two passages situated within the prostate gland and lead from the vas deferens directly to the urethra, through which semen enters the urethra from the prostate and seminal vesicles. See also *"Excretory ducts."*

Enzymes: Proteins that act as catalysts, enhancing a chemical or biochemical process in the body.

Epididymis: A long tubular structure coiled up and attached to the testicles and used to transport sperm, which can be stored there for up to a couple of weeks. It's about 20 yards if stretched out and is wound together for sperm transport.

Epidural: A part of the body inside the spinal canal, separated from the cord and its surrounding fluid.

Epidural Anaesthetic: Used to partially or fully numb the lower body. It is given through a very thin tube (epidural catheter) into the area surrounding the spinal cord within the outer membrane – the epidural.

Epithelial Tissue: Skin and organ linings, made up of cells closely packed and ranged in one or more layers.

Essential Fatty Acid (EFA): A major component of fat, used by the body for energy and tissue development. It cannot be produced by the body and must be supplied from food source

Excretory Ducts: Tiny ducts that accept the prostatic fluid that is secreted from within the prostate gland and, upon ejaculation, shoot it into the prostatic urethra. See also *"Ejaculatory Ducts."*

External Sphincter Muscle: A ring of muscle around the urethra below the prostate which survives radical prostatectomy and helps to control urine flow. See also *"Internal Sphincter Muscle."*

F

Fistula: An abnormal connection between two organs inside the body, that normally do not connect, like the urethra and the rectum. It might occur because of injury, infection, inflammation, or after surgery where some tissues between the two organs have been removed or destroyed.

Flavonoids: A group of chemical compounds naturally found in certain fruits, vegetables, teas, wines, nuts, seeds and roots. Although not considered vitamins, they have a number of nutritional functions that are described as biological response markers. Most act as antioxidants. See also *"Bioflavonoids."*

Foley Catheter: Latex or silicone tube that drains urine from the bladder to an outside collection bag. See also *"Catheter."*

Folic Acid: A B-complex vitamin called folate.

Free Radicals: Highly reactive chemicals that often contain oxygen and are created when molecules are split, a process called oxidation, to produce products that have impaired electrons. They cause oxidative stress through assault on cells, and have been implicated in causing over 100 diseases in humans, including several degenerative diseases such as cancer, heart failure, arthritis and cataracts. Constant assault from free radicals causes a run-down feeling, lack of energy and stamina. It's also widely believed that free radicals are a major culprit in the aging process itself.

Free Radicals Scavenger: A product, such as antioxidant, used to fight off, neutralize or eliminate free-radicals.

Frequency (Urinary): Term to describe the need to urinate more often than every two hours. See also *"Urinary Frequency."*

G

Gastrointestinal: Pertaining to the stomach or intestines.

Genetic: In medical terminology this relates to hereditary factors.

Genitofemoral Nerve: Nerve pulled from the pelvis and used for bridging two ends of the cavernous nerve in a grafting process.

Genitourinary System: The organ system of all the reproductive organs and the urinary system. These are considered together due to their common embryology origin.

Gleason Grading System: A rating scale from 1 to 5 that illustrates the distortion and differentiation of cells in the prostate, and thus helps determine the aggressiveness of the cancer. The higher the number, the more aggressive is the cancer. See also *"Gleason Score"* and *"Grade.."*

Gleason Score: A criteria to determine the official grade of the cancer. It's based on the Gleason grade. Each component is given a grade (1 to 5) and the sum of the two most predominant grades form the Gleason score. See also *"Gleason Grading System"* and *"Grade."*

Gonadotropin-releasing Hormone (GnRH): A decapeptide, consisting of a chain of 10 amino acids. Its key role is the regulation of the reproductive system, acting primarily to stimulate the anterior pituitary gland to synthesize and secrete the follicle-stimulating hormone (FSH) and the Luteinizing hormone (LH), both called gonadotropins. Its secretion at the onset of puberty, triggers sexual development and from then on it is essential for normal sexual physiology of both males and females.

Grade: Term that refers to the rate of growth or aggressiveness of cancer. See also *"Gleason Grading System"* and *"Gleason Score."*

Grafted: Tissue or organ transplanted, from a donor to a recipient, or from one part of the body to another part, in which case the patient is both donor and recipient, to form a working connection or pathway.

H

Harvesting: Extracting organ and tranplanted for use somewhere else.

Hematospermia: A term used for bloody ejaculate, or blood in the semen (ejaculate). Blood in semen can be caused by many conditions affecting the tubes that distribute semen from the testicles (seminal vesicles) or the prostate gland. The most common cause is inflammation of the seminal vesicles or prostate gland. It can also temporarily be caused by injury to the prostate gland, such as from prostate biopsy.

Hematuria: The occurrence of blood in the urine.

Hemiablation: Ablation or destruction limited to one side of a pair of body parts. See also *"Ablation."*

Hemoglobin: A protein in the red blood cells that transports oxygen and carbon dioxide to body tissues and give blood its red colour.

Hesitancy: Delay of several seconds for the stream of urine to begin.

High Dose-rate Radiation: The strength of a radiation treatment given over a period of time. An implant therapy called brachytherapy.

Hormonal Therapy: Therapy based on administering certain hormones that lower the production of, or block the action of other hormones in prostate cancer – those male hormones that promote tumour growth.

Hormone: A natural chemical produced in one part of the body and released into the blood to trigger or regulate particular functions.

Hormone-Refractory: A stage when the cancer does not respond to hormone treatment or it resists the hormone treatment. See also *"Hormone"* and *"Refractory."*

Hot Spots: Areas of increased metabolic activity or disturbances on or in the bones, seen on a Bone Scan via a Gamma camera. These may be due to an old or new fractured bone, other bone infection, arthritis, or cancer on or in the bone.

Hydrogenated: Subjected to the action of hydrogen, through a process called hydrogenolysis, to combine hydrogen with an unsaturated compound, such as oil or fat. When this occurs, a chemical bond in an organic molecule (unsaturated compound – liquid) is broken and simultaneously, hydrogen atoms are added, resulting in a different structural compound that turns solid. See also *"Trans Fat"* and *"Saturated Fat."*

Hypertension: A medical condition, commonly referred to as "high blood pressure," in which the blood pressure is chronically elevated. While it is formally called arterial hypertension, the word "hypertension" without a qualifier usually stands alone.

Hyperplasia: Occurs due to cell division, increasing the number of cells while their size stay the same.

I

Impotence: The inability to have an erection adequate for sexual intercourse. See *"erectile dysfunction."*

Incontinence: Loss of control of the bladder or bowel.

Infectious Disease: Disease caused by a microorganism, bacterial or virus, that can be transmitted from person to person or organism to organism.

Insoluble: Incapable of being dissolved.

Intermittent Androgen Deprivation Therapy: Hormone therapy for prostate cancer characterized by periods of treatment, alternating with periods of rest or no treatment.

Internal Sphincter Muscle: A ring of muscle at the base of your bladder, where it joins with the prostate and helps control urination or the passing of urine. Sometimes called preprostatic sphincter, or urethral sphincter. See also *"External Sphincter Muscle"* and *"Urethral sphincter Muscle."*

Interstitial Radiation: The placing of radioactive material, such as radioactive seeds, directly into the tumour or organ, as oppose to air space.

Intravenous: Into the veins or blood vessels, using thin needle.

Invasive: Surgery via an incision to operate internally. In reference cancer growth, it's moving beyond the organ of origin and into other tissues. See also *"Non-Invasive."*

Isoflavones: Isoflavones are a class of organic compound with strong antioxidants properties, comparable to that of the well known antioxidant vitamin E. They can act as estrogens in the body, although their estrogen effects are much less powerful than the estrogen hormones. Isoflavones and phyto-estrogens exercise a balancing effect when the level of estrogens is low and they can also reduce the effect of the estrogen on cells and skin layers when the hormone levels are high.

K

Kegel Exercise: Pelvic exercises, developed in the 1940s by Dr. Arnold Kegel, an obstetrician/gynecologist, to strengthen the sphincter muscles and help control urinary incontinence in men and women, including men with incontinence following prostate surgery. Widely used by women to regain urinary control after child bearing has overstretched their pelvic floor muscles.

L

Laparoscope: A slim, lighted tube with a tiny video camera on the end, used to look at abdominal tissues.

Laparoscopic: Operating via keyhole type incisions through the abdomen.

Laparoscopy: To look inside the abdomen with a special camera or scope. The insertion of a laparoscope through the abdominal wall, to inspect the inside of the abdomen and remove tissue samples.

Laser *(Light amplification by stimulated emission of radiation):* Very powerful, concentrated beam of high-energy light used in surgery to cut, destroy or fuse cells. Used to operate on delicate tissues.

Local Failure: A situation where the recurrent cancer is evident in the prostate gland or the prostate region, such as seminal vesicles, base of bladder, or peri-prostatic fat and tissues. See also *"Biochemical Failure,"* and *"Systemic Failure."*

Localized: Contained or limited to a specific area within a gland.

Lower Urinary Track Symptoms (LUTS): Irritation in the urinary track resulting from various symptoms of BPH. See also *"Bladder Outlet Obstruction (BOO)."*

Luteinizing Hormone-Releasing Hormone (LH-RH): A hormone produced by the brain that controls production of sex hormones in men and women, including, testosterone.

LH-RH-agonist: A synthetic compound used to alter the brain's control, and subsequently, the body's production of testosterone. These LH-RH-agonist compounds are the most commonly used hormone therapy agents.

Lymph: An almost transparent fluid collected from tissues throughout the body and returned to the blood via the lymphatic system.

Lymphatic System: A complex network of lymphoid organs - lymph nodes, lymph ducts, lymphatic tissues, lymph capillaries and lymph vessels - that produce and transport lymph fluid from tissues to the circulatory system. It is a major component of the immune system. See also *"Lymph Nodes."*

Lymph Nodes: Small, bean-shaped structures scattered along the vessels of the lymphatic system. They act as filtering stations to trap foreign or unwanted cells and toxic materials. It is where the body attempts to "detoxify," "fight," or "eliminate" the unwanted cells. Unfortunately, cancer cells, including prostate cancer cells, often get trapped there and grow. See also *"Lymphatic System."*

M

Macronutrients: Nutrients, such as carbohydrates, protein and fats, in large amounts, that are key sources of energy. See also *"Micronutrients."*

Macular Degeneration: An eye disease caused by deterioration of the central portion of the retina known as the macula. Generally found in people over 60 years of age, it is also referred to as "age-related macular degeneration (AMD)."

Malignancy: A tumour consisting of cancerous cells.

Malignant: Refers to a tumour that's cancerous and may spread to other parts of the body, sometimes resulting in death. See also *"Benign."*

Medical Oncologist: An oncologist who specializes in the treatment of cancer, by chemotherapy. See also *"Oncologist."*

Membranes: A thin, pliable layer of tissue covering surfaces or separating or connecting regions, structures or organs. See also *"Cell Membrane."*

Metabolism: The physical and chemical processes which sustain life, by breaking down food and nutrients into energy the body can use to maintain itself.

Metastasis: The spread of cancer from its original site to other areas of the body via blood vessels or the lymphatic system.

Metastasized: Cancer that has spread from its original domain to other parts of the body.

Micronutrients: Nutrients, including vitamins, minerals and trace elements, provided in small (miniscule) amounts to enable the body to produce enzymes, hormones and other substances that are essential for proper growth and development. See also *"Macronutrients."*

Modality: Certain "way" or "method" to achieve your objective. Often referred to as *"diagnostic modality,"* or *"treatment modality."*

N

Nadir: The lowest consistent level measured after treatment.

Natural Killer Cells: Our cancer fighting cells. They are often one of the first types of cells that a virus or bacteria encounters and have to overcome. If our natural killer cells are effective, the invaders will not be able to infect healthy cells.

Neoadjuvant Therapy: A treatment offered before the main therapy. The main treatment may be surgery, radiation or chemotherapy, and the neoadjuvant treatment may be hormone therapy. See also *"adjuvant therapy."*

Nerve Graft: The bridging of a nerve between, or into, two cut ends of a similar nerve for the purpose of forming a bridge or scaffold for regeneration.

Nerve Sparing: To spare, preserve or protect the neurovascular nerve bundles surrounding the prostate from damage during treatment. Generally refers to a technique to spare the nerve bundles, to allow for continued erectile function.

Neurovascular Nerve Bundles: Fine red cobweb-thin nerves or vessels that originate at the spinal cord, spread out on the surface of the prostate gland and terminate on the shaft of the penis. They include the cavernous nerves that enable the penis to become engorged with blood to achieve erection.

Nocturia: Getting up frequently at night to urinate.

O

Oedema: Oedema is an observable swelling from fluid accumulation in certain body tissues. May sometimes be spelt Edema.

Oncologist: A specialist whose specialty is the evaluation and treatment of cancer. The specialist may be a "Radiation Oncologist," "Medical Oncologist," "Surgical Oncologist," or "Urologic Oncologist." See also *"Radiation Oncologist," "Medical Oncologist," "Surgical Oncologist,"* and *"Urologic Oncologist."*

Optimal: Expressing the best or most favourable of something, for example optimal health.

Optimum: The best, highest or most favourable condition, degree, amount or result for a particular situation.

Orchiectomy: The surgical removal of one or both testicles. See also *"Castration."*

Oxidation: A chemical reaction, when the loss of an electron takes place by a molecule, atom or ion, resulting from exposure to oxygen or other electron-seizing atoms or molecule combination of atoms.

Oxidative Stress: A condition of cell damage and weakened immune system caused by lower than normal level of antioxidant in human beings or a high level of oxidation taking place in the body.

P

Pathologist: A physician who specializes in microscopic evaluation of diseases in tissues and organs. He examines the biopsy samples and surgical specimens to determine the diagnosis, including the nature and extent of disease.

Glossary of Terms

Pathology: The study of changes to body tissues and fluids caused by disease.

Pelvic Bone: Ring of bone forming the skeleton of the pelvis, supporting the vertebral column and resting upon the inferior members. It's composed of the two hip bones, the sacrum, and the coccyx. The pelvic bone is often a point of deposition of escaped prostate cancer cells.

Pelvis: Portion of the human skeleton forming a bony girdle that joins the lower limbs to the body.

Penile Implant: The surgical implantation of a prosthesis (artificial device) into the penis, to overcome erectile dysfunction.

Penile Injection (Therapy): Treatment for erectile dysfunction, involving injection of a drug into the penis.

Perineal: Refers to the space between the legs, scrotum and anus.

Perineal Prostatectomy: Refers to the removal of the prostate gland through an incision in the perineum.

Perineum: Area between the legs, just behind the scrotum, in front of the anus.

Photons: Small packets of energy.

Phytonutrients: Nutrients found in plants and plant products, that are thought to have health benefits.

Pituitary Gland: A small part of the brain that secretes, and controls the production of, hormones.

Plasma: The clear, yellowish fluid portion of blood in which cells are suspended and which contains the proteins that allow the blood to clot. See also *"Serum."*

Pre-Admission Clinic: Advance consultation before admittance to the hospital, to inform patients of procedures and hospital care, policies, pain management and to sort out administrative details, such and method of payment.

Prognosis: The long-term outlook or prospect for survival and recovery.

Prostaglandins: Hormone-like chemical messengers that play many important roles in our bodies.

Prostascint Scan: A nuclear scan using a special compound that seeks out prostate related cells and tissues, used to detect prostate cancer.

Prostate Gland: A walnut sized gland located within the male body just below the bladder, above the scrotum and surrounding the urethra, and secretes a portion of the seminal fluid.

Prostatectomy: The removal of the prostate gland. See also *"Radical Prostatectomy."*

Part VII   Glossary And Resources

Prostate-Specific Antigen (PSA): A chemical substance or protein that's produced only in the prostate. The blood vessels in the prostate cells are porous and become more so in diseased cells. So the prostate cancer cells are more porous than normal prostate cells and therefore more PSA leaks through these more porous cancer cells into the blood stream than for the normal cells. Thus a higher blood PSA level is usually seen in prostate cancers.

Prostatic Bed: A cavity or depression, where the prostate gland lies – sometimes called prostate bed.

Prostatic Fluid: Fluid produced by the prostate gland. It contributes to the make-up of the semen and contains chemical substances contributing to the viability of sperm reproduction. See also *"seminal fluid"* and *"semen."*

Prostatic Massage: Stroking and kneading the prostate using a gloved finger inserted through the rectum. Prostatic massage is used to obtain a sample of prostatic fluid for laboratory examination or to relieve prostate congestion.

Prostatitis: Inflammation of the prostate gland. May be caused by an infection.

Protein: A molecule made up of amino acids that are needed for the body to function properly. Proteins are the basis of the maintenance, growth and repair of body structure and parts such as skin, nail and hair.

PSA Nadir: The lowest PSA reading achieved after any treatment for prostate cancer.

PSA Test: A blood test to determine the level of PSA (Prostate-Specific Antigen), a protein that's often elevated in men with prostate cancer, and other prostate disorders.

R

Radical Prostatectomy: Surgical removal of the entire prostate gland and surrounding tissues, including seminal vesicles, to eliminate cancer. The pelvic lymph nodes are often removed as well, although that's not officially part of the procedure.

Radiation: Energy released in the form of particles or electromagnetic waves. Common sources of radiation include radon gas, cosmic rays from the atmosphere, and medical X-rays.

Radiation Burns: Damages to the external skin as a result of radiation blast during therapy.

Radiation Oncologist: An oncologist who specializes in the treatment of cancer, by radiation therapy. See also *"Oncologist."*

Radiation Therapist: A technologist who specializes in providing radiation treatment under the supervision of an oncologist.

Radiation Therapy: Treatment involving the destruction of malignant tissue growth (cancer) by bombardment with high energy X-ray or other radiation. Radiation may come from a machine outside the body via external beam radiation, or from radioactive material placed inside the body near the cancer cells.

Glossary of Terms

Radioactive: Relating to or making use of substances that emit radiation. Giving off radiation.

Radioactive Seeds Implant: Small, radioactive pellets, seeds or source material placed in or near a tumour inside the body. Cancer cells are killed by the energy given off as the radioactive material irradiates or decays. See also *"Seeds Implant."*

Radiologist: A doctor who specializes in performing and interpreting images of areas inside the body, from X-ray, sound waves (ultrasound) or other methods.

Recovery Room: Area in a hospital to which patients are transferred after surgery for observation and close monitoring, before being sent to their room or home, depending on the type of operation performed. Now often referred to as the Post-Anaesthetic Care Unit (PACU).

Recurrence: Return of an already treated disease such as cancer. Cancer that has returned after a period of time during which the cancer could not be detected. The cancer may return to the same place as the original tumour or in another part of the body.

Refractory: In medicine, it refers to the stage of a disease or condition, such as cancer, when it does not respond to treatment or resists treatment, such as hormone-refractory. See also *"Hormone-Refractory."*

Regimen: A treatment plan of drugs, cycle and schedule.

Remote Afterloading: A machine, used in High dose rate therapy, that stores radioactive source and dispenses them via thin wires strategically inserted through tube (catheters) that are linked from the machine, through the skin, to the patient's cancer location, then retrieves them when the time has elapsed.

Reproductive: Pertaining to reproduction, reproductive system or capability.

Reproductive System: In men, this includes the prostate, testes and penis. In women it includes the ovaries, fallopian tubes, uterus (womb), cervix and vagina (birth canal).

Resectoscope: An instrument, special kind of cystoscope, used to cut out tissue. In the case of the prostate, it's done through the urethra.

Retina: A delicate multi-layered light-sensitive membrane lining the inner eyeball and connected by the optic nerve to the brain.

Retrograde Ejaculation: Ejaculation, during which the semen flows back into the bladder instead of the body via the urethra. May occur after prostate surgery and in particular, after TURP in the treatment of BPH.

Retropubic: Behind the pubic bone.

Robotic-Assisted Laparoscopy: Using robotic equipment to help with a laparoscopy procedure, achieving more precision and better visibility. See also *"Laparoscopy."*

S

Salvage Therapy: The use of an alternative treatment, when the cancer has not responded to previous treatments.

Saturated Fat: Fat, containing all the hydrogen that the carbon atom can accommodate. They are usually solid at room temperature and can normally be dissolved at a given temperature. It tends to raise total blood cholesterol levels. The main source of saturated fat is from animals and some plants. See also *"Hydrogenated Fat,"* and *"Trans Fat."*

Scaffolding: A patch, utilizing material to connect two cut ends of another material or organ, to allow a graft to work as a continuum.

Scar: Area of fibrous tissue that replaces normal skin or other tissue after injury. Scar tissue is not identical to the tissue it replaces. A scar may affect the flow of fluids, particularly in a passage such as the urethra.

Scarring: A biological process of wound repair in the skin or other tissue of the body – healing process. Becoming marked with a scar or sign of damage as a result of injury to a tissue or skin.

Scrotum: External pouch or sac of skin hanging below the penis and containing the testicles and epididymis.

Seeds Implant: Small radioactive pellets, seeds or source material that are placed in or near a tumour inside the body. Cancer cells are killed by the energy given off as the radioactive material irradiates or decays. Also known as Brachytherapy. See also *"Radioactive Seed Implant"* and *"Brachytherapy."*

Semen: A thick, cloudy, white fluid, which is a mixture of seminal fluid, secretion and other fluid from various sex glands within and around the prostate, combined with sperm, which is released through the penis during orgasm and ejaculation. See also *"Seminal Fluid"* and *"Prostatic Fluid."*

Seminal Fluid: The fluid which is released into the ejaculatory ducts of the prostate gland and combines with secretions from the ducts, and sperm, to form semen, at time of orgasm. Seminal fluid contains sugar as an energy source for the sperm. See also *"Prostatic Fluid"* and *"Semen."*

Seminal Vesicles: Two pouch-like glands behind the bladder that produce a thick gel that is one of the elements of semen.

Serum: The clear liquid component of the blood that remains after the solid components of blood cells and clotting proteins have been removed. See also *"Plasma."*

Source: A place or thing from which something originates. In this book it is material used for radiating energy of High dose rate radiation in implanted therapy.

Spasm: A sudden, involuntary contraction of a muscle or group of muscles.

Glossary of Terms

Sperm: Tadpole-shaped cells produced in the testicles and transported out of the body through the urethra by various seminal and prostatic fluids, as semen. Sperm contains the male genetic material for the fertilization of an egg cell for reproduction.

Sphincter: Group of ring-shaped muscles surrounding an opening or tube in the body. They can expand or contract to control the flow of fluid through the opening. See also *"External Sphincter Muscle"* and *"Internal Sphincter Muscle."*

Spinal Anaesthesia: The induction, by injection, of small amounts of local anaesthetic into the cerebro-spinal fluid, usually via the lumbar spine below the level where the spinal cord ends. See also *"Epidural"* and *"Epidural Anaesthesia."*

Stage: Term that refers to the extent of a cancer in the body, whether it's contained within the original site or not, and how far it may have spread.

Staging: The process of determining if the cancer is confined to the original site or whether it has spread. It's based on the size of the tumour and whether lymph nodes contain cancer. Usually determined by doing tests such as blood tests, X-rays and scans.

Stent: Metal tube that connects or provides support to the walls of a structure such as a blood vessel, or the gastrointestinal tract, inside the body and thereby allow blood or waste to flow normally, preventing blockage.

Stricture: Scarring that narrows a channel, such as the urethra, hence urethral stricture. See also *"Scarring."*

Suprapubic: Above the pubic bone.

Sural Nerve: A small nerve located near the ankle and provides sensation to the side of the foot and ankle. May be transplanted to bridge damaged nerve bundles, particularly the cavernous nerves.

Surgical Oncologist: An Oncologist who specializes in the treatment of urologic cancers by surgery, . See also *"Oncologist."* and *"Urological Oncologist.."*

Suture: The process of joining two surfaces or edges together along a line as if by sewing, such as closing a wound or incision, or joining the ends of two tubes.

Synthesis: The combining of separate elements or substances to form a coherent whole.

Synthesized: To combine so as to form a new complex product.

Syringe: A device consisting of a tube and a plunger, used to withdraw fluids from, or inject fluids into, the body.

Systemic Failure: A situation where the recurrent cancer is evident in other areas of the body. See also *"Biochemical Failure"* and *"Local Failure."*

T

Testes (plural): Also known as testicles. They produce sperm and testosterone. Individually they are referred to as testis.

Testosterone: Principal male sex hormone produced largely in the testicles, and in lesser quantity by the adrenal gland. Testosterone stimulates male sexual characteristics as well as the growth of benign and malignant prostatic tissue. It's also responsible for sexual desires and regulation of a number of bodily functions.

Tethering: Binding two severed parts.

Toxins: Poison produced by certain animals, plants or bacteria.

Toxicity: A measure of the degree to which something is toxic or poisonous. It can refer to the effect on a whole organism, such as human or a bacterium, or a plant, or to a substructure such as a cell or organ.

Trace Elements: Chemicals found in very small amounts in substances which contain vital nutrients that are required for the normal functioning of living things. All organisms, creatures, insects, animals, humans, plants and soil and others, need certain trace elements to survive.

Transducer: A device which converts one type of energy to another, or converts one signal from one form to another.

Trans Fat: Fat made from adding hydrogen to vegetable oil, turning liquid oil into solid fat, usually to increase shelf life, a process called hydrogenation. Examples of trans fat are shortening and hard margarine. Trans fat raises the LDL cholesterol level increasing the risk for heart disease and hardening of the arteries. See also *"Hydrogenated Fat"* and *"Saturated Fat."*

Transrectal Ultrasound (TRUS): A procedure in which a probe that sends out high energy sound waves is inserted into the rectum. The sound waves are bounced off internal tissues or organs and produce echoes, forming a picture of body tissue called a sonogram. Used to look for abnormalities in the rectum and nearby structures, including the prostate, and to guide biopsies of the prostate. Also called "endorectal ultrasound." See also *"Ultrasound."*

Transuretheral Resection: The passing of a thin telescope tube up the urethra via the penis so the surgeon may see inside the urethra. The blockage or abnormal area is removed using an instrument that is attached to the telescope

Tumour: An abnormal growth of cells resulting from uncontrolled and disorderly cell replacement. Tumours can be benign or malignant.

Tumour Markers: Chemical substances that can be detected in higher than normal amounts in the blood, urine or body tissue of patients with certain types of cancers.

U

Ultrasound: High-frequency sound waves used for medical diagnosis and treatment. During an ultrasound, sound waves reflected by internal organs produce images. These images are used to assess the absence or presence of cancer, among other things. See also *"transrectal ultrasound."*

Unilateral: Term describing a condition or process that pertains to one side of the body or an organ. See also *"bilateral."*

Unsaturated Oil: Unsaturated oil is usually liquid at refrigerator temperatures. Slightly unsaturated or monounsaturated oil is found in large amounts in foods from plants, including olive oil, peanut, avocado, and canola oil. Highly unsaturated or polyunsaturated oil is found in large amounts in foods from plants, including safflower, sunflower, corn, and soybean oil. Unsaturated oils do not raise blood cholesterol and may actually lower the levels. See also *"Saturated Fat"* and *"Trans Fat."*

Urethra: In males, this is a narrow tube that carries urine from the bladder out of the body and also serves as the channel through which ejaculated semen is transported. Extends from the bladder to the tip of the penis. In females, this short, narrow tube carries urine from the bladder.

Urethral Sphincter Muscle: Sphincter muscle at the junction of the bladder and the prostate which constricts to control urine flow. Most often referred to as internal sphincter muscle. It's destroyed when the prostate is surgically removed. See *"Internal Sphincter Muscle"* and *"External Sphincter Muscle."*

Urgency: An intense need to urinate accompanied by the inability to hold it in.

Urinary Frequency: The need to urinate frequently during the day, more than every two hours.

Urine Retention: Inability to urinate, causing the bladder to fill up and overstretch its muscles. Usually implies the inability to eliminate an adequate amounts of urine.

Urogenital Diaphragm: A sheet of muscle lining the floor of the pelvis.

Urological Oncologist: An Oncologist who specializes in the treatment of urologic cancers by surgery, See also *"Oncologist."* and *"Surgical Oncologist.."*

Urologist: A doctor who specializes in diseases of the male and female urinary systems and the male reproductive system.

V

Vas Deferens: A pair of tubes about two feet long, which transport sperm from the epididymis to the ejaculatory duct, then to the urethra.

Vasectomy: Surgical procedure in which the two vas deferens of a male are severed and tied off to achieve voluntary sterility as a form of birth control.

Virus: A microorganism, smaller than bacteria that cannot be seen with a conventional microscope, but can infect cells and cause disease. Virus multiplies only by attacking living cells.

W

Watchful Waiting: Closely monitoring a patient's condition but withholding treatment until symptoms appear or change. Also called *"observation,"* and *"active surveillance."*

Suggested Additional Books to Read

1. ***Recovering From Prostate Cancer***, by Leonard G. Gomella, M.D., and John J. Fried, Harper paperbacks, New York, N.Y. 1993.

2. ***Benign Prostate Hypertrophy & Prostate Cancer***, by Kurt W. Donsbach D.C., N.D., Ph.D., The Rockland Corporation, 1994.

3. ***The New Nutrition – Medicine for the Millennium,*** by Dr. Michael Colgan, Apple Publishing, Vancouver, British Columbia, 1995.

4. ***Prostate & Cancer*** *– A Family Guide to Diagnosis, Treatment & Survival*, by Sheldon Marks, M.D., Fisher Books, 1995.

5. ***Prostate*** *– Questions you have ...Answers you need*, by Sandra Salmons, People Medical Society, Allenton, PA 1996.

6. ***Man to Man*** *– Surviving* Prostate Cancer, by Michael Korda, Random House, New York, 1996.

7. ***Saw Palmetto*** *– The Herb for Prostate Health*, by Christopher Hobbs, L.Ac., and Stephen Brown, N.D., Interweave Press, Inc., Loveland, Colourado 1997.

8. ***Prostate Health in 90 Days*** *– Without Drugs or Surgery*, by Larry Clapp, Hay House Inc., Carlsbad CA 1997.

9. ***Prostate Cancer,*** by S. Larry Goldenberg, M.D., Intelligent Patient Guide, Second Edition, Vancouver 1997.

10. ***Intelligent Patients Guide to Prostate Cancer***, by S. Larry Goldenberg, M.D., Intelligent Patient Guide, Second Edition, Vancouver 1997.

11. ***Renewal***, by Timothy J. Smith, M.D., St. Martin's Paperbacks, New York, N.Y. 1998.

12. ***Making the Prostate Therapy Decision***, by Jeff Baggish, M.D., Lowell House, Revised Second Edition, Los Angeles, 1998.

Part VII   Glossary And Resources

13. ***Protect Your Prostate***, by Dr. Michael Colgan, Apple Publishing Co. Ltd., Vancouver, B.C., 2000.

14. ***Natural Prostate Health*** *– A Practical Guide to Using Diet and Supplements for a Healthy Prostate*, by Roger Mason, Young Again Products, Wilmington N.C., 1999.

15. ***Taking on Prostate Cancer***, by Andy Grove, Fortune Magazine Time Inc., 1996.

16. ***Prostate Cancer:*** *What it's and how it's treated*, AstraZeneca (1999).

17. ***100 Questions & Answers About Prostate Cancer,*** **by P.** Ellsworth, J. Heaney, C. Gill, Jones and Bartlett, Boston, Mass., 2003.

18. ***Prostate Cancer:*** *A patient's guide,* The Canadian Prostate Health Council (Nov. 2004).

19. ***Sexuality & Cancer:*** For the man who has Cancer, and his Partner, The American Cancer Society, 10/95.

20. *The **World Health Report 1998 – Life in the 21st Century:** A Vision for All*, World Health Organization, May 1998.

21. ***World Health Report 2003*** *– Shaping the Future*, World Health Organization, 2003.

22. ***Prostate Tales,*** *Men's Experiences with Prostate Cancer,* by Ross Gray, Men's Studies Press, Harriman, TN 2003

23. ***National Cancer Institute of Canada:*** *Canadian Cancer Statistics 2005,* Toronto, Canada 2005.

24. ***American Cancer Society:*** *Cancer Facts and Figures 2006.*

Other Resources For Prostate Conditions

The Internet is, among many other things, a medium for scientific and information posting and exchange. It offers much information; however, not all the information is accurate, validated or up-to-date. If you browse the Internet please make sure you validate the information before using it.

Following are some Web sites that provide additional resources for prostate diseases and treatment options. Some of the organizations mentioned may provide contact information about support groups and/or meetings where you can discuss the latest treatments with others who share similar diagnosis.

American Association for Cancer Research
www.aacr.org
The American Association for Cancer Research provides research grants and publishes several medical journals.

American Cancer Society (ACS)
www.cancer.org
The ACS can be a starting point for dealing with family members and other issues that may arise after a prostate cancer diagnosis. The site includes information about the ACS and statistics about prostate cancer incidence rates.

Centre for Prostate Disease Research (CPDR)
www.cpdr.org
The CPDR is a prostate cancer research program funded by the U.S. Army. It conducts research nationwide at U.S. Army, Navy and Air Force hospitals. The site explains the program and provides education and research updates.

Doctor's Guide
www.docguide.com
This site contains the latest medical news for healthcare professionals, patients, family and friends of those diagnosed with enlarged prostate or prostate cancer.

Healing Well
www.healingwell.com
Provides information resource for patients, caregivers, and families coping with diseases, disorders and chronic illness. Their goal is to help people on their way to "healing well," by offering health resources, interactive tools, and community support to enable individual's to take control of their illness and start the healing process.

National Coalition for Cancer Survivorship
www.canceradvocacy.org
The National Coalition for Cancer Survivorship is a grassroots network of individuals and organizations working on behalf of people with all types of cancer.

The National Cancer Institute (NCI)
www.cancer.gov
The NCI is the U.S. Federal Government's principal agency for cancer research and training. It coordinates the National Cancer Program, which conducts and supports research, training, health information dissemination, and other programs with respect to the cause, diagnosis, prevention, and treatment of cancer, rehabilitation from cancer, and the continuing care of cancer patients and the families of cancer patients.

National Institute of Diabetes and Digestive and Kidney Diseases (NIDDK)
www.niddk.nih.gov
The NIDDK, under the auspices of the National Institutes of Health, provides a site with answers to questions about BPH, talks about the lifestyle of a patient with BPH, and provides additional reading.

The Prostate Pointers
www.prostatepointers.org
Here you will find helpful patient education material on prostate cancer, compiled from a wide variety of medical sources.

National Prostate Cancer Coalition
www.fightprostatecancer.org
Aims to educate every American about the risk of prostate cancer, the importance of early detection and the research funding needed to beat the disease.

Prostate Cancer Research Institute (PCRI)
www.prostate-cancer.org
Objective is to educate patients and their families about prostate cancer. This includes new advances in diagnosis, staging, treatments and available resources. They believes that a patient who understands his disease and treatment is empowered to communicate more effectively with his physicians and obtain a better outcome.

US TOO
www.ustoo.com

US TOO helps survivors of prostate cancer and other prostate diseases and their families lead healthy and productive lives. This organization offers fellowship, shared counseling and discussion sessions in both formal and informal settings.

Canadian Cancer Society
www.cancer.ca

A national community-based organization of volunteers, whose mission is the eradication of cancer and the enhancement of the quality of life of people living with cancer.

Canadian Prostate Cancer Network (CPCN)
www.cpcn.org

The Canadian Prostate Cancer Network, a charitable organization, is the national association of prostate cancer support groups, active in creating and maintaining these groups and in promoting early detection testing as the only cure, presently, for prostate cancer.

Prostate Cancer Research Foundation of Canada
www.prostatecancer.ca

The Prostate Cancer Research Foundation of Canada is the leading national organization devoted solely to eliminating prostate cancer. Their mission is to raise funds for research into the prevention, treatment and cure of prostate cancer by engaging Canadians through awareness, education, and advocacy.

Canadian Urology Oncology Group
www.cuog.org

A national alliance of leading academic and community based urologists, medical oncologists, and radiation oncologists, committed to furthering urology research in Canada including pharmaceutical trials. The CUOG, a non-profit, non-share corporation, has a cooperative relationship with the Canadian Urology Association (CUA), and partners with the Canadian Urology Research Consortium (CURC) with respect to mutually held oncology studies.

La Fondation Quebecoise Du Cancer (French only)
www.fqc.qc.ca

A pour mission **d'améliorer la qualité de vie des personnes atteintes de cancer et celle de leurs proches** par des services d'hébergement, d'information et d'accompagnement. Les services sont accessibles à toute la population québécoise par l'entremise du réseau d'hôtelleries situées à Montréal, Sherbrooke, Gatineau et Trois-Rivières.

Index

5-Alpha Reductase, 80, 83, 89

A

Abdominal Ultrasound, 81
Ablatherm, 271-274, 278
Ablation, 83-87, 265, 272-274, 279
Acoustic Ablation, 273
Acute Bacterial Prostatitis, 76, 104 *See also Prostatitis*
Adenocarcinoma, 74
Advanced Cancer, 109, 227, 286
Aggressiveness, 126 *See also Gleason grade*
Alpha Blockers, 83
Alpha1-antichymotrypsin, 117
Alpha2-macroglobulin, 117
Alternative Treatment, 14, 100, 125, 152, 176, 251, 293,
   See also Watchful Waiting, Surgery, External Beam Radiation Therapy, Internal Radiation Treatment,
   Hormone Therapy, Cryotherapy, HIFU, and Chemotherapy
Alzheimer's, 29, 30, 200
Alzheimer's Association (U.S.), 30
Alzheimer's Society of Canada, 30
American
   Cancer Society, 18, 40, 91, 245
   Geriatrics Society, 28, 42
   Heart Association, 37, 38
   Journal of Epidemiology, 32
   Medical Association, 41
   Prostate Society, 192
   Red Cross, 18
Amino Acids, 46, 49, 58, 55
Anaesthetic, 175, 186, 240-242, 262, 298, 303, 312
Androgen, 71, 252, 259, 285   *See also Therapy*
   deprivation Therapy, 252
   suppression Therapy, 252
Angina, 44, 51, 52, 69, 184, 333
Anti-androgen Drug, 255, 258
Antibiotics, 76, 108, 111, 264, 276, 280, 283, 310, 313, 319
Antibodies, 46
Antifolates, 283
Antigen, 60, 81, 1104, 105, 223, 348
Antioxidant, 35, 46, 48, 52, 55-57, 89
Armstrong, Lance, 283
Arnott, Dr. James, 260
Arteriosclerosis, 50
Arthritis, 29, 30, 138
Asthma, 38, 53
Atherosclerosis, 35
Auto-immune Diseases, 31

B

Baby Boomers, 17, 33, 35, 38, 91, 92, 109
Bacterial Infection, 75, 77
Bagchi, D., 57
Bagchi, M., 57
Balanced Diet, 20, 47
Behaviour Tendencies (DISC) *See also Characteristics*, 155-158
Benign Prostatic Hyperplasia (BPH), 15, 18, 74, 78-89
Beta Carotene, 48, 49 *See also Vitamin A*
Bicher, Dr. Haim (James) I., M.D., 271
Bilateral
  extracapsular extension, 134
  nerve-sparing, 21, 24, 124, 214, 224, 294, 303, 305, 332
  procedure, 305
  radical prostatectomy, 21, 214, 224
  retropubic radical prostatectomy, 21, 303
  sural nerve graft, 217
Bioavailable, 20, 21, 327
Biochemical Failure, 344, 345 *See also Recurrence*
Bioflavonoids, 46
Biological Markers, 104
Biopsy
  needle, 112, 115
  procedure, 112
Bladder
  control, 221
  detrusor muscles, 69
  Incomplete emptying of the ..., 79, 86
  Outlet Obstruction (BOO), 80, 87, 267
Blana, A., 276
Blood Test, 60, 81, 93, 98, 102-105, 109, 142, 199, 338, 340
Bone Scan, 15, 60, 98, 109, 123, 125, 137-139, 205, 262, 295, 343, 348
Bortz II, Dr. Walter, 28, 41
Bostwick Laboratories, 119, 120
Brachytherapy, 175, 191, 199, 203, 236-239, 245-249, 257, 268, 278, 293, 347, 350
  See also Internal Radiation Treatment, Seed Implant, and High Dose Rate
Briefs, 329, 330

C

Calcium, 50, 53, 54
Canadian Cancer Society, 18, 51, 91, 200
Canadian Heart & Stroke Foundation, 37
National Centre for Chronic Disease Prevention and Health Promotion, 42
Capillary Fragility, 57
Capsular Penetration, 141-146, 305
Carbohydrates, 21, 45-49, 169
Carcinoma, 306
Cardiovascular Disease, 29, 33, 37, 50, 51, 55
Carlson, Richard, Ph.D., 167
Carter, H.B., (Dr.)
Castration, 193, 252-256 *See also Orchiectomy*
Catheter
  Foley ..., 264, 276, 306-309
  suprapubic ..., 263, 264, 276, 309, 314, 318
  urinary ..., 206, 240-242
  warming ..., 262, 266
Cavernous Nerves, 67, 69, 204, 206, 213, 218, 305
Cell
  membrane ..., 47, 52
  Leydig ..., 71
Changes
  in Penile Morphometrics, 218,
  physiological ..., 40
Characteristics, 22, 155-158 *See also Behaviour Tendencies (DISC)*
  Conscientiousness, 157
  Dominant, 66, 129, 156
  Influential, 156
  Steadiness, 157
Check-up
  medical ..., 12, 14, 16, 58-60, 101, 103, 136, 182, 337-343

Part VII   Glossary And Resources

post-surgery ..., 335, 338-340
Chemotherapy
　advantages, 288
　side-effects, 287
　disadvantages, 289
Chin, Dr. Joseph, 8, 10-13, 211
Cholesterol, 19, 21, 34, 42, 44, 50, 52, 56, 60, 258
Chronic
　degenerative diseases, 15, 27, 29, 31, 47-57
　bacterial prostatitis, 76, 77   *See also Prostatitis*
Clapp, Larry, 175
Climacteric, 78
Clinical Stage, 132, 141-146, 205, 274, 280
　See also Stage
Clinical Trial, 106, 278, 281, 285
Coagulation Necrosis, 273
Coefficients, 149
Coenzyme Q10 (CQ10), 50, 170
Cold Sore, 21
Cold Spots, 248, 249
Colgan, Dr. Michael, 35, 37, 115, 169, 175
Colon, 34, 41, 42, 48, 56, 170
Conclusive Evidence, 108
Conversations with God, 132
Cooper, Dr. Kenneth, 42
Critz, Dr. Frank, 195
Cryoablation, 260, 269   *See Cryotherapy,*
Cryosurgery, 193, 260, 261, 265-268, 278, 296, 328, 343, 350   *See Cryotherapy*
Cryotherapy, 260-269, 293, 343
　advantages, 268
　side-effects, 267
　disadvantages, 268
CSTAR, 211
CT Scan, 123, 295, 223, 241-243, 262, 343, 348
Cure Rate, 195, 196, 207, 211, 245
Cystoscopy, 81, 98, 113, 240, 266, 338

D

Dairy, 22, 33-39, 46, 49, 169, 171
Das, D.K., 57
da Vinci Surgical System, 210, 211
Death Rate, 40, 41, 92, 255
Decreased Urinary Flow, 79
Degenerative Disc Disease, 138
Denial, 6, 12, 16, 119, 150, 160, 161, 174, 218
Detectable PSA, 118, 279
Detoxifying, 33
Diabetes, 41, 42, 44, 56, 122, 184, 200, 215
Diabetic Retinopathy, 57
DiagnoCure, 120
Diagnosis
Diagnostic Process, 108, 117, 183
Differentiated, 128-130   *See also Gleason grade*
Digital Rectal Examination (DRE), 15, 59, 80, 98, 101, 103, 120, 182, 343
Dihydrotestosterone (DHT), 80, 83, 89
Diphtheria, 28
Disraeli, Benjamin, 312
Dissects the Prostate, 306
Distant Disease, 344   *See also Recurrence*
DNA, 226
Dorsal Lithotomy Position, 208, 240, 243, 262, 274

E

Ear, 319
Early Detection, 91, 105, 108, 224, 238
EDAP Technomed, 272
Edouard Herriot Hospital, 272
Eggleton, Regional C., 272
Eisenberger, Dr. Mario, 206
Ejaculatory Ducts, 65-69
EndoWrist Instruments, 210, 211
Enema, 111, 274
Enlargement of the Prostate, 74, 78
Enucleanation, 88
Environment, 27, 31, 38, 39, 155-158, 247
Enzymes, 46, 53, 202

Epididymis, 67-69
Epidural, 84, 274
Epithelial
  cells, 106
  tissue, 48
Epstein, Professor Jonathan, 106
Erasmus, Dr. Udo, 35
Erectile Dysfunction, 12
Erection Capability, 215, 218-220, 265, 267, 294, 305
Essential Fatty Acid (EFA), 35, 52
Excretory Ducts, 66, 68, 69
Extended Nursing Care, 333
External Beam Radiation Therapy, 193, 226
  See also Radiation Therapy
  advantages, 234
  after-effects, 232
  disadvantages, 235

F

Farber, Sidney, 283
Fat
  hydrogenated ..., 170, 187, 326
  saturated ..., 30, 35, 36, 38, 56, 170, 326
  trans ..., 30, 35, 326, 327
Fibre
  water-insoluble, 34
  water-soluble, 34, 35, 49, 50
Fistula, 267, 268, 275
Flour
  enriched, 34
  refined, 34
  white, 169, 170
  whole wheat, 54, 170
Focus Surgery, 271
Folic Acid, 48-50, 283
Food and Drug Administration (FDA), 210, 277, 285,
f-PSA, 117-120
Fradet, Dr. Yves, 120
Free Enterprise System, 179-191
Free-PSA, 115, 117
Free Radicals, 47, 48, 52, 57, 73, 175
Free-Radicals Scavenger, 51
French National Institute for Health, 272
Fructose, 33, 68
Fruits, 57, 89, 171, 195
Fry, Francis, 272
Fry, William, 272

G

Gamma Camera, 138
Gastrointestinal, 48, 56
Genetic, 19, 36, 37, 119, 226, 233, 283
Genitourinary System, 75
Gilman, Alfred, 282
Giovannucci, Dr. Edward, 56
Glands
  adrenal, 252, 255
  Bulbourethral, 68, 69, 333
  Cowper, 333
  fluid producing, 65, 68
  pituitary, 255, 256
Gleason, Dr. Donald F., 127
Gleason
  grade, 126-131, 143-146 *See also Differentiation*
  grading system, 127
  score, 127-131, 137, 140-142, 161, 257
Gold, 198, 244
Goldenberg, Dr. S. Larry, 352
Gonadotropin-releasing Hormone (GnRH), 256
Goodman, Louis, 382
Goodwin, Dr. Pamela, 51
Grade of the Cancer, 22, 111, 126, 197, 306, 349 *See also Aggressiveness*
Grapefruit, 37, 55.
Grape Seed Extract, 57, 89, 170
Grove, Andy, 352
Guiliani, Rudy, 99

Part VII   Glossary And Resources

H

Harvard Medical School, 55, 56, 283
Hazardous Substances, 27, 31
Health Canada, 277
Health Care
  centres, 159, 191
  counsellors, 193
  facilities, 296
  plan, 197, 225, 235, 251
  professionals, 179, 222, 301
  providers, 152
  system, 124, 191, 251
Healthy Lifestyle, 19, 46, 326
Heart Disease, 26, 30, 35, 40-42, 44, 56, 201, 258
Hematospermia, 80
Hematuria, 80
Hemi-ablation, 279
Hemoglobin, 316-319
Hertz, Roy, 283
High Blood Pressure, 26, 42, 44, 51, 53, 254
High-density Lipoprotein (HDL), 19, 42
High Dose Rate, 175, 193, 231, 237, 241   *See also Internal Radiation Treatment*
High-frequency Sound Waves, 112, 270
High Intensity Focused Ultrasound (HIFU), 270-273, 275-281
  advantages, 280-281
  after-effects, 280
  disadvantages, 281
Hodges, Dr. Clarence V., 254
Homeopathic, 194
Hormone Therapy, 238, 244, 252-259, 284, 296, 347
  advantages, 258
  after-effects, 258
  disadvantages, 258-259
Hormone-Refractory, 285
Hot Spots, 60, 138
Huggins, Dr. Charles Brenton, 254
Hydrogenated Oils, 33   *See also Fat*

Hypertension, 29, 30, 35, 37, 41, 42, 215

I

Immunization, 28
Impotence, 65, 80, 212   *See also Erectile Dysfunction*
Incision, 83, 86, 87, 204-212, 234, 248, 260, 263, 268, 270, 273, 280, 303-309, 318, 323, 336
Incontinence
  overflow …, 222
  stress …, 222
  urge …, 222
Induration, 102, 116
Infectious Disease, 33
Infertile, 206
Informed Treatment Decision, 150
InSite 3-D Vision System, 210
Intermittent Androgen Deprivation, 256
Internal Radiation Treatment (IRT)   *See also Radiation Therapy and Brachytherapy* 236-239, 241, 243, 251, 196
  advantages, 247-248
  disadvantages, 248-249
  high dose rate, 237, 241
  seed implant, 237, 239
  side-effects, 249
International Osteoporosis Foundation, 30
International Prostate Symptom Score (IPSS), 81
Interstitial Radiation, 230, 231
Intravenous (IV), 81, 137, 299, 301, 309
Invasive
Iodine 125, 244
Iodine 129, 244
Iridium 192, 244
Iridium 194, 244
Irrigating Fluid, 84
Irrigation System, 309
Isoflavones, 46

Index

J
John Hopkins University, 55, 106, 140, 207, 286
Joshi, S.S., 57

K
Kegel, Dr. Arnold H., 331
Kegel Exercises, 71, 222, 324, 331, 334
Kilto, Harriet, 283
Klotz, Dr. Laurence, 200, 201
Kramer, Dr. Barnett, 201
Kuszynski, C.A., 57

L
Landers, Ann, 40
Langevin, Paul, 272
Laparoscopic Radical Prostatectomy, 209, 210, 303
   See also Radical Prostatectomy
Laparoscopy, 209
Laser, *83, 87,* 88
Lederle Laboratories, 283
LH-RH, 255
LH-RH Agonists, 255, 256, 259   *See also Therapy*
Libido, 85, 186, 219, 220, 253, 258, 333
Li, Min Chiu, 283
Local Failure, 344, 345   *See also Recurrence*
London Health Sciences Centre, 8, 211, 308
Loss of Sexual Desire, 65
Low-density Lipoprotein (LDL), 19
Lower Urinary Track Symptoms (LUTS), 80
Lupus, 31
Luteinizing Hormone-Releasing Hormone (LH-RH), 255
Lycopene, 55, 56, 88-90, 170
Lymphatic System, 92
Lynn, John G., 272

M
Macronutrients, 45, 49

Macular Degeneration, 57
Magnesium, 53, 54
Malignancy, 72, 113, 114, 141, 283
Malnourished, 26
Membranous Urethra, 69-71, 206, 222
Merkin, Gabe, M.D., 77
Metabolism, 42, 46, 49, 54
Metastasis, 122, 135, 206, 208, 262, 305
Micronutrients, 47, 57
Microscopic Analysis, 111, 304
Microwave Energy, 86
Minerals, 13, 19, 20, 35, 47, 48, 50, 53-55, 57, 88, 175, 326, 327
Minimally Invasive, 86, 209, 210, 236, 260, 261, 279
Monotherapy, 238, 244-251, 256
Multiple Sclerosis, 31
Muscular Sphincters, 70

N
Nutritional, 13, 20, 26, 31, 35, 47, 54-56, 60, 71, 89, 138, 168, 175, 185, 194, 317, 321
Nadir, 195, 207, 233, 245-247, 266, 279
   See also PSA Nadir
Nasal Cannula, 309, 311
National Cancer Chemotherapy Services Centre (U.S.), 283
National Cancer Institute (U.S.), 18, 34, 35, 200, 283
National Institute of Health (U.S.), 30
National Osteoporosis Foundation (U.S.), 30
Natural Killer Cells, 33
Naturopathic, 176-178, 195
Neoadjuvant Therapy, 238, 255 *See also Therapy*
Nerve
   bundles, 66-69, 204-223, 230, 249, 263-267, 275, 280, 305, 332, 337, 349
      Genitofemoral …, 217
   graft, 216, 217, 301
   sparing, 124, 207, 211, 214-224, 265, 271, 294, 303-306, 332, 337

383

Neurovascular Nerve Bundles, 66, 69, 213, 249, 305 *See also Nerve Bundles*
Nickel, Dr. J. Curtis, 75
Nitrogen Mustard, 282
Nocturia, 79
Non-bacterial Prostatitis, 76, 77 *See also Prostatitis*
Non-conventional remedies, 110
Non-invasive, 83, 190, 227, 270-273, 279, 280, 288 *See also Invasive*
Nutritional Supplement, 20, 47, 138, 168, 176, 317, 321, 327
Nutritionally Sufficient, 20

O

Obesity, 29, 35, 208, 215
Oedema, 276
Oligomeric Proanthocyanadins (OPCs), 56, 57 *See also Proanthocyanadins*
Omega-3, 52, 170
Omega-6, 170
Oncologist, 94, 194-199, 202, 228-231, 242, 284, 343, 345, 348, 350
Open Prostatectomy, 83, 87
Optimum Health, 21, 48, 49, 51
Orchiectomy, 193, 252, 255
Organ-confined, 141-146
Orgasm, 65, 125, 186, 191, 196, 203, 212, 215, 268, 333
Osteoporosis, 29, 30, 53, 54, 258, 285
Osteoporosis Canada, 30
Oxidation, 19, 47, 50-52
Oxidative Stress, 27, 31, 38, 48, 52, 57, 73

P

Pain During Ejaculation, 80
Palladium 103, 244
Partin, Dr. Alan W., 140
Partin Tables, 15, 140-145, 149, 274, 294, 304, 337
Pathologist, 93, 111, 127, 129, 133, 1411, 149, 208, 207, 223, 283, 306
Pathology, 106, 130, 259, 266, 337, 346
PCA3, 120
PCA Pump, 310, 314, 317
Pelvic Bone, 139, 229, 304
Pelvis, 68, 76, 92, 119, 134, 199, 217, 239, 262, 331, 344
Penile
  implant, 221, 334
  injection, 333
  length, 218, 219
  shortening, 212, 219
  urethra, 69-71
Penis, 67-71, 77- 84, 93, 114, 125, 184, 191, 206, 212-221, 240, 253, 262, 305-323, 332-340
Perineal Radical Prostatectomy, 208, 303
Perineum, 77, 204, 208, 240-242, 248, 261, 264
Pesticide DDT, 38
pH, 53, 175
Photons, 227
Physical
  activity, 41-44
  condition, 22, 294
Physiotherapist, 312, 317
Phytonutrients, 56
Plant, Jane (Professor), 36
Plasma, 106,
Polio, 28
Popp, Nancy, 169
Pre-Admission, 297
Preprostatic Sphincters, 70 *See also Sphincter*
Primary Tumour, 134
Proanthocyanadin, 56, 57, 89, 170 *See also Oligomeric Proanthocyanadins (OPCs)*
Probability, 141-149, 190, 197, 294, 345
Prognosis, 126, 127, 132
Prostaglandins, 47, 52
Prostascint Scan, 348, 349
Prostate

Index

disorder, 12, 20, 22
problem, 8, 12, 13, 59, 60, 64, 74, 163
Prostate Cancer Research Foundation of Canada, 18
Prostatectomy *See Radical Prostatectomy*
Prostate-specific Antigen (PSA), 15, 81, 91, 98, 104
Prostatic
  adenocarcinoma, 74
  bed, 224, 349
  fluid, 65, 68, 69, 74, 77
  massage, 77
  urethra, 66-71, 80, 84, 85, 204, 206, 221, 240, 275
  utricle, 68
Prostatitis (Tpyes)
  acute bacterial ..., 76, 109
  chronic bacterial ..., 76, 77
  non-bacterial ..., 76, 77
  prostatodynia, 76, 77
Protein, 21, 46, 49-52, 56, 117, 118, 169
Pruess, H.G., 57
PSA-ACT, 117, 118
PSA-AMG, 117
PSA Nadir, 195, 196, 207, 233, 246, 247, 266
PSA Test, 93, 119, 201
Pubic Bone, 64, 205
Public Health Agency of Canada, 30
Pumpkin Seed, 89, 170

Q

Quality of Life, 13, 64, 99, 122, 152, 158, 172, 192, 259, 277, 296, 305, 325, 334, 341

R

Radiation Burns, 226
Radiation Oncologist, 124, 179, 223, 228-233, 239-247
Radiation Therapy *See also Treatment Options and Therapy*
  Combined ..., 238
  External Beam ..., 193, 226
  Conformal Proton Beam ..., 227, 228
  Intensity Modulated ..., 227, 228
  Three-dimensional Conformal ..., 227, 228
  Internal ... (Brachytherapy), 226 *See also high dose rate and seed implant*
Radical Prostatectomy *See also Surgery*
  Laparoscopic ..., 209, 210, 303
  Perineal ..., 208, 303
  Retropubic ..., 21, 205, 207, 303
  Robotic-assisted Laporoscopic ..., 210, 211, 224
Radioactive Tracer, 137
Radiologist, 111-114, 138, 149, 235, 262, 264
Rapid Interstitial Therapy, 237, 241, 246
Rectum, 274-276, 280, 306, 331, 349
Recurrence *See also Salvage Therapy*
  biochemical ..., 344, 345
  distant ..., 345, 347
  local ..., 344-348
  systemic ..., 345, 346
  treatment, 345
Refractory, 285
Regimen, 41, 282, 284
Remote Afterloading, 237, 242, 243
Repeat-PSA, 115
Reproductive
  capability, 64, 341
  system, 52, 54, 67, 150
Resectoscope, 84
Retina, 57
Retrograde Ejaculation, 69, 70, 85, 87, 196, 333
Retropubic Radical Prostatectomy, 21, 205, 207, 303
Rewcastle, John C. Ph.D., 276
Rogenhofer, S., 276
Rudolph, Gaale Ph.D., 45

S

Salt, 37, 38, 260, 263

Salvage Therapy after failure of: *See also Recurrence*
  Cryotherapy, 350
  EBRT, 349
  Radical Prostatectomy, 349
  SI or HDR, 350
Saturated Fat, 30 *See also Fat*
Saw Palmetto, 88, 89, 110, 170, 202
Scarring, 232, 267
Scar Tissue, 102, 209, 218, 221, 230, 268, 273, 338
Schwartz, David, Ph.D., 167
Screening, 18, 102, 105-108, 177, 201, 277, 285
Scrotum, 77, 114, 125, 208, 268, 303
Second Hand Smoke, 38, 39
Second Opinion, 23, 94, 124, 129, 149, 151
Seed Implant, 148, 193, 237, 239, 293 *See also Internal Radiation Treatment*
Selenium, 51-54, 89, 90
Semen, 113, 247, 248, 333
Seminal Fluid, 68
Seminal Vesicles, 223, 229, 248, 262, 306, 333, 343, 349
Serum, 106, 254, 256, 307, 309
Sexual Intercourse, 125, 186, 215, 218, 247
Shrunken Penile Tissue, 65
Simulation, 228, 229
Smallpox, 28
Smith, Timothy J., M.D., 32, 167
Sonablate (SB500), 271, 272
Sonar Signals, 112
Soy, 56, 89
Specimen, 81, 111, 114, 129, 131, 223, 306
Sphincter Muscle
  external ..., 69, 204, 210, 221, 263, 329, 331, 333
  internal ..., 71, 83, 85, 221, 222, 328
  urethral ..., 79, 134, 248
Spinal Anaesthesia, 86, 87
Staging
  Method of ..., 132
  T-N-M ..., 134
  Whitmore-Jewett A-B-C ..., 133
Surveillance Therapy Against Radical Treatment (START), 200
Statistics, 41, 91, 187, 207, 234, 245, 247
Stent, 50
Sterility, 65, 85
Stohs, S.J., 67
Stress, 27, 31, 32, 38, 41-52, 57, 60, 73, 77, 212, 218, 222
Stricture, 232
Sugar, 33, 34, 89, 94, 123, 169, 170, 185, 326
Supplement, 20, 21, 27, 53, 55, 89, 168, 170, 220, 326, 327
Sural Nerve, 217
Surge, 109, 225, 255
Surgeon General's Report, 43
Surgery *See also Radical Prostatectomy*
  risks and after-effects, 212
Survivors, 7, 151, 152, 161, 175, 181, 212, 220
Sutures, 206, 210
Synthesis of Prostaglandins, 47
Systemic Failure, 344, 345 *See also Recurrence*

T

Taxotere, 284-286
Testes, 68, 71, 253
Testicles, 67, 69, 71, 76, 252-255, 258
Testimonials, 249
Testosterone, 71, 80, 83, 89, 252-258
Tethering, 220, 221
Therapy *See also Treatment Options and Radiation Therapy*
  adjuvant ..., 255
  androgen-deprivation ..., 252
  androgen suppression ..., 252
  drug ..., 83, 84, 254
  freeze ..., 260
  intermittent ..., 257
  interruption ..., 257

Index

LH-RH agonists ..., 255, 256, 259
neoadjuvant ..., 238, 255
palliative radiation ..., 257
primary ..., 266, 279
rapid interstitial ..., 237, 241, 246
salvage ..., 261, 346-350
smart bombed ..., 241
triple modality ..., 238, 239
Tiplisky, Dr. Michael, 53
Toxicity, 48, 49, 52, 229, 255
Trace Elements, 13, 20, 47, 48, 53, 57, 327
Traditional Treatments, 139, 179, 192-194, 328
Transducer, 112, 272-275
Trans Fat, 30, 35, 326, 327   *See also Fat*
Transrectal Ultrasound (TRUS), 111, 237, 261, 272, 348
Transurethral
  Incision of the Prostate (TUIP), 83, 86
  Microwave Thermotheraphy (TUMT), 83, 86
  Needle Ablation (TUNA), 83, 86
  Resection of the Prostate (TURP), 83, 84
Treatment Options   *See Watchful Waiting, Surgery, External Beam Radiation Therapy, Internal Radiation Treatment, Hormone Therapy, Cryotherapy, HIFU, Chemotherapy*
Trials, 51, 272, 277, 284-286, 293, 329
Tuberculosis, 28, 283
Tumour Marker, 110

U

Uchida, Dr. Toyoaki, 276
Ultrasound
  probe, 112, 240, 242, 263, 272, 274
  transducers, 272
  waves, 271-275
Unilateral Extracapsular Extension, 134
Unsaturated Oil, 170   *See also Saturated Fat*
uPM3TM, 119, 120
Urinary   *See also Lower Urinary Track Symptoms (LUTS)*
  bladder, 69
  catheter, 206, 240-242
  control, 70, 79, 211, 223, 247, 294, 341
  frequency, 79
  function, 64
  obstruction, 76, 232, 255, 268
  problems, 59, 74
Urine
  Flow Study, 81
  Retention, 328
  Test, 116
Urogenital Diaphragm, 68

V

Vas Deferens, 67, 69, 204, 206, 209, 306
Vasectomy, 69, 206
Vegetarian, 22, 194
Virility, 93
Virus, 33
Visual Image, 111
Vitamin
  A, 48
  B1, 49
  B2, 49
  B3, 49
  B5, 49
  B6, 49, 54
  B12, 49
  C, 50, 51
  D, 50, 51
  E, 19, 20, 48, 51, 52, 54, 60, 90, 170

W

Waitley, Dr. Denis, 167, 168
Walsch, Neale Donald, 312
Walsh, Dr. Patrick, 207, 216, 222, 223
Walter, B., 276
Watchful Waiting, 16, 23, 82, 82, 148, 190 203, 261, 347
Weidner, W., 75
Wentz, Dr. Myron, 34, 58, 187

Western Methods of Treatment, 125
Western World's Lifestyle, 29
Wheeler, Dr. Harold, 76
Wieland, W.F., 276
Whittemore, Dr. A., 35
Wood, Tim Ph.D., 45
World Health Organization, 23, 36
World Health Report, 29

X

X-Rays, 138, 226-229, 239, 262

Y

Yoo, Dr. J., 140
Your Health, 5, 13, 19, 26, 42, 59. 202, 225, 235, 251, 287, 334

Z

Zinc, 53, 54, 89, 110, 170
Zone
 central ..., 66, 80
 peripheral ..., 65, 66, 80
 periurethral ..., 66, 80
 transitional ..., 66

ISBN 1412089944-1